Planning Clinical Research

G000068163

This book teaches how to choose the best design for your question. Planning a clinical study is much more than deciding on the basic study design. Who will you be studying? How do you plan to recruit your study participants? How do you plan to retain them in the study? What data do you plan to collect? How will you obtain this data? How will you minimize bias? All these decision must be consistent with the ethical considerations of studying people.

Drawing on their many years working in clinical research, Robert A. Parker and Nancy Greene Berman guide readers through the essential elements of study planning to help get them started. The authors offer numerous examples to illustrate the key decisions needed, describing what works and what does not work, and why. Written specifically for junior investigators beginning their research careers, this guide will also be useful to senior investigators needing to review specific topics.

Dr. Robert A. Parker has been a consulting biostatistician for nearly 40 years. He has worked in academia, medicine, industry (a Top 25 global pharmaceutical company), and government (World Health Organization; US Centers for Disease Control). In industry, he was the arbiter of statistical methods for more than 100 statisticians at the company that employed him. Having worked with junior investigators for most of his professional life, he is dedicated to mentoring the next generation of medical researchers. This book reflects his passion to train junior investigators in the art of clinical research.

Dr. Nancy Greene Berman has been a consulting biostatistician for more than 35 years. She has worked in private consulting for NIH and other government studies. In Los Angeles, she was chairperson of the annual Statistical Workshop and treasurer for the Southern California Statistical Association. As the General Clinical Research Center (GCRC) statistician and consultant at the Harbor-UCLA Medical Center, she worked with both junior and senior investigators developing protocols for clinical studies. Doing this work she identified the need for a book that would provide details of clinical design in an accessible format for all investigators. This book is intended to fulfill that need.

Planning Clinical Research

Robert A. Parker
Harvard Medical School

Nancy Greene Berman
School of Public Health, UCLA Los Angeles

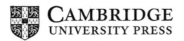
CAMBRIDGE
UNIVERSITY PRESS

CAMBRIDGE
UNIVERSITY PRESS

One Liberty Plaza, 20th Floor, New York NY 10006, USA

Cambridge University Press is part of the University of Cambridge.

It furthers the University's mission by disseminating knowledge in the pursuit of education, learning, and research at the highest international levels of excellence.

www.cambridge.org
Information on this title: www.cambridge.org/9780521840637

First published 2016

Printed in the United Kingdom by Clays, St Ives plc

A catalogue record for this publication is available from the British Library.

ISBN 978-0-521-84063-7 Hardback
ISBN 978-0-521-54995-0 Paperback

Cambridge University Press has no responsibility for the persistence or accuracy of URLs for external or third-party Internet Web sites referred to in this publication and does not guarantee that any content on such Web sites is, or will remain, accurate or appropriate.

To Laurie, for everything (R.A.P)
To my family (N.G.B)

Contents

Preface

This book is entitled *Planning Clinical Research*. We call it "planning" because much of what we do is not the design – in the strict statistical sense – but the overall planning of a study. This includes, of course, the actual design of the study, but planning begins much earlier, with the initial decision: What questions will you ask and how will you ask them? The questions you ask have an impact on the basic design – can you do an interventional study or not? What type of interventional study are you using? Or must you do some type of observational study? But planning a study is much more than choosing the basic design. So even if you have decided on the design (say, a randomized, double-blind, placebo-controlled parallel group study [see Chapter 5 for more about this]), you still need to plan all the details of the study. Who will you be studying? How do you plan to recruit them? How do you plan to retain them in the study? What data do you plan to collect? How will you obtain this data? How will you minimize bias in all aspects of the study? All these decisions must be consistent with the ethics of studying people. This book will help you understand these questions, gain insight into approaches to making these decisions, and understand some of the ethical problems involved in clinical research.

This book is intended to provide the essential concepts and elements of study planning to help you get started. Although we occasionally mention analysis techniques, our focus is on what to do before you have started collecting data. We tried to anticipate the needs of junior investigators who are beginning their research careers, but we hope the book will also be useful for more senior investigators needing to review a specific topic.

To do this, we have used a lot of examples. Often examples are presented multiple times, with refinements or additional information, reflecting how we actually plan a real study. We consider options and keep refining them as we develop the study. We have found that it is best to sketch out options rather than to write out a detailed plan. It seems that once a lot of effort has been put into writing the detailed plan, it becomes an anchor, and making changes to the basic plan becomes very difficult – even when other alternatives are better. We urge you to limit your plan to a single page – preferably a bulleted list – to keep your mind open about possible changes until you really have fully defined the study and have obtained critiques on the idea, so that you are open when a suggestion is made for a radical revision. If you remember nothing else from this book but that you need to always be thinking about refining your design and sharing the plan with your colleagues and (most importantly) actually considering the suggestions they make, we have helped you.

The book is organized in 6 parts containing a total of 30 chapters and 2 appendixes. The organization of the book reflects the basic organization of the research protocol for a study. A study is any systematic investigation intended to answer a question. Since our focus in this book is on clinical research, the questions answered will involve people. However, much of the material, particularly for the design of interventional studies and control of bias, applies to all biological research, whether molecular pathways, cell cultures, or animal studies. The book is not intended to be read cover-to-cover, but rather for you to dip into it as needed.

Clinical studies can only begin after approval by your local Institutional Review Board (IRB), also called an Institutional Ethics Committee (IEC). Thus, Part I of the book (Chapters 1–3) is an introduction to both the fundamental questions you should be asking yourself and ethics and consent issues in clinical research. Some readers may feel that Chapter 1 is quite pretentious. Most statisticians feel that this is the heart of what we do. We discuss ethical issues at length in Chapters 2 and 3. These issues are so fundamental to clinical research that we end each subsequent chapter with a brief discussion of the ethical issues that are relevant to the technical material in the chapter.

The research protocol provides the IRB with the information it needs to decide whether to approve your study. There are many components of the protocol, including the aims of the study, background as to why the study is needed, and the basic study design. Part II of the book (Chapters 4–10) is intended to help you determine the appropriate design for your study. We recommend that all readers read Chapter 4, which provides an overview of all the designs discussed. Then, if you think you are doing an interventional study (meaning that you are doing something to the participants and seeing what happens), you would probably want to go to Chapter 5 for more details of the different types of interventional designs possible. If you are considering an observational study, you would probably want to go to Chapters 6–8, selecting the appropriate one(s) based on the overview material in Chapter 4. We know that many readers may be planning to do record reviews. Although Chapter 9 does discuss this, the chapter – and the design of your record review – will make much more sense to you after reading Chapters 6, 7, or 8, depending on the design used for the record review. Finally, Chapter 10 attempts to synthesize how to select the basic design to be used for your study.

Your protocol also needs details about the participants being studied, the types of data being collected, and how you are intending to control bias. Part III (Chapters 11–18) discusses a number of core concepts that we believe apply across all study designs. These include such basic ideas as generalizability and validity (Chapter 11), practical issues about recruiting and retaining participants (Chapters 12 and 13), the types and uses of data that you will be collecting (Chapters 14–16), and bias and methods to avoid it (Chapters 17 and 18).

Depending on the study design, additional details are needed. Parts IV and V help with these details. Part IV (Chapters 19–24) discusses practical issues relevant to interventional studies, such as how one actually defines the intervention (Chapter 19), how one actually does randomization (Chapters 20 and 21), the hierarchy of blinding and how one does it (Chapters 22 and 23), and how to improve participant adherence (Chapter 24). Part V (Chapters 25–28) discusses the practical issues for observational studies, such as identifying appropriate populations for cohort studies (Chapter 25) or case-control studies including matching (Chapters 26 and 27) and blinding in observational studies (Chapter 28).

The last part (Chapters 29 and 30) discusses the practical issue of data collection methods and data quality.

Two appendixes complete this volume. One discusses the basic ideas behind hypothesis testing, while the second discusses the ideas underlying calculation of an appropriate sample size. A word of warning on this last part of the book: We do not provide formulas, but there are formula in the supplementary material on the book's website (www.cambridge.org/9780521840637) to help you understand sample size calculations and links to appropriate software.

Our examples may reflect real studies we have read, studies planned with colleagues but never done, studies that were completed or may have been completed by the time you read this book, or studies invented solely to make a specific point. We do not include references to any real examples since we have abstracted what we consider the key features illustrating the design point we are trying to make and never present results. Moreover, we often have presented wrong decisions or used hyperbole in the descriptions to help make our point clear.

Of course, just reading a book will not make you an expert in study design or planning. You need to find some mentors – experienced investigators who can help you become a better investigator. We would also recommend that you identify a statistician to work with in developing your study plan.

Given our focus on the ethical aspects of all the topics discussed in the book, although the term "subject" has been used historically for participants in research studies, throughout the book we use terms such as "participant" or "individual" to remind us that the *"subjects" are human beings*, with their own rights and needs. You never have the right to use, or treat, or think of participants as objects in your research.

To you, our reader, and all your staff and associates, we wish success as a researcher.

Acknowledgments

I thank all the investigators I've worked with, and all the students who have taught me so much. It has been a pleasure working with you.

(R.A.P.)

I would like to thank my husband, Arnold Berman, and our children for their encouragement and support as I worked on this book. I also would like to thank the many investigators who I have worked with both in Washington and at the Harbor-UCLA Medical Center for giving me insight into the investigators' needs in planning clinical studies and providing me with interesting studies to work on.

(N.G.B.)

Part I

INTRODUCTION

Questions before Starting on the Details

The later chapters in this book discuss details. These details matter: we have spent most of our professional lives helping researchers improve details. These details determine whether a grant will be funded and increase the chance that an investigation, once begun, succeeds in obtaining the data needed with acceptable accuracy so that valid conclusions can be drawn from the research. There are, however, broad questions that you should consider *before* you worry about the details. These questions are so fundamental that they are rarely even recognized, let alone addressed. At times these questions may seem too personal, but they are intended to force you to think carefully about yourself, your motivations, ideas, and goals before you invest your time, energy, and effort in doing clinical research. It is important that you answer the first question (Why are you doing research?) for your own benefit, while you need answers to all the other questions to convince others that you can do the research you propose.

1.1 What Are the Broad Issues?

We have identified five questions you must consider before developing a detailed research plan. Although most questions focus on the specific project, the first question is broader:

Question 1. Why are you doing research?

You must understand why you are doing research to decide how important research is to you. Doing good research is very, very hard.

Doing good clinical research is even harder: you have to deal with human beings on top of everything else. To do research at all, you must invest your energy, effort, and time in the project. You should answer this question before doing your first project – and at least briefly consider it every time you are thinking about starting a new project. For each project requires you to invest part of your life in it – and that is a trade-off that you should consciously be making, not drifting into it because you "ought to do some research."

To this, we add four more questions, based on ideas in Cochran and Cox (1957), which are usually posed by funding agencies as part of a grant application. There questions are:

Question 2. What is your question?

Specifically, what do you hope to learn once the project is over? In grant language, these are the specific aims of the project and may include innovation aspects as well.

Question 3. Why does answering this question matter?

This is the justification for someone to pay you to answer your question (if resources are needed), and part of your rationale for investing your time, energy, and effort into the project. In grant language, this is the significance section, which needs to be buttressed by the background information, and again may include innovation as well.

Question 4. Why are you the person to answer this question?

This is a demonstration that you are capable of achieving your goal. In grant language, this is the investigator and the environment aspects of the grant.

Question 5. How will you know whether you have answered your question?

This provides an objective measure, when the project is over, to assess whether you have succeeded. Grants do not seem to consider this as part of the evaluation at all – but if you cannot succinctly state this, others will wonder whether your approach is actually complete.

1.2 Question 1: Why Do You Want to Do Research?

This question would seem to be none of our – or anyone else's – business. But it is a lot of other people's business, including your coworkers and especially your family. You are taking time away from all of them to indulge yourself in doing research. For research *is* an indulgence. You are planning to invest a considerable amount of your effort, energy, and time in doing research. Research takes time – far more than you would expect. Even experienced researchers find that research almost always takes more effort than they expected.

We have no desire to make you feel good or bad about your reasons, nor do we actually care why our collaborators are doing research. But it is only by knowing your reasons for doing research that you can decide how much of your energy, effort, and time you should invest in doing research. We emphasize that you are spending precious resources on research: your emotional energy, your physical energy, and your time. Your time has value both in terms of what you can achieve and how you focus your life. You have other responsibilities, a personal life and interests, perhaps students or a family. The time you spend on research is taken from these other areas. Generally, your responsibilities stay the same even when your research commitments increase. Thus, the cost to you of doing research is being paid, at least in part, by reducing the time available for your personal activities and your relationships. There may not be a dollar cost associated with this loss, but there is a cost, a cost that might not be apparent to you today but a real one nonetheless.

It may be that the real reason you are doing research is one or more of the following, which focus on specific projects:

- I want to do this research project studying this disease because I want to find a cure for a specific disease which has affected me personally in some way.
- I want to do this research project studying this disease because the disease fascinates me.
- I want to do this research project because I want to know the answer to this question.
- I want to do this research project because it would be a challenge to pull it off.

- I want to do this research project because it would be fun.
- I want to do this research project because if I am right, it would be exciting and maybe have an important impact.

Some of our favorite colleagues do research for these very reasons. We work in medical research because of some underlying altruism (we want to "help humankind" through better health), but on a day-to-day basis we work with medical researchers because it is (usually) a challenge, it is (sometimes) fun, and it is (often) neat. Unlike many physicians, however, neither of us feel "called" to study a specific disease, or do a specific research project, although we have both been "called" to be biostatisticians.

Sometimes, though, the reasons for doing research, while still very personal, are more generic or professional, such as:

- I would like to do a research project because I have never done research and would like to try something new.
- I would like to do a research project because I want to expand human knowledge.
- I would like to do a research project because I want to develop, maintain, or enhance my professional reputation.
- I would like to do a research project because I want to cut back on clinical hours or on administrative responsibilities.

Finally, you may need to do research for some external reason, such as:

- I need to do a research project as part of my fellowship program.
- I need to do a research project because my mentor wants me to.
- I need to do a research project because my advisor wants me to.
- I need to do a research project because I am at an academic institution and I am expected to do research.
- I need to do a research project because I need it for a promotion (or retention).
- I need to do a research project because I need to bring in salary support for my staff.
- I need to do a research project because I need to bring in salary support for myself.

Often there is a combination of the "want," "would like," and "need" issues. One common combination among our successful colleagues is:

"I want to study this disease because ..." and "I need external support to keep all my staff."

1.3 Question 2: What Is Your Question?

It is only after you have some background in an area that you can hope to develop the goals for your study. The reality is that every study has several specific goals, some scientific and technical, and some personal to the investigators. Question 1 should have helped you identify the personal goals for this and all your studies. Question 2 should help you focus on the scientific and technical goals of your study.

A standard framework of science – taught in many elementary and secondary schools – is that science is hypothesis-driven, that is, observations leads to an idea (a hypothesis), and one then conducts experiments to test the hypothesis by collecting new data, which allow one to provide support for or evidence against the hypothesis. This fits the current notion of hypothesis-driven research as essential for funding. Although successful grant writers will honor the conventions and frame their grants as hypothesis-driven research, the reality appears to be that investigators start by asking interesting questions. What happens if ...? Why does this ...? Does this affect ...? We believe that the scientific goal of a study is to answer one or more such questions. The hypothesis-driven approach formalizes this approach into a testable question and is discussed in Section 1.6.

Although no one can be certain of the outcome of research, and the most interesting and important results are frequently serendipitous, you should be able to be specific and unambiguous in terms of the major questions that the project is intended to answer. One of the most effective ways to do this is to draft an abstract for a paper addressing each of the major questions. Putting your ideas down on paper is the most effective way we know to help define the questions concretely, to ensure that you express what you hope to achieve. Investigators often have an idea of what they hope to find. By drafting the abstract you are communicating a clear idea of the aims of your study, even if you have question marks for all the numbers. The abstract helps you identify the primary endpoints for the study, which dictate the data you need to collect. This abstract is for personal use when planning the study; it is not for publication. It provides you a framework for developing the study design and implementation.

Doing the study is a necessary step in answering your questions, but it is not the goal itself. The goal is not to do, for example "a randomized double blind clinical trial of two specified treatments to assess the effect of the treatments on a specific outcome," although many investigators initially describe their goal in these terms. The goal is to find the answer to a specific research question, in this case, probably, "Which treatment works better?"

You may not be able to formulate the research question immediately. It may be helpful to work with others while you develop clear and concrete goals. Others can help by providing you a sounding board, an opportunity for you to talk through your ideas, by pointing out to you when your ideas are fuzzy or vague. Sometimes, others can even help you figure out what you are attempting to do, providing an initial version of what your abstract might be. Eventually, however, you have to be able to identify your questions, otherwise you will never be able to design a study to answer them. If you undertake a study without a clear idea of what you are trying to achieve – and both of us have worked with investigators who have done this – you run a major risk of achieving nothing, of having nothing to show despite the effort you spent on the study. We do not want this to happen to you.

If you really do know the questions you are attempting to answer, you should have little difficulty in stating these questions clearly. Since you do not have to hone the language and fit within a 250 word limit, writing an abstract should not be very hard, if you know what you are trying to do. It should help you identify the reasons why a sponsor should fund the study (Section 1.4). In our experience, investigators who know what they want to do have little trouble actually writing such an abstract, while those most resistant to doing so often have no clear idea of what they are planning to do.

On occasion, investigators feel that this "prejudges" the study and prevents them from being "objective" when assessing the results from the study. Nonsense! The results you hope to find are the reason you undertake a study. The results from the study are what you report, whether they match your hopes or not.

1.4 Question 3: Why Does Answering This Question Matter?

This question is addressed in the Significance and Background sections of a grant application. We assume that you know enough about the research area to know that the question has not already been answered or, if there is a conventional answer, that you can put together a persuasive argument that the conventional answer might be wrong or inadequate. Here we focus on another aspect of whether the project is worthwhile: Who cares?

No matter what question you are trying to answer, we hope that you feel that the question is important. But if no one else would care what the result was, why are you spending your time and effort doing the study? Given all your investment in a research project, you must feel that the results will matter to others and possibly will matter a lot. If not, should you be doing the study?

The Significance section of the proposal hopefully convinces someone that such research should be funded. Although wanting to do it "because it will be fun" might be adequate for you, regrettably payers who fund studies, whether internal or external, rarely find fun fundable. Thus, you must tell why the question matters to other people. Without some type of support, it usually is impossible to complete any but the simplest studies. Except for a record review, some resources are likely to be needed for any study; even for a record review, there may be charges associated with record retrieval, data abstraction and management, analysis, and publication. You must know why your question matters if you hope to get support to answer it.

Although it may be difficult to accept, knowledge per se is not always valued. Possible ways to show the value of the knowledge include the magnitude of the problem being addressed (in human or financial terms, preferably both) or a display of how this new knowledge may lead (directly or indirectly) to new or improved therapies (more effective, less expensive, or more cost-effective approaches).

Personally, we have a lot of problems with such questions. We started writing this book because we thought that writing a book would be fun (naive, innocent biostatisticians that we were) and that it would be useful. We still hope it will be useful.

1.5 Question 4: Why Are You the Person to Answer the Question?

The fact that the question is important is not in itself sufficient. In addition to being important, is it reasonable to expect that the question can be answered? And is it reasonable to expect that *you* can answer the question?

You might have a fantastic idea that is clearly worthwhile. To answer the question, however, you might need a large number of participants, need a large number of expensive measurements, or need to follow participants for many years. Thus, the study cannot be done without substantial resources. Even if you have the financial resources, do you have the other resources needed for the study? Do you have access to the participants you need, in the quantity you need? Do you have access to the personnel you will need for the study team, the measuring instruments and assays you need, access to sufficient infrastructure for the study (such as a place to meet participants), and sufficient time to do the study? If you have all the necessary resources, is the study feasible? Even with an adequate number of potential participants, is it possible to recruit enough participants into the study? Recruiting and retaining participants becomes increasingly difficult as the length of the study increases and as it becomes more difficult for a participant to be involved in your study, whether because of the frequency of visits, invasiveness of procedures, duration of measurements, or challenges in following an assigned intervention. If the study will require many years to complete, are you willing to make that commitment? What impact will the inevitable personnel changes have? Will the funding agency be willing to wait so long for results? Sometimes the ideal study cannot realistically be done by you or anyone else.

You also need to consider whether you are the right person to do the study. Even small studies usually require a variety of skills and abilities. Do you have the skills necessary to complete the study single-handedly, or have you put together a team that could answer the question? Without such skills and knowledge, it is very unlikely that you can successfully complete a project; learning skills on the fly while doing research is hardly optimal, and at best might lead to having to redo much of your initial work. Possession of the necessary knowledge and skills – either by you or by the study team – is thus a prerequisite to carrying out a project successfully, of achieving your goal and answering your question.

If you are seeking support for the research, moreover, you must have more than knowledge. You are asking someone to give you support, provide you with *their* resources. They usually will expect some evidence that you will use their resources appropriately, that by giving you resources the research will be successful. If you are requesting only a relatively small amount of resources, sponsors may settle for "potential" as adequate proof. For more substantial support, however, you will have to provide evidence that you can complete the project and achieve the goal. At the highest levels of support, you will have to show that you have previously carried out work of a similar complexity successfully and that you have the experience to perform the necessary procedures.

You must be able to answer this question – at least to yourself – before you start a study, and must present your answer persuasively in the grant application if you submit one.

1.6 Question 5: How Will You Know Whether You Have Answered Your Question?

At the end of the study, you will have some information. If the study were designed appropriately (which we hope this book will teach you), and your study worked out reasonably well, you should have enough information to answer your question. After the study is done, will the answer to your question be:

- clear-cut?
- precise?
- reliable?
- convincing?

It is in this context that we feel that the hypothesis-driven view of research makes sense. This view implies that there is an underlying hypothesis being tested, which then allows the machinery of statistics, particularly the formal framework of hypothesis testing, to quantify statistically how clear-cut your answer is. (Appendix A provides an introduction to hypothesis testing.) Statistics also provides tools to quantify the precision of your answer. But statistical methods cannot assess how reliable your answer is – how free your answer is from bias and confounding – nor can statistical methods assess whether your answer is convincing or useful to others.

You may feel that you yourself can judge the validity and credibility of your study, so that you will be the ultimate arbiter of this question. Even if you could do this objectively (which we question), what possible use would the information be *unless* you disseminate it to your peers? We believe that information must be used, must be incorporated into the pool of knowledge, before it can be considered reliable and convincing. Thus, we do not believe that you can know whether your study is reliable and convincing unless you disseminate your results and see whether the study you have done and the answers you have obtained are accepted by your peers as convincing. By disseminating the results of your study you have a concrete result that you and others can use to assess whether or not you have answered the question. This might be a final report on a project to the sponsor, a presentation at a scientific meeting, or publication in a peer-reviewed journal. We use presentations and publications because they are the most common means of disseminating results we encounter, but in other environments your answer might help develop a patent application or marketable product, improve a process with specific measurable objectives such as reducing cost or downtime, or fill in specific gaps in knowledge required for one of these achievements.

1.7 Ethical Issues

You might think that there are no ethical issues involved in any of these questions, since these questions really do not involve any of the details of what you might propose. If you think this, you are wrong.

First, unless it is likely that you will be able to achieve your goal, you have no right to impose anything, no matter how trivial it may seem to you, on any participant. Second, if your goal does not matter, you have no right to impose anything, no matter how trivial it may seem to you, on any participant. If you cannot define your goal, or tell why the idea is worthwhile, you have no right to do anything, no matter how trivial it may seem to you, to any participant. Finally, if you do not know why you are doing research, then why should you expect a participant to help you to do research?

KEY POINTS

- You have to consider the following issues before you begin the detailed design of a study:
  - Why do you want to do research?
  - What is your question?
  - Why does answering this question matter?
  - Why are you the person to answer the question?
  - How will you know whether you have answered your question?
- If you can successfully answer these questions, then you can proceed to the next step: designing the study, which is what the rest of the book is about.

References

William G. Cochran and Gertrude M. Cox, *Experimental Design*, 2nd edition, New York: John Wiley & Sons, Inc., 1957.

2

Ethics

In the following chapters we describe many of the important technical procedures and methods in clinical study design. Every chapter focuses on a single topic. Because clinical research is research on human beings, there is one consideration that is basic to any study: it must be ethical. If it is not ethical, then it should not be done. This is of such importance that in each of the individual chapters there is a section addressing the ethical issues relevant to that chapter. Here we give an overview of the important codes of ethics that have been developed in the past century, the principles that should guide your research and some of the regulations that embody these codes and practices. We do not include many details of these regulations because they are frequently amended.

Oversight of research conducted on human subjects is carried out by the Institutional Review Board (IRB) or Institutional Ethics Committee (IEC). In addition, in an interventional study, there may also be a Data Safety and Monitoring Board (DSMB) that monitors the progress of the study. We discuss the composition and responsibilities of the IRB in Section 2.3 and of the DSMB in Section 2.4.

2.1 How Ethical Guidelines Developed

Concern with the ethics of medical practice has a long history, beginning with the Hippocratic Oath. The focus was on medical treatment until the 20th century, when news of extraordinary violations of human rights in the name of research led to international and national codes of ethics for medical research. We discuss the international codes first and then specific events in the United States, but obviously these events are intertwined.

2.1.1 International Codes

In 1948, the first major international document to provide guidelines on research ethics, the Nuremberg code, was developed in response to the Nuremberg Trials of Nazi doctors who performed unethical experiments during World War II. The Code made voluntary consent a requirement in clinical research studies, emphasizing that consent can be voluntary only if:

- participants are able to consent;
- they are free from coercion (outside pressure); and
- they comprehend the risks and benefits involved.

The Code also states that researchers should minimize risk and harm, make sure that risks do not significantly outweigh potential benefits, use appropriate study designs, and guarantee participants' freedom to withdraw at any time.

The Council for International Organizations of Medical Sciences (CIOMS) was founded in 1949 under the auspices of the World Health Organization (WHO) and the United Nations Educational, Scientific and Cultural and Organization (UNESCO). Among its mandates was that of maintaining collaborative relations with the United Nations and its specialized agencies, particularly with UNESCO and WHO. CIOMS guidelines were developed in association with WHO to develop procedures for carrying out the principles outlined in the Declaration of Helsinki. The guidelines were published in 1982 and updated in 1993 and 2002. Guidelines for epidemiological studies were published in 2009.

In 1964, at the 18th World Medical Assembly in Helsinki, Finland, the World Medical Association adopted 12 principles to guide physicians on ethical considerations related to biomedical research. Known as the Declaration of Helsinki, it emphasizes the distinction between medical care that directly benefits the patient and research that may or may not provide direct benefit. These guidelines were revised at subsequent meetings in 1975 (Tokyo, Japan), 1983 (Venice, Italy), and 1989 (Hong Kong). The code was revised extensively in 2000 (Edinburgh, Scotland) to reflect the concerns of developing nations, which emphasized the need that research should benefit the communities in which the research is performed, to avoid the ethical problem of experimenting on individuals who could not benefit from the research because of cost or logistic requirements. The Declaration of Helsinki was revised again in 2008 (Seoul, Republic of Korea). The most recent revision was in 2013 (Fortaleza, Brazil), focusing on increased protection for vulnerable subjects, compensation for harm from research, and access to the results and beneficial treatments post study.

2.1.2 The United States

In the United State, the revelations of the Tuskegee Syphilis Study from 1932–1972, in which participants were followed and not offered effective treatment even after the availability of penicillin in 1947, led to the National Research Act that was signed into law in 1974. This law created the National Commission for the Protection of Human Subjects of Biomedical and Behavioral Research. The Commission was charged with identifying the basic principles that should govern medical research on humans and then recommending steps to improve the currently existing regulations. The Commission also identified the Institutional Review Board (IRB) as one mechanism through which human subjects would be protected. IRBs had been in place at the U.S. National Institutes of Health (NIH) prior to this date, but the National Research Act and subsequent regulations defined the role of IRBs and their legal necessity for ethical research. Further legislation delineated some of the details of what the IRB is expected to accomplish and some of the procedures it must follow.

In 1979, after four years of work, the National Commission issued "The Belmont Report: Ethical Principles and Guidelines for the Protection of Human Subjects of Research." The report sets forth three principles underlying the ethical conduct of research:

1. respect for persons: recognizing the autonomy and dignity of individuals, and the need to protect those with diminished autonomy (that is, impaired decision-making skills), such as children, the aged, and the disabled;
2. beneficence: an obligation to protect persons from harm by maximizing benefits and minimizing risks; and
3. justice: fair distribution of the benefits and burdens of research.

The Belmont Report led to the ongoing development of federal policies and regulations on the ethical use of human beings in research. These are described as "The Federal Policy for the Protection of Human Subjects," generally known as the Common Rule.

These regulations were based on recommendations included in the National Research Act of 1974 and updated in 1981, 1991, 2005, and 2009. The current version of the Common Rule contains five subparts. Subpart A is the basic set of protections for human subjects issued in 1975 and updated since then. Sometimes just this subpart is referred to as the Common Rule. Subparts B, C, and D add protections for special populations involved in research: pregnant women, fetuses and neonates; prisoners; and children. These are discussed in more detail in Chapter 3, which discusses informed consent. Subpart E required registration of Institutional Review Boards.

In 1996, Congress enacted the Health Insurance Portability and Accountability Act (HIPAA). The main purposes of the act were to enable better access to health insurance, reduce fraud and abuse, and lower the overall cost of health care in the United States. The act did not include standards for use of health information, and Congress asked the U. S. Department of Health and Human Services (HHS) to develop these standards. The regulations (Standards for Privacy of Individually Identifiable Health Information) were developed in the next several years. Compliance with these regulations, known as the Privacy Rule, was required as of April 14, 2003.

The Privacy Rule establishes a category of health information, referred to as "Protected Health Information" (PHI), which may be used or disclosed to others only in certain circumstances or under certain conditions. PHI is a subset of what is termed "individually identifiable health information." With certain exceptions, the Privacy Rule applies to individually identifiable health information created or maintained by a covered entity, which are health plans, health care clearinghouses, and health care providers that transmit health information electronically in connection with certain defined HIPAA transactions, such as claims or eligibility inquiries. Researchers are not themselves covered entities, unless they are also health care providers and engage in any of the covered electronic transactions. If, however, researchers are employees or other workforce members of a covered entity (e.g., a hospital or health insurer), they may have to comply with that entity's HIPAA privacy policies and procedures. Researchers who are not themselves covered entities, or who are not workforce members of covered entities, may be indirectly affected by the Privacy Rule if covered entities supply their data. In addition, researchers are required by HHS and U.S. Food and Drug Administration (FDA) regulations to take measures to protect personal health information from inappropriate use or disclosure.

We will not go into the complexity of these regulations, but two things are important to know. First, the Institutional Review Board (IRB; Section 2.3) has a major role to play in assuring that the privacy standards described later in this chapter are met. Second, an Authorization Form that describes the uses of the data and requires the participants' agreement has been added to the consent process. Although investigators have often included data use as part of the consent process, this act makes it a formal procedure. This is described in more detail in Chapter 3.

2.2 Principles of Ethical Practice

The following material has been based on various NIH sources (see Section 2.5 for suggestions on reliable resources). Seven main principles are described as guiding the conduct of ethical research:

- Social and clinical value;
- Scientific validity;
- Fair subject selection;
- Favorable risk-benefit ratio;
- Independent review;
- Informed consent; and
- Respect for potential and enrolled subjects.

2.2.1 Social and Clinical Value

An answer to the research question should be important or valuable enough to justify asking people to accept some risk or inconvenience.

In other words, answers to the research question should contribute to scientific understanding of health or improve our ways of preventing, treating, or caring for people with a given disease. Only if society will gain useful knowledge – which requires sharing results, both negative and positive – can exposing human beings to the risk and burden of research be justified.

Example 2A: An investigator has an extensive history of research projects, but the results of most of the investigator's studies are never published. The investigator's personal website shows a large number of studies having been done, but results are shown for only a fraction of the completed studies. The rest are all shown as "analysis in process," even though some of the studies were completed more than a decade earlier. Studies for which results are shown are always positive, supporting the investigator's underlying research program, and these are the only studies that have been reported in the medical literature.

Although editors are often reluctant to publish negative studies, there is no justification for not providing the results of all the studies that are completed on the investigator's website. We believe that this behavior borders on unethical. In fact, the perception that this is routinely done by certain commercial enterprises has led to registries of clinical studies (such as clinicaltrials.gov), which require that (a) the design of the study be posted before the study is started; and (b) a summary of the results be posted within 12 months of the close of the study. Many journals now will publish clinical studies only if they have been registered prior to the start of the study.

2.2.2 Scientific Validity

A study should be designed in a way that will get an understandable answer to an important research question. This includes considering whether the question researchers are asking is answerable, whether the research methods are valid and feasible, and whether the study is designed with a clear scientific objective, using accepted principles, methods, and reliable practices. It is also important that statistical plans be of sufficient power to test the objective (Appendix B). Invalid research is unethical because it is a waste of resources and exposes people to risk for no purpose. We have addressed this issue in each chapter of the text in the last section titled Ethical Issues.

2.2.3 Fair Subject Selection

Who does the study need to include to answer the question it is asking? The primary basis for recruiting and enrolling groups and individuals should be the scientific goals of the study – not vulnerability, privilege, or other factors unrelated to the purposes of the study. Consistent with the scientific purpose, people should be chosen in a way that minimizes risks and enhances benefits to individuals and society. Groups and individuals who accept the risks and burdens of research should be in a position to enjoy its benefits, and those who may benefit should share some of the risks and burdens. Specific groups or individuals (for example, women or children) should not be excluded from the opportunity to participate in research without a good scientific reason or a particular susceptibility to risk.

Example 2B: An investigator is studying a new liposuction device under an investigational device exemption. Although the study has no inclusion or exclusion criteria based on race or ethnicity, the investigator has focused all recruitment efforts on several lower socioeconomic status areas, to speed up the rate of recruitment. These areas consist largely of minority populations who for financial reasons have minimal access to cosmetic surgical procedures except through participation in the study. As part of the inclusion criteria, all participants need to be "healthy" at the time of randomization, so the investigators provide participants who join the study a complete physical, and the study will provide any needed medications or other medical care to ensure that all participants are healthy prior to randomization in the study. This recruitment strategy is problematic for several reasons. We will only mention here that the population being studied is unlikely – except for the study participants themselves – to be in a position to enjoy the benefit being provided if the new device is successful. As such, it would appear that they are being recruited because of their availability and willingness to participate, and that the potential beneficiaries of the study, those who can afford to have cosmetic surgery, are not bearing any of the risks of the study.

2.2.4 Favorable Risk-Benefit Ratio

Uncertainty about the degree of risks and benefits associated with a drug, device, or procedure being tested is inherent in clinical research – otherwise there would be little point to doing the research. And by definition, there is more uncertainty about risks and benefits in early-phase research than in later research. Nonetheless, everything possible must be done to minimize the risks and inconvenience to research subjects. Ultimately, the potential benefits to individuals and society need to be proportionate to, or outweigh, the risks for the study to be ethical.

Example 2C: Studies are often done at multiple different institutions, each with its own IRB. In that case, a study might be considered to have an acceptable risk-benefit ratio by one IRB but not by another. As an example, a study involving a frequently sampled IV glucose tolerance test (FSIVGTT) being done solely for research purposes in children was considered acceptable at Institution A where FSIVGTT was frequently done for clinical reasons, but not at Institution B where it was used only as a research procedure. At Institution A, where several members of the IRB used FSIVGTT in clinical care, it was considered a low-risk procedure, possibly because of their familiarity with the procedure. At Institution B, the IRB considered it a higher-risk procedure, potentially reflecting their lack of routine use of the procedure. The risk-benefit ratio is a subjective decision: there is no objective standard to determine whether Institution A or Institution B is correct.

2.2.5 Independent Review

To minimize potential conflicts of interest and make sure a study is ethically acceptable before it starts, an independent review group with no vested interest in the particular study should review the proposal and ask important questions, including: Are those conducting the trial sufficiently free of bias? Is the study doing all it can to protect research volunteers? Has the trial been ethically designed and is the risk-benefit ratio favorable? In the United States, independent evaluation of research projects is done through granting agencies, local IRBs, and DSMBs. These groups also monitor a study while it is ongoing.

2.2.6 Informed Consent

For research to be ethical, individuals should make their own decision about whether they want to participate or continue participating in research. This is done through a process of informed consent in which individuals (1) are accurately informed of the purpose, methods, risks, benefits, and alternatives to the research, (2) understand this information and how it relates to their own clinical situation or interests, and (3) make a voluntary decision about whether to participate. We give more information about informed consent in Chapter 3.

Example 2B (continued): Recall that as part of the study procedures, participants need to be "healthy" at the time of enrollment, and can receive all needed medical care without charge prior to randomization. Since potential participants who need medical care and are unable to afford it have a strong incentive to participate, these practices would raise issues about how "voluntary" the decision to participate truly is.

2.2.7 Respect for Potential and Enrolled Subjects

Individuals should be treated with respect from the time they are approached for possible participation – even if they refuse enrollment in a study – throughout their participation and after their participation ends. This includes:

1. Respecting their privacy and keeping their private information confidential.
2. Respecting their right to change their mind, to decide that the research does not match their interests, and to withdraw without penalty.
3. Informing them of new information that might emerge in the course of research, which might change their assessment of the risks and benefits of participating.
4. Monitoring their welfare and, if they experience adverse reactions, untoward events, or changes in clinical status, ensuring appropriate treatment and, when necessary, removal from the study.
5. Informing them about what was learned from the research.

2.3 The Institutional Review Board (IRB)

In the United States, by 1953 the NIH required that all proposed clinical research projects at its center in Bethesda obtain approval from a protection-of-human-subjects review panel. In 1966, the U.S. Public Health Service issued its first set of regulations extending this review requirement to all extramural research supported by the agency. These rules were further revised in 1971 and 1974 and led to the establishment of IRBs at hundreds of institutions receiving federal funding for research. Legislation in 1981 and 1991 (the Common Rule; Section 2.1.2) delineated some of the details of what the IRB is expected to accomplish and some of the procedures it must follow. Subpart E of the Common Rule established the need for IRB's to be registered.

The IRB is a committee that has been formally designated by the institution to approve, monitor, and review biomedical and behavioral research involving humans with the aim to protect the rights and welfare of the research participants. The Federal Policy for the Protection of Human Subjects requires that all research involving human subjects conducted, supported, or otherwise subject to regulation by any federal department or agency be conducted under the auspices of an IRB. The federal regulations specify detailed requirements for the membership and responsibilities of the IRB. Most IRBs are established within academic and medical institutions, although private, for-profit IRBs are also accepted if they meet the federal requirements. The responsible IRB has the power to approve, require modifications in (to secure approval), or disapprove research within the institution. This implies that studies may require approval from multiple IRBs if multiple institutions are involved in a study.

There are detailed federal regulations on the composition of the IRB, which must contain at least five members, although most contain considerably more members to cover a broad range of scientific studies. IRBs must include both scientific reviewers, at least one nonscientific reviewer, and at least one person who is not affiliated with the institution. IRBs are expected to be sensitive to cultural backgrounds and community attitudes as well. In addition, if the IRB has oversight of studies that include special populations, such as children, it should have members who have experience working with these groups.

The purpose of an IRB review is to assure, both in advance and by periodic review, that appropriate steps are taken to protect the rights and welfare of people participating in a research study. A protocol cannot be initiated without receiving IRB approval. For most grant supported studies, the IRB reviews research protocols and all related materials when it is likely that a submitted protocol will be funded. The members will pay particular attention to participant selection, informed consent, and methods of recruitment to assure that participation is truly voluntary and participants are aware of their choices. Before and during the study, they will continue to monitor the study to make sure that things are going as planned and there are no unforeseen risks to the participants.

The IRB is responsible for making sure that investigators comply with the requirements of the Privacy Rules. It can advise the investigator how to develop an Authorization for a study. Specifically, when an Authorization to use participant data is part of the Informed Consent, which is the usual case, the IRB will review them together. It also has the authority to grant a waiver or an alteration of the Authorization.

As an investigator, you may sometimes find the requirements of the IRB a little burdensome, but they are necessary. You can also turn to your IRB for information on the details and changes in federal regulations.

Example 2D: Although the usual perception is that IRBs always delay research, an IRB can on occasion act quite quickly to allow research to proceed. Following an industrial accident involving a chemical exposure, an investigator wanted to study which of two FDA approved treatments was more effective in treating the accident victims. The IRB provided temporary approval on the night of the accident, so patients could be enrolled in the study immediately, with a formal protocol submitted for review and approval at a special committee meeting the following day.

The preceding paragraphs may sound like there are a lot of regulations, and you might think you will have a difficult time satisfying all of them. In most institutions there are people who will help you navigate the regulatory landscape and keep you from being the next scientific scandal in the popular press or even worse – harming participants in your study.

2.4 The Data Safety and Monitoring Board (DSMB)

If the study is a Phase 3 clinical trial and subject to federal regulation, there must be a group responsible for monitoring the study data to ensure subject safety. This is often called the Data and Safety Monitoring Board (DSMB), but other names are also used. The DSMB is an impartial group that oversees a clinical trial and reviews the progress and safety issues to see if they are acceptable. This group determines if the trial should continue as planned, be modified, be closed to enrollment, so existing participants can continue on study, or be stopped. The DSMB complements the preliminary work of the IRB by monitoring the ongoing safety (and sometimes efficacy) results of a study in detail.

Each study must report to a specific DSMB, although one DSMB may serve for several protocols or members may overlap. The members include at least one expert in clinical aspects of the study, one or more biostatisticians, individuals with expertise in current clinical trial conduct and methodology, and, sometimes a member of a community organization. The members must have no intellectual or financial ties to the investigators.

During the course of a study the DSMB meets at least once annually, but sometimes more frequently. They review the progress and current status of the study. This includes data documenting adverse events, the adherence to the protocol, monitoring actual recruitment and retention compared to initial goals, maintenance of confidentiality, and factors external to the study that may impact the ethics of the study or the safety of the participants. The DSMB may also perform or have performed interim analyses of the data according to a predetermined schedule. The DSMB may recommend modifications of the study based on the safety data or problems in recruitment. It may also recommend suspension or termination of the study based on the results of the interim analysis. If recruitment problems seem intractable, it may recommend that a study be closed.

2.5 Resources for Further Reading

Because the regulations and guidances that explain the regulations are subject to change, we recommend that you use reliable websites for additional information. Although your institution may have information available, for investigators based in or working under U.S. regulations we recommend websites of U.S. government agencies. Because of our focus on grant funded research, the National Institute of Health (NIH) is our primary source for this information (www.nih.gov). We do not list specific pages within that website, as the location of material is often changed, but a search for "ethical guidelines" within the NIH website should get you to the right location (at least as of the date we wrote this!). Another reliable website would be the Office for Human Research Protection (OHRP) of the U.S. Department of Health and Human Services (HHS) (www.hhs.gov/ohrp). Although we are confident that the information available from the U.S. Federal Drug Administration (FDA) (www.fda/gov) is reliable, our limited review found the information harder to locate than on the other two websites.

For investigators working under other national regulations, we would suggest that your first source of information be the website of your national counterpart to the NIH, HHS, or FDA. For a truly international perspective, we recommend the World Health Organization (www.who.int).

KEY POINTS

- Clinical research involves human beings.
- The first and overriding requirement for clinical research is that it must be ethical.
- Ethical issues include (but are not limited) to
  - independent ethical review and approval of the research;

- informed consent from participants;
- scientific validity of the study; and
- favorable risk-benefit ratio.
- If a study is not scientifically valid, then doing research is not ethical.
- Despite the common view of IRBs as hindrances, IRBs are there to help you!

3

Informed Consent

No investigator may involve a human being as a subject in research … unless the investigator has obtained the legally effective informed consent of the subject or the subject's legally authorized representative. An investigator shall seek such consent only under circumstances that provide the prospective subject or the representative sufficient opportunity to consider whether or not to participate and that minimize the possibility of coercion or undue influence. The information that is given to the subject or the representative shall be in language understandable to the subject or the representative.

From the Code of Federal Regulations, Title 45, Public Welfare, Department of Health and Human Services, Section 46.116.

3.1 The Consent Process

When you read this book, you will notice that in many chapters we say that one of the most important ethical issues is that an individual who is invited to participate in a clinical study must be able to understand and willing to sign an informed consent. You may feel we are putting too much emphasis on this. We are all good people and would never deliberately do anything to harm anyone. But in the terms that the public sees it, you are planning to experiment on human beings. We all know of instances in the past when "researchers" have experimented on human beings without their consent and sometimes without their knowledge, and we all find this reprehensible. So you, as a scientist, want to be sure that anyone who participates in your study understands everything about the study and is a willing participant. The two requirements, understanding and willingness, are the basis of a process in which the investigator provides information to the potential participants, answers all their questions and concerns, and, when individuals have been provided all the necessary and requested information, asks for their consent to participate in the study. The process is based on the Informed Consent document and an interview or discussion between a member of the study team and the potential participant to ensure that understanding is complete.

3.1.1 The Consent Document

In this section we describe the items that must go into an informed consent document. Most importantly, the document must be comprehensible to the participant. It should contain as little medical jargon as possible. It should not be in the style of a publication for a journal, nor a literary essay. Most experts agree that the language level should be designed at the eighth grade reading level. If you use a medical or technical term, you should explain it in lay language. For example, many people do not know that a "bolus" is an amount given all at once or that "malaise" means feeling lousy. If you use acronyms, such as "CNS" or "CSF," spell them out and explain what they are. If you use metric measurements, try to give an approximate equivalent value in common units; for example, 2 cc is slightly less than half a teaspoon. Use concrete language rather than general statements that can be ambiguous.

Example 3A: A standard way to judge whether the reading level of an informed consent is appropriate is to use one of several different reading level tests, which most word processors can generate automatically. Here are two ways of saying similar things. "During the course of the study, we will collect blood samples during the experimental infusion of up to 240 ml on each of 5 separate occasions, including baseline and at your visits every 3 months through month 12. This volume of blood drawing is consistent with safety guidelines." This has a Flesch-Kincaid reading level corresponding to about the end of the second year of college, so it is far too complicated for a consent form. A simpler way of conveying the same information would be: "We will collect blood samples while giving you the experimental drug over three hours. This will be done the first time you get the drug, and then at the visits at 3, 6, 9, and 12 months. The volume of blood (240 ml, about 8 ounces or 16 tablespoons) each time is about half of what you would donate at a blood drive, so it is consistent with the safety rules." This has a eighth grade reading level, generally considered appropriate for a consent document.

The following are the basic elements of informed consent. We intend this to be an overview of the general contents rather than an exact template for your study. Every study is unique, regulations governing clinical research may be altered over time, and almost every institution has its own required material as well. If the study is not an interventional study, then perhaps some of the items on the following list are not required in the consent document. However an observational study may involve some intervention, for example blood drawing for testing, and this procedure and its risks would need to be in the consent document.

When you write your proposal, you will work with your mentors and your Institutional Review Board (IRB; Section 2.3) to determine the exact requirements. Most institutions have templates available which provide the starting point for writing the informed consent document.

The consent document should include the following:

- A statement that the study involves research and a description of the purposes of the research.
- A detailed description of what the individual's participation entails, including the procedures that will be followed and the expected duration of participation. This could be the longest part of the consent document, since you should explain every procedure, the timing, special requirements (e.g., fasting prior to a test), questionnaires that may be administered, and other details. This section should indicate which procedures are experimental and which are standard.
- A description of any risks or discomfort that might be a result of participating in the study, with an indication of severity. If one of the interventions tested is a placebo, then this normally must be explicitly stated in the consent form.
- If the research involves more than minimal risk, then an explanation of whether medical treatment will be available and, if so, what it is and where it will be obtained and how to obtain further information.

The document must state what the institution is voluntarily willing to do under such circumstances, such as providing for compensation beyond the provision of immediate or therapeutic intervention in response to a research-related injury, but the participant should not be given the impression that they have agreed to and are without recourse to seek satisfaction beyond the institution's voluntarily chosen limits.

- If the study would involve risks to a fetus or other adverse outcome should the individual become pregnant, this should be explicitly stated (Section 3.4.4).
- A description of the possible risks to the individual of providing data for the study. This could be discomfort or embarrassment at addressing the issues.
- A statement describing the extent to which confidentiality of records identifying the individual will be maintained. This includes a list of which personnel will have access to the identifiable data, how it will be protected, and how the information will be destroyed or securely archived at the end of the study. This is described in Section 30.6.
- A similar statement of confidentiality for any specimens that may be collected during the study, including whether they will be destroyed or saved at the end of the study, and what additional use can be made of them by other studies.
- A description of what, if any, treatment or interaction with the investigator will occur at the end of the person's participation in the study, which may occur before the study has been completed for all participants.
- A description of the potential benefits to the individual or to society in general.
- A statement of alternate procedures or treatments, if any, that may be used by the individual if they do not participate in the study.
- An explanation of who to contact for answers to pertinent questions about the research and the rights of the participant, as well as who to contact in the event of an adverse reaction or injury to the participant.
- Authorization for use and disclosure of their data as required for the study. This authorization is required by the Health Insurance

Portability and Accountability Act (HIPPA) of 1996 (Section 2.1.2). It may be part of the informed consent form or a separate document. In either case it must include the information described in Section 3.2.

- Most important, a statement that participation is voluntary, that refusal to participate will involve no penalty or loss of benefits to which the individual is otherwise entitled, and that the participant may discontinue participation at any time without penalty or loss of benefits to which the individual is otherwise entitled. If there are significant consequences of the participant's decision to withdraw, these should be stated and a procedure for termination described.
- A statement that if new findings develop during the course of the study that could affect the individual's willingness to participate, the individual will be informed and advised on his or her possible options.

That is a very long list of items, and one of the problems of writing a consent document is that it can be quite lengthy yet should be easy to read, preferably below an eighth grade reading level. We again encourage you to contact your local IRB to obtain the basic template which you need to follow, as some of the material will have to be followed exactly. We give a couple of brief examples of various points to illustrate the level of detail necessary, recognizing that we have personally seen consent forms that are well over 20 pages long.

Example 3B: The following illustrates the level of detail expected in a consent form. For brevity we have only said "tests" in the document, although you would actually need to list all the tests and details in the consent form. The reading level is Grade 8.4, between eighth and ninth grade, a little higher than one would like for a consent form.

"You will be followed for a total of 9 visits over the course of one year, including this visit (enrollment) and at 1, 2, 3, 4, 6, 8, 10, and 12 months after enrollment. At the first visit we will collect a detailed medical history and perform a physical exam, as well as collecting blood (about five tablespoons) to make sure you are healthy enough to participate in the study. We will also perform some standard tests to assess your condition. We will then give you study medication to last through the next visit. This visit will take about three hours. At each of the follow-up visits, you will bring back all your unused study medication. We will perform a brief physical examination and ask about any new medical problems or symptoms you have. At each visit we will also collect blood (about three tablespoons) both for your safety and to assess whether the drug is working. We will then give you study medication to last through the next visit. At the 3, 6, and 12 month visits we will perform the tests listed above as well. Your 1, 2, 4, 8, and 10 month visits should take less than one hour each. Your 3, 6, and 12 month visits should take less than 3 hours each."

Example 3C: The following illustrates the interactions an investigator might have with a participant at the end of a study and distinguishes between the end of an individual's participation and the end of the study.

"At the end of your participation in the study, if you wish, we will give the results of your final tests to your personal physician to help guide your future medical care."

"After the study is completed for all participants:

- We will tell your personal physician which treatment you received during the study.
- We will tell you when the results of the study are presented at a meeting or published and provide a summary of the results to you.
- If you ask us, we will send you a full copy of the results when they are available."

Example 3D: For a study that involves cognitive and personality effects of alcohol consumption in adults, the local IRB required that the investigators implement specific procedures to protect participants' safety as a condition of approving the study. These procedures have to be described in the consent document when discussing that the participant has the right to withdraw at any time. For example:

"You can withdraw from the study at any time, for any reason. However, we must make sure that you can get home safely if you are under the influence of alcohol when you withdraw. If you drive to your appointment for one of the visits in which you are drinking alcohol, we will have to get your car keys before the experiment starts. If someone comes to drive you home, we will give them the keys. After drinking any alcohol, if there is no one to drive you home, we cannot give you back your car keys for at least six hours, or until your serum alcohol level is below the legal limit, whichever is longer. If you withdraw before we can give you back your keys, you will need to leave your car here and take a taxi home. We will pay for the taxi. You can return the next day to pick up your car keys and get your car. We will pay the costs of your coming back here and the fees for parking your car overnight."

Example 3E: Typically, confidentiality is maintained through several mechanisms. These procedures are described in the human subjects section of a grant submission, and have to be described in the consent document when discussing that the participant has the right to withdraw at any time. Typical procedures would be described as follows. (The references to different sections of the book would not be in the consent form for the participant).

"We will do everything possible to keep your data private. You will be assigned a Study ID (Section 29.1) not related to you by name or other personal information. All the data we collect will have the Study ID, not your name on it. The form connecting your Study ID to you will be kept in a locked cabinet in a special area where only research staff can go. The computer files containing study information are protected just the same way as we protect your medical record. We will never include any information that could identify you when we present or publish the results of the study. The group funding us makes us allow other researchers to obtain our data after we publish our results (Section 30.6). Before we share the data with other researchers, they have to promise to make no attempt to try to use the information to identify you. We also remove any information that could potentially identify you before giving study data to other researchers."

3.1.2 The Consent Interview

The consent process begins with an interview between the potential participant and a member of the study team authorized to obtain informed consent; for convenience, we will call this study team member the "interviewer" here. The interviewer will show the person the consent document (and HIPAA Authorization, if separate) and go over the contents of the document. The interviewer will explain the details of the study objective and the requirements of the participant in clear terms, stating the possible risks and benefits in language that the layperson can understand. The potential benefits should never be overemphasized: a study may help the individual, but there is no guarantee that it will. There should be no attempt to "persuade" the individual to participate even when the interviewer thinks that participating in the study would really be in the person's best interests. (Section 3.3). The interviewer should also describe alternatives to participation and ensure that the individual understands that there will be no penalty for refusing to participate. The potential participant must be assured that his privacy will be respected. All this information will be in the Informed Consent document. The participant should be encouraged to ask questions and not worry about whether they may seem "dumb." The interviewer should make sure that all questions are answered completely and that the potential participant understands the answers.

The potential participant will also be given a way to contact study representatives if he or she thinks of more questions.

At the end of the interview, the potential participant may be asked if he or she wishes to participate and given the option to think about it for some interval of time. The potential participant should be reassured that no legal rights will be surrendered and that he or she can withdraw from the study at any time without penalty.

At this point, in some instances, the interviewer may make an assessment of whether the individual is capable of understanding the study and can legally give informed consent. Usually these problems are identified before the consent process begins. If the individual's age is below the legal limit, or if the individual is incapable of understanding, then an appropriate agent should be selected to represent the participant in the consent process (see Sections 3.4.1 and 3.4.2). If the individual is not fluent enough in English to understand the document, then a qualified, unbiased translator may be required (see Section 3.4.3). If these conditions cannot be met, it may be necessary to reject the potential participant. If the individual or the agent agrees to participate, then the consent document should be signed by the participant or the agent, the interviewer obtaining the consent, and a witness. To avoid the appearance of conflict of interest, the witness should not be the same person who obtained the consent, nor should it be the investigator. The participant must be given a copy of the completed consent form. The time and date of the consent and the person doing the interview must be documented in the study records and a copy of the signed consent form filed as specified by your institutional policies. On occasion, such as when the study only involves a survey with no identifiable information (discussed in Section 8.4), the IRB may waive the requirement for a signed consent form. The appropriate consent information must still be given to the participant, however.

3.2 The Authorization Form for Protecting Data

This form, which is specified in the HIPPA Act (Section 2.1.2) in the United States, should contain the following information:

- The name and a brief description of the study for which the data will be collected.
- A description of the data or information to be used.
- The person or persons that are authorized to release the data. This may be a specific person by name or a title, such as a study coordinator, or a group of people, such as the data coordinating center staff.
- The person or persons who are authorized to receive and use the data.
- A description of each purpose of the requested use of the data. This should be research study specific or, in some cases, will be for future approved research until consent for use of the specimen (e.g., a blood sample for DNA extraction) is withdrawn.
- Expiration date or expiration event for the authorization of the use of the data, which may be related to an individual's schedule (e.g., five years after enrollment data or the end of the study) or to the purpose or use of the disclosure (release) of the information.
- Signature of the individual and date. If the Authorization is signed by an individual's personal representative, a description of the representative's authority to act for the individual is needed.

- A statement that the individual has the right to revoke the Authorization in writing. This should include a description of the consequences of revoking the authorization, such as discontinuation of participation in the study.

3.3 Coercion and Undue Influence

The U.S. Code of Federal Regulations (45 CFR 46.116) states: "An investigator shall seek such consent only under circumstances that provide the prospective subject or the representative sufficient opportunity to consider whether or not to participate and that minimize the possibility of coercion or undue influence."

Coercion occurs when an overt or implicit threat of harm is intentionally presented by one person to another to obtain compliance.

Example 3F: One of the more difficult issues in obtaining consent is when you are attempting to recruit your own patients into a study. For example, if you specialize in a rare disease, then it may not be possible to identify other patients with the disease for your study. In this case, you have to be especially careful when obtaining consent to make it clear to your patients that their participation is voluntary, that they can refuse to participate, and that the participant may discontinue participation at any time without penalty. This may be very difficult for your patients to actually do, as they may feel that you will be annoyed with them or disappointed with them if they refuse to participate. You should make sure that they are comfortable refusing to participate in the study. Many of our colleagues in these circumstances have sent the patients letters describing the study to them, and ask them to contact the investigator if they are interested in participating, rather than discussing the study during a visit for care. Even then, however, our colleagues are aware that some patients are participating only to please their physician, and try to ensure that the patient realizes that they are free to refuse to participate. Often they had someone not involved in any patient care actually obtain consent from their patient.

Undue influence is much more subtle than direct coercion. It can occur when recruiting material is available in a physician's office or a clinic, implying that the clinic wants them to participate. Sometimes patients may feel they have to participate because their physician is a study investigator. Although it may be reasonable to offer a small reward for participation, to reimburse the participant for time or related expenses for transportation or child care, excessive reimbursement can be considered undue influence. If an investigator assigns students to a study promising extra credit and does not offer an alternative way to achieve it, then the investigator is unduly influencing potential participants. If the investigator offers comparable non-research alternatives for earning extra credit, the possibility of undue influence is reduced but not eliminated. Because undue influence may depend on the individual's situation, knowing when undue influence occurs is difficult. You must work with your IRB (Section 2.3) to determine which circumstances give rise to undue influence. For example, an IRB might consider whether the informed consent process will take place at an appropriate time and in an appropriate setting, and whether the prospective participant may feel pressured into acting quickly or be discouraged from seeking advice from another source.

3.4 Special Populations

The participants in your research may be special populations such as children, pregnant women, or prisoners. Often research involving these populations will require additional input from the IRB, and some (e.g., prisoners) require review and recommendations from the Secretary of HHS. We recommend that you consult your IRB if you are considering enrolling any of these special populations.

In the following sections we describe some important considerations for working with common special populations.

3.4.1 Children

By regulatory definition, children are persons who have not attained the legal age for consent to treatments or procedures involved in the research, under applicable law of the jurisdiction in which the research will be conducted. Generally in the United States, any person younger than 18 years is considered to be a child. In these cases the consent is usually provided by one or both parents or by the legal guardian. However, the agreement of the child to participate is still required, unless the investigator can determine that the child is too young or otherwise not able to understand and agree to the treatment. The form that documents the child's agreement is called an "assent form." If the study involves a range of ages, an investigator may have multiple assent forms, one for young children, one for somewhat older children, and one for teenagers.

The assent form is similar to the consent form. The child should know what he is getting into and what effects participation could have on him. For an older teenager, it will include the same information and the wording may be similar to that in the consent form, whereas for a younger child it would be much simpler. The amount of detail may vary with the age and understanding of the child. It will often be in a more conversational form than the consent document. Some scientists suggest writing it in question and answer form for younger children, beginning with "Why am I here" and including such questions as "Will it hurt?" and "Will I get paid?" The child should be informed of his parents' or guardians' approval of his participation. Female participants at or near the age of menstruation should be told of the risks to the fetus if she becomes pregnant. An interviewer who is good at talking with children should conduct or be involved in the assent interview to explain the study and listen to the child and answer her concerns to ensure that she understands what will be done. Children of appropriate age should be given the name of a study team member that they can contact personally with questions.

3.4.2 Persons Unable to Understand and Agree to the Study

The situation of a person who is not capable of full understanding and consent because of cognitive limitation, dementia, lack of awareness, or other debilitating condition is similar to that of a child. The consent process should be directed to the individual's legal guardian, but if possible, the individual should still be asked for an assent. Depending on the degree of impairment, this may require a very special version of assent with perhaps less detail but enough to feel that the individual has some understanding and has been able to agree to participate.

3.4.3 Speakers of Other Languages

If the potential participant is not fluent enough in English to understand the terms and conditions of the study, then there are several steps which should be taken. Ideally, there should be a copy of the consent document in the individual's language, which has been back-translated to assure that it agrees with the original document. There should also be either a study staff member who is fluent in the language and authorized to obtain consent, or a qualified translator to answer questions and discuss the details of the consent. The translator should be trained for this task. Just calling upon someone in the institution who speaks the language is not adequate, as the person may not have an understanding of the requirements of the consent process or of the study. Family members are not appropriate, since they may want to add their own views to the process and bias the participant into agreeing or not agreeing to participate in the study. Moreover, someone fluent in the language must be available during the term of the study, to continue to speak with the participant. Sometimes it is necessary to reject a potential participant because there is no one who can adequately handle obtaining informed consent in the participant's language.

3.4.4 Pregnant Women, Fetuses or Neonates

The use of pregnant women, fetuses, or neonates in research potentially involves a very high level of risk for these populations. Not surprisingly, the regulations regarding their inclusion and treatment are very complex and subject to modification over time. Again, the best place to begin is with your local IRB for current information. Therefore, we will not try to present the details of this. Some things that are important to know:

- Pregnant women are excluded from studies that do not relate to meeting the health needs of the mother or that pose more than minimal risk to the fetus. The consent of the pregnant woman must be obtained for this research. Individuals engaged in the research will have no part in any decisions as to the timing, method, or procedures used to terminate a pregnancy, and no inducements, monetary or otherwise, will be offered to terminate a pregnancy.

- If research is on a neonate of uncertain viability, individuals engaged in the research must not make the decision about the viability of the neonate. If necessary, an individual not involved in the study will be asked to make that decision.

3.4.5 Prisoners

The use of prisoners as participants in a study introduces a large opportunity for coercion or undue influence. For this reason, the U.S. regulations have limited the type of studies that may recruit from prison populations and issued regulations on these studies and specific criteria relating to prisoners.

The risks involved in the research should be less than or equivalent to risks that would be accepted by non-prisoner volunteers. To avoid coercion, any possible advantages the prisoner would get through his or her participation in the research must not be so great as to induce the prisoner to agree to the study without adequate consideration of the risks. Moreover, each prisoner must be clearly informed in advance that participation in the research will have no effect on parole.

3.5 Use and Retention of Tissue Samples

A study may sometimes require the use and retention of biological specimens for various purposes. Some studies may use only tissue samples and not perform any intervention on the participant, for example using discarded umbilical cords for studies of tissues or cells. In other studies, material obtained as part of the intervention may be used for other purposes. A patient obtaining a transplant or having a tumor removed may donate the diseased organ or tumor for study. In general, material may be used only for the intended purpose and then appropriately destroyed, or stored for use in future studies.

Even if the material is obtained as part of normal health care and not part of a study, or even if it will be pooled with other similar material and the donor will not be identified or stored for future use, the participant should be requested to review and sign an informed consent, which may be simpler than one for a full research study. An important question is whether the future use of the specimen is limited to those uses described in the initial request or may be used for new research and technologies. This entire area is currently controversial, so you should consult your IRB for the most recent standards.

3.6 Situations When Consent Is Not Required or May Be Postponed

There are special circumstances in which consent is not required. The most common of these is in an observational study where all the information comes from existing records that are not identifiable. Within an institution, the source may be institutional records from which all identifying information such as name, date of birth, address, social security number, hospital number, and all other pieces of protected health information has been removed. Survey files where the informant was never identified do not require a consent. Data files from other sources, such as pathology results and other documents or tests, where the individuals cannot be identified either directly or through other identifiers linked to the individual do not require consent.

If you think your study may be exempt for the requirement of informed consent, talk to your IRB. Sometimes, under special circumstances, the investigator may be able to waive the consent signing so that the individual may be enrolled and treatment may start immediately. This sometimes is allowed if the initial presentation of the individual would be in an emergency room in an unconscious or befuddled state and treatment should be started immediately. If a responsible family member is present, they may sign an emergency consent, or in some cases the investigator or a member of her staff may sign it. A full consent should be obtained if and when the individual is capable or an agent is available. Emergency consent must be approved by the IRB. The IRB will require frequent review of how this power has been used.

3.7 Ethical Issues

This chapter is about a major ethical issue. To use a participant in a study without their consent, except in extraordinary circumstances, is not only unethical but will almost always be illegal. You do not just obtain consent. You must obtain an Informed Consent. You cannot just give a brief description or talk to an individual and then say, "Sign here." You must give the potential participant full information, including all procedures, the risks and benefits, and time to think about it. You must not coerce or unduly influence the individual to participate. Special populations, such as children, require special methods. In exceptional cases, approved by your IRB before the study begins, such as an unconscious patient in the emergency room, treatment may be started before obtaining consent but consent must be obtained at an appropriate time if possible.

KEY POINTS

- An individual who is asked to participate in a research study must be provided enough information to understand the study and enough time to decide whether to participate or not.
- The information is contained in a document called the Informed Consent, which the individual is asked to sign. The document should be complete and understandable.
- The individual should have opportunities to ask questions and to think about whether he wishes to participate.
- There should be no explicit or implicit coercion to agree to participate.
- Persons who are unable to understand the information or below legal age must be represented by an agent who can consent to the study for them. The participants' assent to the study should also be obtained.
- Written consent may not be required if the IRB specifically waives this requirement before the study begins.
- There are extraordinary circumstances in which informed consent can be postponed if the IRB approves this before the study begins.
- The specific procedures used in a study, including the Informed Consent document, must be approved by the IRB (or an exemption waiver be obtained) prior to beginning any research.

Part II

STUDY DESIGNS

4

Overview of Study Designs

In this chapter we introduce the two basic approaches to clinical research: interventional studies and observational studies. In an interventional study, the primary focus is the effect of the intervention under the investigator's control. In an observational study, however, the main focus is on collecting data. No matter how extensive the data collection procedures might be, the information collected is the focus of the study. Although we present these descriptions as if there are clear boundaries between the two types of studies, often a single study will involve both interventional and observational components.

4.1 Interventional Designs

In an interventional study, the investigator does "something" to the participants. We deliberately use "something" here, because although an interventional study may be giving a treatment to a patient for a condition, other interventions are possible. The treatment is most often a drug but may also be something else, such as exercise, diet, or surgery. Measuring physiological changes under a variety of conditions determined by the investigator (such as an insulin clamp) is an example of an interventional study not involving treatment.

There are two basic approaches to interventional studies. Either all participants receive the intervention, normally an active treatment, or only some of the participants receive the intervention and others receive a different intervention (normally another treatment or a placebo).

In a single arm study, also called a case series, all participants receive the active treatment (Figure 4.1). The effect of the intervention could be determined by the changes over time within a participant or by the

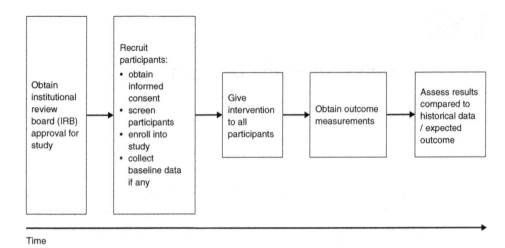

Time

Figure 4.1. Interventional Study: Single Arm (Case Series) Study Design.

outcome at the end of the study period. In both situations, the effect is interpreted based on historical data or assumptions about the results expected.

In a parallel group study (Figure 4.2), only some of the participants receive the intervention. The allocation of the intervention is done by the investigator. This allocation should be random, unless there are compelling reasons against randomization. We have never heard a "compelling reason" from an investigator that did not reduce to randomization being too much work, so we have included it as an essential feature in Figure 4.2. Randomization is discussed in detail in Chapters 20 and 21. The effect of the intervention is determined by differences between the effects in the two groups.

In a crossover study (Figure 4.3), all participants also receive the intervention. However, in a crossover study, participants are studied for two periods: one period with the intervention and one period without the intervention, usually with a placebo or alternate treatment. The allocation of the order of the interventions is done by the investigator and should be random, unless there are compelling reasons against randomization. Given that we have never heard a "compelling reason" from an investigator that did not reduce to randomization being too much work, we include randomization as an essential component in Figure 4.3.

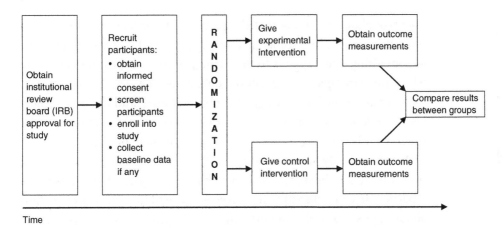

Figure 4.2. Interventional Study: Parallel Group Study Design.

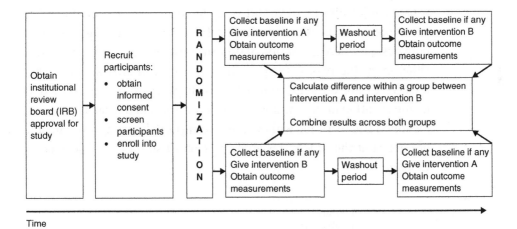

Figure 4.3. Interventional Study: Crossover Study Design.

The effect of the intervention is determined by pooling the difference between the two treatment periods across the different treatment orders. Interventional study designs are discussed in detail in Chapter 5.

4.2 Designs for Observational Studies

In an observational study, the treatment, usually referred to as the "exposure," is not assigned by the investigator. For convenience, we say throughout this book that the participant selects the exposure, but often it is assigned by someone else (e.g., an employer assigning jobs), or something that happens to the participant (e.g., exposures caused by where the participant lives) without deliberate choice by the participant.

There are three basic designs for observational studies. Two designs test the relationship between exposures and outcomes over time, while the third is best thought of as the clinical equivalent of a survey.

A cohort study involves studying a specified group of individuals over time. The cohort may be formed based on a particular exposure or a particular characteristic. The investigator would collect information about exposures and outcomes and see if there is a relationship. The study may be a prospective (or concurrent) cohort study in which the participants are followed after they are identified (Figure 4.4), or a retrospective (or historical) cohort study in which information about the past is obtained either from records or from participants (Figure 4.5). In both designs, there is a period of time over which the cohort is followed, either in the future or in the past. The key feature in these studies is that the investigator does not control the participant's exposures, so there is no intervention under the investigator's control, and the participants are identified and recruited without the investigator's knowing any outcome of interest at the time of recruitment. Cohort studies are discussed in Chapter 6.

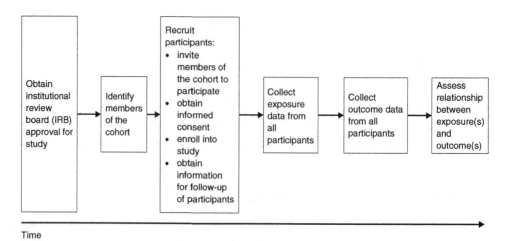

Figure 4.4. Observational Study: Prospective (Concurrent) Cohort Study Design.

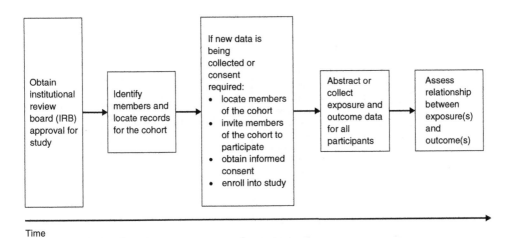

Figure 4.5. Observational Study: Retrospective (Historical) Cohort Study Design.

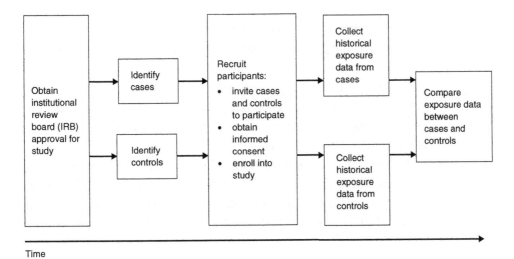

Figure 4.6. Observational Study: Case-Control Study Design.

A case-control study (Figure 4.6) is the other basic design for an observational study assessing the relationship between an exposure and an outcome. The investigator selects two or more groups based on the outcome: a group of cases who have an outcome of interest (e.g., multiple sclerosis), and a group (or groups) of controls who do not have the outcome of interest (e.g., do not have multiple sclerosis). The investigator then collects data on potential exposures. Again, since

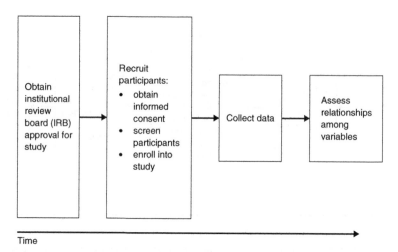

Time

Figure 4.7. Observational Study: Cross-Sectional Study Design.

the investigator does not control the participant's exposure, there is no intervention under the investigator's control. We discuss case-control studies in Chapter 7.

A cross-sectional study (Figure 4.7) is similar to a survey, describing some characteristic of a group at a point in time. There is no attempt to assess an exposure-outcome relationship in such a study. Chapter 8 is about cross-sectional studies.

A record review is an observational study. Depending on the specific question asked, the record review could be a retrospective (or historical) cohort study (Figure 4.5), a case-control study (Figure 4.6), or a cross-sectional study (Figure 4.7). Record reviews are discussed in Chapter 9.

4.3 Clinical Trials

Often, the term "clinical trial" is used when referring to any interventional study assessing the efficacy or effectiveness of a treatment, but in reality this term covers a range of different studies, with different purposes, in the drug development process. The ultimate goal in drug development is to obtain regulatory approval for a new treatment (or use of an existing treatment in a new indication). In the initial stages of drug development, when one is studying the pharmacodynamics and pharmacokinetics of a drug (sometimes called Phase 0), or early studies attempting to determine a safe dose range (Phase 1), a single arm study (case series) might be appropriate. In later stages, when attempting to get preliminary evidence of efficacy and further safety date (Phase 2), or attempting to show definitive evidence of efficacy (Phase 3), randomized studies (either parallel group or crossover studies) are almost always required. Phase 4 studies (sometimes called post-marketing studies) may be required by regulatory authorities to show clinical effectiveness or efficacy on a long-term endpoint or provide additional safety data. Usually these would be cohort studies of patients taking the drug, but sometimes parallel group studies are used as well.

4.4 Different Questions May Represent Different Designs in the Same Study

Given how difficult it is to do a study, often an investigator will try to use the data collected for multiple research questions, each with a different focus. These different research questions might represent different study designs, as shown in the following example.

Example 4A: To study the effect of a new therapy in individuals with a specific disease, individuals were randomized to receive either the new therapy or standard of care (SOC) until death from any cause. The primary endpoints of this study were time until death from the disease of interest (with deaths from other causes being considered a censoring event) and adverse events from the new therapy. This study, when published, will be a randomized parallel group interventional study (Figure 4.2; Chapter 5).

As part of the study, baseline data were collected on all participants before therapy. Specific baseline characteristics could be summarized and reported in a separate publication – for example, a study of the nutritional status of participants with this disease. This reflects a cross-sectional design (Figure 4.7; Chapter 8).

The detailed course of the disease in those participants receiving SOC could be described in another publication. Such a publication could include the duration from diagnosis until first hospitalization for the condition, the number and duration of hospitalizations, palliative care needs of participants, and so forth. Here, all participants have the same exposure, so one is describing the outcome for the total population. Such a report would reflect a prospective (or concurrent) cohort design (Figure 4.4; Chapter 6).

In the SOC group, there might be some participants who have long-term survival despite the disease. This group could be compared to those who succumb quickly to the disease, to identify prognostic factors predicting long-term survival with the disease, which could be analyzed as if the data came from a case-control study (Figure 4.6, Chapter 7).

This example illustrates that the paradigms that we use in this book are just that: ideals of a pure form. Clinical research often does not fall into these neat designs. Particularly for larger, long-term studies, there will often be a dominant feature (in Example 4A it is the randomized parallel group interventional design), but in addition some of the data may be used in other ways for other purposes, and would be interpreted as if it came from a different design altogether. This is not inappropriate or misleading. Indeed, given the difficulty in recruiting and retaining participants in studies, it would be wasteful not to attempt to gain as much information as possible.

In an observational study, however, there is no intervention that can be compared in a secondary study. Some of the data in a cohort study could perhaps be treated as if it was collected as part of a cross-sectional study, and a subset of the data could be used for a case-control study. This is called a nested case-control study since the case-control study is nested inside the cohort study. The ability to use data as if it arose from multiple designs is less likely to occur in a case-control study or a cross-sectional study.

4.5 How You Frame the Question Affects the Types of Studies Possible

An important point when planning a study is defining the question to be studied. The way in which the question is asked can affect whether an interventional study is ethically permissible.

Example 4B: An investigator wants to determine whether exposure to specific chemicals in a large factory increases the risk of various adverse long-term health outcomes, despite the routine safety precautions being used. Given that the study is being done because of concerns about the safety of these chemicals, it would be unethical for the investigator to study the effect of the chemical by randomly allocating participants to exposure or not. Therefore, the investigator must follow a group (cohort) of individuals all of whom work in the factory at a certain time. The investigator would then follow these individuals long term and compare results between those who are exposed to the chemicals as part of their job and those who are not exposed. The results would show the effect on long-term health between those who are exposed to the chemicals and those who are not exposed.

Example 4C: An investigator wants to assess whether there are beneficial effects on long-term health outcomes in reducing the exposure to specific chemicals in the factory. Because there are no ethical concerns about reducing the exposure to these chemicals, it would be ethical to randomize individuals who are exposed into a group allocated to follow the routine safety precautions and a group receiving additional safety precautions. These additional safety precautions, such as using piped-in external air rather than using face masks, are intended to further reduce the potential risk from the chemicals. The investigator would then follow these individuals long term and compare results between those who are randomized to follow the additional safety precautions and those who are randomized to follow the standard safety precautions. The results would show whether there are beneficial effects from these additional safety precautions on long-term health.

To some degree, both of these studies will compare the effect of exposure to these chemicals on long-term health effect of participants, but there are major differences between the studies, which are summarized in Table 4.1. These two examples show that different study designs – an observational study or an interventional study – are possible for what appears to be the same underlying question. One study asks if there is a long-term effect, whereas the other one asks if this effect can be

Table 4.1. Comparison of Two Study Designs to Assess the Impact of Exposure to Certain Chemicals on Long-Term Health

	Example 4B	Example 4C
Investigator's question	Effect of chemical exposure on long-term health	Effect of safety procedures designed to reduce chemical exposures on long-term health
Basic design	Observational (cohort) study	Randomized study
Population studied	Cohort of current employees in the factory at time study starts	Group of current employees in the factory working with the chemicals agreeing to participate in the randomized study
Outcome measurement	Long-term health measures	Long-term health measures
Comparison made	Comparing cohort members who are exposed to the chemical to cohort members who are not exposed to the chemical	Comparing a group randomized to follow routine safety precautions and a group randomized to use additional safety precautions. Groups compared independent of whether they follow the assigned safety precautions.
Major potential problems	Those willing to have long-term exposure may be tolerant of them (e.g., do not have side effects from the chemicals), so that potential adverse outcomes are underestimated	Substantial fraction of those assigned to routine precautions decide they want to follow the additional safety precautions
	Those willing to have long-term exposure may be induced to do so because of pay differentials and other benefits for doing the specific jobs, which might confound results	Substantial fraction of those assigned to additional safety precautions may not follow them because they are too onerous
Question answered by study	Does exposure to the chemicals affect long-term health outcomes?	Do safety methods designed to reduce exposure to the chemicals affect long-term health outcomes?

reduced by reducing the exposure. Therefore, there would be differences in the interpretation of the results even when the studies appear to be similar.

Finally, it would be possible for the company itself to dictate the improved safety procedures for all employees.

Example 4D: The company decides to reduce its potential risk due to the exposures to specific chemicals. To do this, it introduces stringent safety precautions at a new factory and requires that all employees at the new factory follow these precautions. The old factory continues to follow the old safety procedures, because it would be too hard to retrofit the factory, and it is going to be closed after the new factory is fully operational. The company will collect data both on those exposed in the old factory with the old safety precautions and in the new factory with the new safety precautions and compare results between these two cohorts to assess whether the long-term health outcomes are better with the new safety precautions.

4.6 Advantages of Interventional Studies

Interventional studies are generally stronger designs than observational studies as they provide more convincing scientific evidence. When an interventional study is randomized (see Chapters 20 and 21), it provides the best evidence of an effect of an intervention. In Example 4C, by comparing two groups of participants in the same location at the same time, the investigator is controlling to some extent for temporal changes in the behavior of individuals, seasonal effects, the effect of participating in a study, and so on to demonstrate more convincingly the effect of the new safety procedures. In contrast, in Example 4D, the investigator is observing what happens between groups whose exposure is related to which factory they were working in, so that it is more difficult to sort out the effect of the new safety program itself from other effects of being at the old factory itself, especially if the factories are in different locations. Having two separate factories means that workforce characteristics unrelated to the factory (such as residence area air pollution) might be confounding any relationship observed.

4.7 Difficulties of Interventional Studies

Although a randomized interventional study is the strongest design possible, there are often problems in using this design. First, it is unethical to assign participants to an intervention that may harm them unless there are strong potential benefits for the participants. We discuss this point further in Section 4.8.

Even if studying a specific intervention is ethical, there are often significant logistical issues involved in doing an interventional study. First and foremost, although almost all studies need approval from the appropriate institutional review board (IRB; Section 2.3), interventional studies usually receive more scrutiny than observational studies do. In an interventional study, the investigator is doing something to participants to see what happens (in addition to making measurements). Unless the intervention is considered innocuous or recognized to be beneficial, the risk-benefit ratio for using the intervention in participants will be carefully considered by the IRB.

After the study is approved by the IRB, the investigator then faces the problems of implementing the study. Recruiting individuals for an interventional study is difficult for many reasons. First, often very rigorous inclusion and exclusion criteria are used for an interventional study to ensure a homogeneous population and increase validity (Section 11.3). This can severely limit the number of individuals who might be eligible to enroll in the study. It is not unheard of for a study to screen 10–20 individuals to identify just one who is suitable for enrollment. Inclusion and exclusion criteria are discussed further in Section 12.2. Second, the person must agree to participate in the study and receive (or potentially receive) the intervention. In contrast, in an observational study, the investigator is observing what happens to individuals who choose a specific exposure – and thus only needs permission to collect data, which requires less effort from the participants and makes it easier to recruit individuals.

Once participants are recruited, they must be retained in the study – and often have to follow an intervention – for the duration of the observation period. Often, several years are required to observe a sufficiently big difference for the interventional study to be feasible. Thus, for the investigator, an interventional study on the efficacy or effectiveness of an intervention may be a demanding multiyear project. Some strategies for retaining participants in studies are presented in Section 13.4 and Chapter 24.

4.8 Ethical Issues

In Chapter 2 we discussed the basic ethical issues applying to all clinical research, including the appropriateness of procedures used to collect data, issues of participant privacy and confidentiality, and impact of results on participants. Here we focus only on the specific issue of deciding whether one can intervene to study a specific question. This is fundamentally an ethical issue. Only if it is ethically permissible to intervene can you consider the practical issues of whether and how to implement the intervention. Even if it is acceptable to intervene, you cannot intervene without full informed consent from the participant or legal representative (Chapter 3).

The overriding principle about whether or not an intervention is ethical is that it is unethical to do harm to a person. You may never knowingly do something to a participant that will cause harm, unless it is intended to mitigate or stop a greater harm already occurring to that specific person (e.g., you can give very toxic drugs to certain cancer patients with end-stage disease, because you hope that the drug will directly benefit the patient).

The issue is much less clear when the intervention would produce short-term harm that would not be expected to leave long-term consequences. For example, starting participants on an exercise program would be expected to lead to delayed muscle soreness following exercise. Normally, such soreness resolves over a day or two and is relieved by additional use of the muscles. However, an exercise program might produce sprains and strains, or even significant injuries on occasion (e.g., dropping a weight on a foot).

The principle that the study cannot do significant harm to an individual also applies to the selection of a control intervention if one is used in the study. If the study involves a new treatment for a condition, then if a standard therapy exists for the condition, the question arises whether all participants will receive:

- the standard treatment plus the intervention or the control treatment, assuming this is medically sensible;
- the intervention or the standard treatment; or
- the intervention compared to a placebo control treatment.

There are important ethical issues with the use of placebo controls in a study when there is a standard therapy for the condition. If the condition causes significant morbidity, then both the severity of the morbidity and the reversibility of the morbidity become critical issues. There is a general consensus that a placebo control cannot be used if the morbidity is serious or if it is irreversible. For less severe morbidities, the question arises as to how long the standard treatment will be delayed by the study. The concepts of "serious" and "too long" are not well-defined. Investigators and IRBs regularly grapple with these issues.

Many research studies may involve more than minimal risk interventions for research purposes, for example comparing different drugs in a chemotherapy or HIV trial, or additional radiation exposure for nondiagnostic purposes, such as when developing a new approach to diagnosis of a disease. In these cases, one must consider the risk-benefit ratio for the participants. Does the potential benefit of the intervention (either directly to a participant or benefit to society) justify the potential risk of the intervention to the participant? This can lead to what at best is a gray and murky zone for IRBs: one site might approve a study that would be rejected at another site, because the assessment of the risk-benefit ratio differs at the different institutions as in Example 2C. Because individuals might include the payment that they receive for participating in a study in their personal calculation of benefit, many IRBs have very definite rules about what is and is not allowed in terms of payment for a study procedure. These rules are intended to minimize any potential coercive effects of payment on participation.

Although societal benefit enters into this calculation, it is always a secondary consideration. Societal benefits alone are often considered adequate to justify a relatively low risk to an individual provided the individual is fully informed of this and voluntarily gives fully informed consent. As the anticipated risks from a study increase for a participant, however, societal benefit is less and less a justification for the intervention on a participant.

KEY POINTS

- There are two basic types of studies:
  - an interventional study in which the investigator does something to the participants to see what happens; or
  - an observational study in which someone other than the investigator (usually the participant, but sometimes a participant's personal physician, employer, or even the environment) affects what is done and the investigator observes what happens.
- The term "clinical trials" covers a range of studies: most are interventional studies, but some may be cohort studies.
- How you frame the question affects whether you can even consider an interventional study.
- Even though they appear to be asking the same question, an interventional study and an observational study may actually answer different questions.
- The most important question when considering whether an interventional study can be done is whether the intervention can ethically be given to a participant. If giving the intervention would be unethical, then only an observational study can be done.
- Decisions about the ethics of an intervention focus primarily on risk-benefit ratio for the participants.
- Societal benefit is a secondary consideration in this risk-benefit assessment.

5

Designs for Interventional Studies

In this chapter we discuss the basic designs for interventional studies. In an interventional study, the investigator studies an intervention that can be given to either some or all of the participants in the study. This provides the strongest scientific evidence that the intervention causes an effect. Because the investigator is deliberately giving the intervention to the participants, the ethical issues associated with use of the intervention are extremely important.

5.1 Summary of Interventional Designs

In an interventional study, you are doing something to the participants. The something may be a treatment for a disease. It may be an intervention to try to improve the health of the participants in general, rather than for a specific disease, such as nutrition counseling to improve diet. It can be something used to study a physiological process, like an insulin clamp.

There are four basic interventional study designs:

1. a study in which all participants receive only the intervention and the interpretation is based on the results within individuals, usually with an explicit or implicit comparison to data outside the study (a single arm or case series study);

2. a study in which some participants receive the active intervention and some receive a different intervention, which may be a placebo, and the results are compared between the intervention groups (a parallel group study);

3. a study in which each participant receives both the active intervention and a different intervention in some order, and the results are compared between the two interventions within individuals (a crossover study); and

4. a study in which all participants receive only the intervention and the interpretation is based on the changes within individuals without an explicit or implicit comparison to data outside the study (a pre-post study).

5.2 The Question Being Studied

If you are doing an interventional study, there are two different questions you might attempt to answer: (1) What is the effect of the intervention overall? or (2) How does the effect of the intervention differ between participants with different characteristics? For the first question, all participants are considered to come from a single population, although they may receive different treatments, and the primary analysis focuses on the results in the whole group. To answer the second question you need to target your recruitment to have sufficient participants with each of the specific characteristics in which you are interested, and the primary focus of the study will be on how the results differ between these groups. Even in the first case, although many factors will vary between individuals, you are not selecting participants based on these factors. However, you can and should examine whether common factors such as sex, age, and ethnicity impact the effect of the intervention.

The distinction between the two questions may affect which design is selected. If the study is primarily focused on the overall impact of an intervention compared to other interventions or a placebo, it is likely that either the parallel group study (Section 5.4) or crossover study would be preferred (Section 5.5.1). These designs are appropriate independent of whether you are hoping to find the new intervention superior to the control (a superiority study), similar to the control (an equivalence study), or even not too much worse than the control (a noninferiority study). If the study is primarily focused on differences between groups in their response to an intervention, it is possible that a single arm study with multiple groups might be best (for example, the continuation of Example 5A in Section 5.3.2), since then the effect of the intervention could be assessed in all the participants in the study. However, either a parallel group or crossover design can be used to assess differences between groups as well.

5.3 Studies in Which All Participants Receive the Intervention

5.3.1 Single Group of Participants

The basic design of a single arm study, also called a case series, is shown in Figure 5.1. We prefer the term "single arm study" to "case series" as this makes it clear that it is a prospective interventional study design. A group of participants is identified. After they have consented to the study, any necessary screening procedures are done to ensure eligibility. Following this, all participants who meet the enrollment criteria receive the new intervention, and the results of the intervention are observed. The major drawback of this design is that the interpretation of the results depends on assumptions about what would have happened in the absence of the intervention. This type of design would commonly

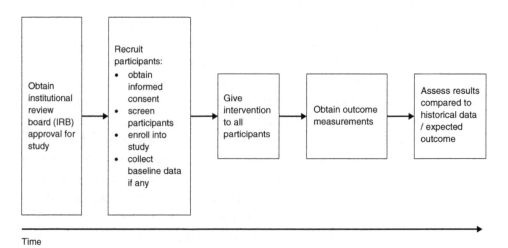

Figure 5.1. Single Arm (Case Series) Study Design.

be used as an initial assessment of a new treatment, such as to assess whether there is any evidence to suggest that a new therapy works as intended (sometimes called a "proof of concept" study). In the clinical trial context, the Phase 0 or Phase 1 study might have this design. This design could be extended to assess differences between prespecified groups of participants (Section 5.3.2).

Example 5A: An investigator wants to assess the weight loss of obese individuals after participating in an exercise program focusing on a specific type of weight training. The participant's weight and percent body fat is measured before and after they have been in the exercise program for a given amount of time. The fact that participants lose weight during the exercise program suggests that the program may be effective in weight loss.

Interpreting the clinical importance of weight loss in Example 5A requires that assumptions be made about the change that would have occurred without the intervention. As such, it will provide little information about how useful the exercise program would actually be in practice, since the participants may have lost weight solely because of participation in the study. For example, knowing that someone else will be weighing them, the participants might have eaten less, to avoid being embarrassed at the end of the study. Such a study design, however, can be very useful to assess how participants react to the program and to help refine the program before formally testing it as a weight loss program in a parallel group study.

Example 5B: One of the best uses of a single arm study is for a rare disease with a uniformly poor outcome. Hurler's syndrome, or Mucopolysaccharidoses (MPS) 1, is a congenital metabolic disorder that results in deterioration in young children and, if untreated, is usually fatal by age 10. Enzymatic and genetic treatments are being studied. Because the syndrome is rare and because the outcome is certain, most studies use a single group of patients, all of whom receive the treatment.

Sometimes a single arm study is done in sequential groups, possibly with the intervention being changed after each group.

Example 5C: New drugs are often initially tested in a group of healthy normal controls. Section 12.2 discusses how difficult it is to actually specify what this means. For drugs that are expected to have significant side effects, these initial studies may be done in patients who have failed standard therapies. The initial studies, called "Phase 1 studies" in the clinical trial literature, usually focus on determining the safety of doses with some preliminary evidence of effect (e.g., a biochemical marker of effect). There are several standard dose-escalation designs, but many are simply a set of single arm studies (Figure 5.1) at different dose levels in which all participants are given active treatment and both safety and efficacy are measured. The first group receives the lowest dose. After safety is shown at this lowest dose, another group receives the next higher dose, and the study continues with increasing doses until the maximum tolerated dose, which is the dose causing a specified amount of toxicity, has been reached or exceeded. Although there are multiple groups (dose levels) in such a study, participants are not randomized – safety at a lower dose must be established before new participants are recruited and exposed to the higher dose. At the end of the study, results are compared across groups to determine an appropriate dose or doses (considering both the preliminary efficacy information and the safety results). Although studies in which all participants receive the new drug are not uncommon, there are advantages to doing even these early studies as parallel group studies with some participants (usually a small fraction) receiving placebo treatment at each dose level.

5.3.2 More Than One Group of Participants

Figure 5.2 shows how the simple design in Section 5.3.1 can be expanded when results are being compared between several groups of participants. As in the single arm study, all participants receive the intervention, but there are two or more different groups being studied. These groups are specified before the study begins. This characteristic can be something the participant is born with (e.g., sex; current age when comparing older vs. younger participants), something that the participant chooses (for example, whether to drink alcohol or not; whether to diet or not), or something that has happened to the participant (such as whether the

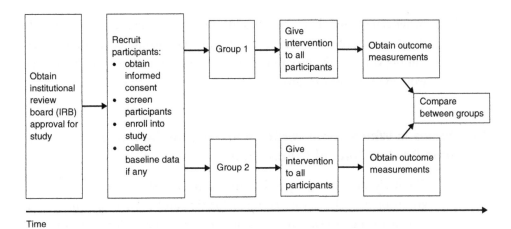

Figure 5.2. Single Arm Study Design with Group Comparisons.

participant has a prior history of myocardial infarction or not; whether the participant has been diagnosed as a diabetic or not). Note that although there is more than one group in the study, the investigator cannot allocate participants to the different groups: the groups are defined by the participant's characteristics.

Example 5A (continued): The investigator wants to assess whether the results of the weight training exercise program are beneficial both in men and in women. The investigator has to systematically recruit the needed number of men and women to ensure that both groups are adequately represented. Change in weight and body fat is calculated for each group. Because men and women have substantially different baseline weights and body compositions, the investigator must carefully consider precisely how to quantify changes to ensure that assessments in each group are meaningful. Because of the differences in baseline weight and percent body fat, the investigator decides to use percent changes rather than absolute changes. The investigator also decides not to formally compare the two groups, but only to look at whether it appears that only one sex benefits from the program or whether it appears that both sexes can benefit.

In this example, the primary focus is on whether changes in weight and body fat at the end of the exercise program appear to be clinically beneficial separately in men and in women, not the average response to the exercise program. The results of this study would be useful in determining whether the program should be studied further in both men and women or in just one group.

5.4 Studies in Which Some Participants Receive the Intervention and Some Do Not: Parallel Group Studies

The basic design for a parallel group study is shown in Figure 5.3. A group of participants is recruited for the study. After they have consented to the study, any necessary screening procedures are done to ensure eligibility. Following this, participants meeting all the enrollment criteria are allocated to one of the two (or more) interventional groups. The allocation to intervention group should be randomized to minimize bias (see Chapters 20 and 21 for more on randomization and Chapters 17 and 18 for a general discussion of bias). Since statisticians are loathe to say something is impossible, it is conceivable that there would be some overwhelming reason why randomization is impossible for a specific study. However, we cannot imagine a reason that would justify compromising the basic scientific integrity of an interventional study. The group receiving the intervention of interest is generally referred to as the intervention group. The group not receiving the intervention – who may be receiving a different intervention or, in some cases, no intervention – is called the control group. One of the important considerations in a parallel group study is that the differences in intervention between the two groups may cause differences in outcome that are not due to the intervention, but due to the participant's and sometimes the rater's feelings about the intervention, if it is known. Therefore, it is important to blind the true intervention whenever possible, or use the most objective methods available to collect endpoint data to minimize the potential for bias. However, when participants or raters are aware of the intervention received, this knowledge alone can affect how the participant responds during the study or how the rater assesses outcome. Blinding, also known as masking, is an important feature in interventional studies and is discussed in detail in Chapters 22 and 23. The following multipart

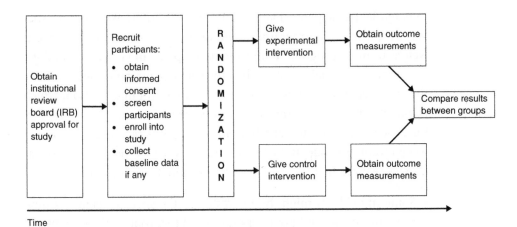

Figure 5.3. Parallel Group Study Design.

example illustrates some of these issues when the intervention cannot be blinded.

Example 5D: Basic Design: The preliminary studies in Example 5A showed that weight training did help both men and women lose weight and reduce percent body fat.

The change in percent body fat was much more dramatic, so the investigator decided to focus on this measurement for future studies. The investigator then decided to do a parallel group study to see whether or not the specific weight training program reduces percent body fat. The investigator decided to include both men and women in this study, and used stratified randomization (Section 21.3.1) to assure that the sex distribution would be similar in the two groups. The investigator proposed to study two interventions and randomize participants to one of two groups:

- Group 1: a conventional weight loss program giving diet counseling and weekly meetings; or
- Group 2: a conventional weight loss program giving diet counseling and weekly meetings plus the special weight training program.

The investigator realized that there was an obvious problem with the basic design: the basic interventions are very different. This would be known to the participants, since the informed consent must mention to potential participants that they may or may not be assigned to a special weight training program. In addition to the benefits of the special weight training program, if any, the participants in Group 2 would get much more personal attention than the participants in Group 1. Initially the investigator considered that there be a control intervention, which is intended not to affect the outcome but rather to control for other factors, such as the additional attention participants receive in the special weight training group. In further discussion the investigator and his colleagues realized that there are potential dropout issues as well:

- Some individuals might be interested in the special weight training program. If they did not get randomized to Group 2, they might not bother to participate, biasing the comparison.
- Other individuals might be interested only in the conventional program and do not want to exercise. If they were randomized to Group 2, they would not bother to participate, biasing the comparison.
- Some – possibly many – individuals in Group 1 might decide to start exercising on their own, potentially affecting the validity of the comparison.

For all these reasons, the investigator decided to modify the design and have both groups have some exercise program.

Example 5D (continued): The investigator decided to modify the intervention in the first group and randomize participants either to:

- Group 1: a conventional weight loss program giving diet counseling and weekly meetings plus a conventional aerobic exercise program; or
- Group 2: a conventional weight loss program giving diet counseling and weekly meetings plus the special weight training program.

When the investigator discussed the design with his colleagues, they pointed out two other alternatives for the intervention: (1) using a conventional weight training program instead of an aerobic exercise program for the control group; or (2) using a combined exercise program (aerobics plus the special weight training program) as a third group. In addition, the investigator's colleagues pointed out some potential problems: some participants might already be exercising; and the amount of exercise might differ between the two groups, which would affect the validity of the conclusions.

Example 5D (continued): The investigator carefully considered all these suggestions. He decided to reject using a conventional weight training program instead of an aerobic exercise program, because conventional weight loss programs generally talk about aerobic exercise, particularly walking, so he wanted to have an aerobic exercise component. The investigator also rejected the combined aerobic and weight training program because he was worried about how hard it might be to recruit participants who were not regularly exercising to begin so much exercise. The investigator realized that the other two issues were major concerns, and revised the design further:

- adding a new exclusion criteria for participants who were regularly exercising, for two reasons: (1) they might be unwilling to change their exercise routine for the study; and (2) they were likely to benefit less than individuals who were not exercising at all;
- estimating the amount of calories burned in the two exercise programs, and adjusting the duration of the aerobic exercise so they should be equal; and
- adding an exercise and calorie diary for participants to record how much exercise they do, to better assess any potential differences that these confounders might have at the end of the study.

This is an example of a standard parallel group study. There are two intervention groups being compared. The goal is to see whether the new intervention is better than the standard intervention (formally, a superiority study), and the results are based on one well-defined primary endpoint.

There are, however, other parallel group study designs that are not as simple. We describe them in the next two examples to give you a feel for the range of designs and some of the variations possible.

Example 5E: Current therapy for drug-sensitive tuberculosis is long and complicated, involving a four-drug regimen for two months followed by a two-drug regimen for at least four more months. There are many variants based on the frequency of treatment, whether treatment is observed, and the duration of the second stage of treatment. A fairly high fraction of patients beginning treatment are not cured by the scheduled end of the treatment course. Many new regimens are being developed, and eventually there will likely be multi-arm studies comparing several different experimental regimens to the standard therapy. The goal of these studies would be to identify all new regimens that are "adequate" compared to the standard of care. This criterion would incorporate multiple factors including the cure rate, the completion rate of therapy (which would reduce the danger from drug-resistant TB strains), side effect profile, and even the ease of administration. For each individual measurement, the results cannot be "too much worse" than the standard of care, but overall the results need to be "better."

Example 5E shows several differences from the straightforward study in Example 5D, including multiple intervention groups and multiple endpoints. Also, no one endpoint defines "better" between groups. This is what is formally called a non-inferiority study for each individual endpoint. What "not too much worse" really means is defined in the design phase of the study. In this type of study, the overall results can be considered "better" if the clinical outcome(s) meet(s) the "not too much worse" criterion and the intervention has other types of benefits, such as ease of use, improved adherence, or reduced side effects.

Example 5F: An investigator wants to study the effect of a specific exercise regimen on physical performance. The investigator starts with a standard parallel group study design, with one group given the specific exercise regimen initially and a second group having the intervention deferred. The second group is actually a placebo control group for the comparison, but receives the intervention in a subsequent period, called an "extension phase" (Figure 5.4). By offering an incentive to stay in the study during the control period, the investigator is attempting to minimize dropouts from the control group.

Example 5F illustrates how one can add additional observations and interventions around a core study. This type of deferred treatment study is frequently done in the later stages of drug development, termed a "Phase 3 study" in the clinical trial literature, when the goal is to show

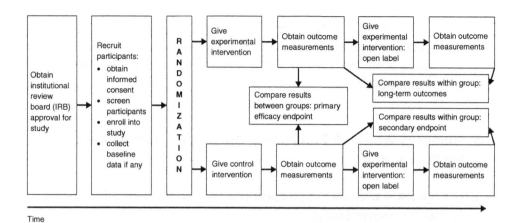

Figure 5.4. Parallel Group Study Design with Extension.

treatment efficacy to obtain regulatory approval for the therapy. In an open-label extension, participants in both groups receive and know that they are receiving the experimental intervention after the formal parallel group study ends. Such an open-label extension helps improve participant retention during the parallel group study and provides the opportunity to gather additional safety data during the open-label phase. Using only data from participants in the deferred group at the end of the parallel group study and at the extension phase is an example of a pre-post study, discussed in Section 5.5.2

In Examples 5D, 5E, and 5F randomization is possible and should be done (Chapters 20 and 21). However, there are some parallel group studies in which individual randomization is not possible.

Example 5G: Studies assessing the effect of informational and community interventions (such as television advertisements) need to be done with the intervention being assigned to a community or a large area rather than to specific individuals. Although there is, again, some element of randomization, the randomization unit is communities, not individuals. Sometimes, different treatments may be used in different clinics for logistical reasons, and comparison of the effectiveness of the treatment in practice assessed between clinics. The results for these special cases are the outcomes in the randomization units (the community or the clinic, respectively), rather than the results for each individual.

Try as we might, we have been unable to develop an example of a parallel group study in which randomization at some level cannot be done. Moreover, randomization should always be done to enhance the validity of the study.

5.5 Studies in Which All Participants Are Studied with and without the Intervention

5.5.1 Comparison within a Single Participant with Intervention in Random Order (Crossover Study)

The basic design of a crossover study is shown in Figure 5.5. A group of individuals is recruited for the study. After appropriate consent is obtained, and any necessary screening procedures are done to ensure eligibility for the study, those who meet all the enrollment criteria are then randomized to one of two or more intervention orders. By far the most common design (shown in Figure 5.5) is what is termed an AB/BA design. Participants are randomized either to receive intervention A followed by intervention B (AB) or intervention B followed by intervention A (BA). Between the two interventions there is often a period without any intervention, termed a "washout period," as it allows the effect of the first intervention to dissipate. Normally one of the two interventions is considered a control for the intervention of interest, although that does not imply that a placebo must

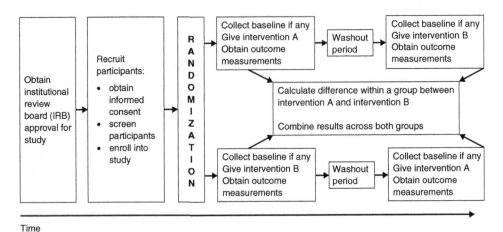

Time

Figure 5.5. Crossover Study Design.

be used. After outcome is assessed with both interventions, the effect of the intervention is defined as the difference (within each person) between intervention A and intervention B. This is not the only design possible, however, and other crossover designs have been published, involving additional intervention orders or additional interventions.

The main advantage of the crossover design is that differences are measured within an individual. Normally, differences within individuals are less variable than differences between individuals, so that a smaller sample size would be needed for the study (Appendix B). This usually is assumed to mean that recruitment for the study would be easier, but this is not necessarily true. For example, participants might be more willing to be involved in a parallel group study that lasts three months than in a crossover study that lasts six months.

There are three special problems with crossover studies, which always must be considered. The first two issues relate to the interpretation of the results of the study, while the last affects the feasibility of a crossover study. First, there is the problem of the stability of the underlying condition over time. In the study of a disease, this implies that the disease condition is stable, or relatively stable, over the duration of the study. In a physiological study, it implies that the underlying physiology is stable.

Example 5H: An investigator wants to study a treatment for the common cold. Given how quickly cold symptoms change, a crossover study is not appropriate.

Example 5I: An investigator wants to study a treatment for osteoarthritis. Although the condition does change and is slowly progressive, it would be possible to study the effect of a treatment on symptoms in a crossover study because the condition does not change rapidly.

The second major problem is the duration of the effect of the initial intervention, usually called the "carryover effect." With the AB intervention order, does A somehow affect the underlying process (disease or physiology), making a washout period necessary before starting to assess intervention B? This is almost always a question that can be raised about a crossover study, and there is frequently inadequate information to answer the question or to determine how long the appropriate washout period should be.

Example 5I (continued): One problem with studying osteoarthritis is potential carryover from the initial treatment. Suppose that you are studying a new therapy against a standard of care control intervention. If the therapy were very effective, it might also affect the severity of the underlying osteoarthritis over an extended time, in addition to short-term benefits while it is being taken. If this is a concern, then a parallel group study (Section 5.4) would be preferable.

Finally, there is an important practical issue when considering a crossover study. If participants do not complete the study, they provide relatively little information about the study question, and standard methods for the analysis of crossover studies do not incorporate their results in the analysis. If the dropout rate is high, therefore, a large number of participants might be required for the crossover study. This becomes a major problem when the intervention or the measurements in the study are so unpleasant that participants are likely to drop out before the second phase of the study. Such a situation also raises ethical issues.

Example 5J: An investigator wants to assess the effect of a single 30-minute exercise session on metabolic pathways. To do this, the investigator has to collect muscle biopsies both in the absence of an exercise session and after an exercise session. This requires that muscle biopsies be collected on two separate days, since it would be very painful to exercise immediately after a biopsy is taken. Muscle biopsies, however, are not pleasant. Therefore, many participants might refuse to come back for the second biopsy, so they will only provide data for one period (either before exercise or after exercise).

Although fewer participants are normally required for a crossover study than for a parallel group study, this does not mean it will be completed sooner. If the study is sufficiently long or complicated, it may actually be easier to recruit a larger number of participants for a shorter parallel group study than for the longer crossover study. In addition, the crossover study will take at least twice as long for each participant to complete as the parallel group study does. Thus, the parallel group study might be completed earlier, and results available earlier than for the crossover study, which potentially benefits the entire community.

Example 5K provides a fairly typical example of the situation when a crossover study would be used. The disease is relatively stable over time, it is unlikely that there will be long-term carryover effects, and the procedures are not particularly onerous.

Example 5K: An investigator wants to study the effect of adding a second lipid-lowering medication in patients already on one medication. The effect on lipid levels would be assessed as the change between the lipid panel collected at baseline and the lipid panel collected after 8 weeks of treatment. Since lipid levels generally return to baseline levels quickly after lipid-lowering medications are discontinued, it would be possible to do this as a crossover study to eliminate any temporal factors or changes in diet over time.

5.5.2 Comparison within a Single Participant with Intervention in Fixed Order (Pre-Post Study)

In a pre-post study (Figure 5.6), a participant is studied before the intervention, sometimes with a placebo or standard of care, and then with the intervention. The effect of the intervention is determined as the difference between outcomes in the pre-intervention period and the intervention period. Often the period of the pre-intervention phase is very short. It may be just the time required to prepare the participant and take measurements, or a washout period to allow the effects of previous treatments to dissipate.

This type of study is actually a single arm study with baseline data collection prior to the intervention. By making the comparison internal

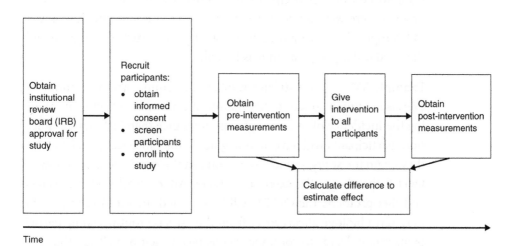

Time

Figure 5.6. Pre-Post Study Design.

to the study, it attempts to avoid the major concern of the single arm study, that the interpretation depends on data outside the study. The interpretation of a pre-post study depends on the critical assumption that no change would be expected in the participants during the study in the absence of the intervention. This may or may not be reasonable. Although the pre-post study appears to avoid the need to use data outside the study to interpret the study results, it actually makes the external data an assumption in the interpretation.

The crossover study is generally considered preferable to the pre-post study since it prevents confounding of intervention effect with intervention order, but a fixed intervention order may be necessary when there is a long-term effect of the intervention.

Example 5L: Instead of examining the effect of a single 30-minute exercise program on metabolic pathways (Example 5J), the investigator decides to assess the effect of a long-term exercise training program lasting multiple weeks on metabolic pathways. To do this, the investigator needs to collect muscle biopsies in a systematic order: prior to the exercise training and after the training program is completed, since there is likely to be a lengthy carryover effect of the exercise program.

In Example 5J a crossover study might be possible – some participants could have a muscle biopsy taken after an exercise session, and several weeks later have a muscle biopsy taken without an exercise session, while other participants have biopsies collected in the reverse order if there were no concerns about a high dropout rate. In contrast, in Example 5L studying the effect of a long-term exercise program, only the fixed order pre-post study is feasible.

Example 5M: An investigator wants to determine whether a moderate exercise regimen added to diet modification is more effective in reducing the incidence of impaired glucose tolerance than just diet modification. Participants will have an oral glucose tolerance test (OGTT) when they begin the study, spend 8 weeks on just the restricted diet, repeat the OGTT, then begin the exercise protocol. After 8 weeks on the exercise and diet protocol, the OGTT will be repeated. In addition to possible long-term biological carryover from the exercise routine, some participants might decide to continue exercising on their own. Thus, the order of interventions cannot be randomized.

This is actually two pre-post studies, done in sequence: the first study assesses the effect of the diet modification on OGTT comparing the first and middle measurements, and then the second study assesses the effect of adding the exercise program by comparing the middle and final measurements.

A recent innovation, called a "stepped wedge design" attempts to mitigate the concern about temporal effects affecting the results of a pre-post study. It is actually a series of pre-post studies started at different sites over time. The idea is that the participants are grouped by the time of starting the intervention (the "stepping"), so that the pre-intervention measurements can control for temporal changes occurring while the intervention is being tested. As more and more sites implement the intervention over time, the diffusion of the intervention is like a wedge, small at first, but steadily spreading. The order in which the groups begin should be randomized to minimize any bias in the trend of the pre-intervention measurements across the sites.

Example 5N. A program is attempting to train primary care physicians (PCPs) to better screen for autism spectrum disease in toddlers. The program is being implemented at a number of sites, with the sites randomized to begin the intervention at different times using a stepped wedge design. PCPs are recruited by each site. Each PCP's screening practices are measured prior to the start of the training program and again after the training program ends. The analysis of pre-test measurements over all the sites is an attempt to assess whether other factors, such as changes in pediatric practice guidelines or insurance quality assessment measures, are affecting the autism screening rates over time. If the pre-test measurements are stable across sites over time, this would suggest that the pre-post changes are caused by the training program. If the pre-test screening rate is increasing over time across the different sites, however, this would suggest that at least some of the improvement seen in the pre-post comparison might be due to factors other than the training program. Similarly, if the pre-test screening rates were decreasing over time, this might explain why the observed effect of the training program was not as large as had been hoped.

Stepped wedge designs are often used pragmatically when assessing the impact of a policy intervention in a large health care system, when the intervention is rolled out over time. This might occur when a country implements a new program, but can only afford to implement it slowly over time. In this case, the pre-post comparison is based on summary measures at each site, rather than results for individuals as in Example 5N.

5.6 Ethical Issues

The very real ethical considerations about doing any kind of interventional study are discussed in Section 4.8. One major issue, the selection of the control intervention in either a parallel group study or a crossover study, is included in that section. However, once an investigator has concluded that it is ethical to use the intervention and determined the control intervention, there are still several ethical issues involved in selecting the design. If all participants receive the intervention (the single arm study), then there are significant limits as to how the results of the study can be interpreted, and very likely the results would be considered weak. If such a study is done to justify a more extensive study, then it would probably be useful. If the study is intended by itself to change actual practice, however, the study is questionable as it is very unlikely to achieve its goal except in exceptional circumstances. It is important to note, however, that exceptional circumstances do exist, for example for a disease with a known uniform poor outcome (Example 5B).

Doing a parallel group study or a crossover study reduces this concern, but raises others. As mentioned in Section 5.5.1, there are basic scientific questions involved in interpreting the results of any crossover study. There are also potential ethical issues about enrolling people in crossover studies. If the study is so invasive that many participants are likely to drop out – such as Example 5J, which requires muscle biopsies close together – then it is essential that participants only be enrolled if the investigator is confident that the participant understands what is involved at screening and also believes that the participant will complete the entire crossover study. Otherwise, the participant's effort in the initial phase of the study does not contribute to the outcome of the study, so it is wasted. In addition, if a participant is doing very well on the initial arm of a therapeutic crossover study, then it becomes questionable whether the intervention the participant is receiving should be stopped so that the participant can crossover to the alternate therapy in the study.

KEY POINTS

- There are four basic designs for interventional studies:
  - a study in which all participants receive the intervention and the interpretation is based on information external to the study (a single arm study);
  - a study in which some participants receive the experimental intervention and others do not (a parallel group study);
  - a study in which all participants receive the experimental and the control intervention, but in different orders (a crossover study); and
  - a study in which all participants receive the intervention and the interpretation is based on changes within participants (a pre-post study).
- The major disadvantage of a single arm study is that the results can only be interpreted based on information external to the study.
- A single arm study may be used to compare the effects of an intervention in two separate groups, both receiving the intervention.
- The parallel group study allows for comparing the effects of the intervention in concurrent groups of participants avoiding the need to refer to external data to interpret the results.
- The crossover study allows for comparison of the effect of the intervention within participants, so there should be less variability of results than for a parallel group study.
- The validity of the crossover study can be questioned because of concerns about the stability of the disease condition in participants over time and concerns about the possibility of a carryover effect from the initial intervention.
- A pre-post study is a single arm study which is interpreted based on changes within the study participants.
- A stepped wedge design is a series of pre-post studies done at multiple sites

6

Cohort Studies

A cohort study follows a group of people over time. This allows multiple outcomes to be observed and the natural history of the entire group to be followed. The purpose of the cohort study is to determine if there is a relationship between specific exposures and later outcomes. A cohort can be selected based on convenience (for example, all nurses in certain states) or based on a particular potential exposure (for example, all employees in a factory). Cohorts can be formed and then followed over time – like the Roman legions from which the name comes – or identified retrospectively. The cohort study is the only way to determine the range of adverse outcomes from a potentially harmful exposure, since it would be unethical to use a potentially harmful exposure in an interventional study to see what happens. In addition, a series of cohort studies may provide sufficient evidence for an association to justify an interventional study to determine whether a relationship is causal or not.

6.1 Basic Designs

There are two basic designs in a cohort study:

- a prospective (also called concurrent) cohort study, in which the cohort is identified and exposure determined as it occurs, and cohort members followed over time to determine outcome (Figure 6.1).
- a retrospective (also called historical) cohort study, in which the cohort is identified and historical exposure information collected (Figure 6.2). The historical cohort study also may collect historical outcome data, so that all the data is abstracted at a single time point.

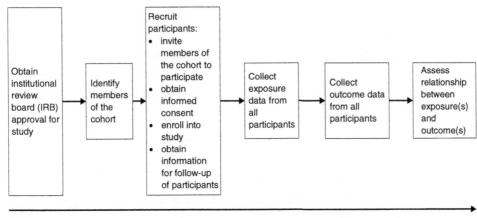

Time

Figure 6.1. Prospective (Concurrent) Cohort Study Design.

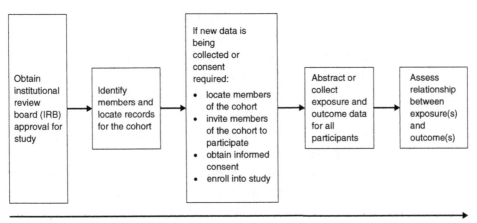

Time

Figure 6.2. Retrospective (Historical) Cohort Study Design.

As such, many record reviews (Chapter 9) are actually retrospective cohort studies. Once a retrospective cohort has been identified, additional outcome information may be collected as well.

Example 6A: The Nurses Health Study is a large-scale, long-term prospective cohort study, begun in 1976, with subsequent waves started in 1989 and 2010. In the original cohort, nurses in 11 states were contacted by mail and asked whether they would be willing to participate.

Those agreeing to participate were asked detailed questions about multiple potential exposure factors. Periodically, exposure information is updated, new exposures assessed prospectively, and outcomes, such as major adverse events, updated. Information about participants who have died is collected from contacts identified by the participants and public records.

Example 6A is a prospective cohort study of a large population. Such an approach allows the cohort to be divided based on any of the exposures for which the investigators have collected data. These exposures can then be assessed against any of the outcomes queried (e.g., cardiovascular disease, cancers of various types, strokes). As the cohort has aged (and many individuals have now been followed for almost 40 years), the study has systematically collected additional exposures (such as hormonal replacement therapy for menopausal symptoms and detailed diet records), while ongoing exposures can be updated (e.g., smoking history), and new adverse events can be collected. The study has established a specimen bank that also allows for genetic studies and validation of putative markers of subsequent disease. Ultimately, the data collected could be used to assess the association of any of the potential exposures collected with any of the potential outcomes collected leading to a plethora of publications.

There are very few such cohort studies, however, because of the money and time involved in forming and following the cohort. Other noteworthy large cohort studies include the Framingham Heart Study (started in 1948 and now following the third generation of participants and expanded to include additional cohorts from the area) and the Honolulu Heart Program (started in 1965). However, most cohort studies focus on a smaller group and fewer outcomes, and occur over a shorter period of time.

Example 6B: An investigator reviewed the records of all patients hospitalized with Crohn's disease who were treated in a single institution over a 10-year period to obtain an adequate number of participants. Such a retrospective cohort study can assess the impact of various factors (e.g., patient characteristics, prior medical history, different treatments used when treating these patients during this admission, etc.) on outcomes such as complications, time to recovery, and others during the hospitalization.

Example 6C: An investigator decides to summarize the data on all patients seen in a specialty pain clinic during the previous calendar year. Such a retrospective cohort study can describe the population coming to the clinic, including their diagnosis, prior treatments, , and the treatment offered to them. The outcome of treatment can also be assessed among those with follow-up data.

In both these examples, the population is selected for a specific characteristic. Both examples are retrospective cohort studies – that is, the cohort was formed and both exposure and outcome information obtained retrospectively. This allowed both these studies to be completed relatively quickly. However, it would be possible to do either study as a prospective cohort study, although this approach would require a much longer period of time.

Example 6B (continued): Instead of abstracting data from medical records for the last 10 years of admissions for Crohn's disease, the investigator could systematically collect data on patients admitted for Crohn's disease until an adequate number of participants had been identified. Based on the number admitted to the hospital (about 15 per year for the age group of interest), this would require about 10 years before there would be adequate data for analysis.

A prospective cohort study can also be done on routinely collected data.

Example 6D: As part of a hospital quality improvement program, routine data is prospectively collected on all patients receiving outpatient surgery. This data included basic demographics and risk factors on each patient from the pre-admission anesthesia assessment, the type of surgery (which was then classified by surgical severity for the analysis), staff involved in care, the duration of the surgery from administrative records, and outcome (e.g., need for postoperative admission into the hospital, emergency room visit within 48 hours of surgery, etc.). This is a prospective cohort study attempting to identify risk factors for adverse outcomes so that they can be reduced.

Cohort studies with the same design and protocol may be done on different groups of individuals to determine if the exposure-outcome relationships are the same in each group. For example, an investigator might want to determine if the effects of chemical exposures are influenced by other environmental factors, so the investigator might study cohorts in different factories around the country. These studies are called comparative cohort studies and are usually done at about the same time to avoid temporal effects.

6.2 Advantages of Cohort Studies Compared to Interventional Studies

There are three major advantages to cohort studies compared to interventional studies. Perhaps most important is that cohort studies are the only way to assess all the effects of an exposure that could not ethically be used in an interventional study.

Example 6A (continued): In the Nurses Health Study, information on cigarette smoking was collected concurrent with use. Subsequent studies have assessed the effect of smoking on breast cancer. The exposure information could also be used to assess the impact of smoking on any of the other outcomes collected. One could not do an interventional study of smoking because it would be unethical to deliberately expose individuals to an intervention that is known to be harmful. Even before there was a general acceptance that smoking was harmful, an interventional study of smoking would have been impractical: recruiting a population that agrees to be randomized to smoking or not would for all practical purposes be impossible.

Another advantage of the cohort study is that results can be rapidly available. By using a retrospective (historical) cohort design, a long interval of time between exposure and outcomes can have already elapsed before starting the study. Thus, results could be obtained rapidly rather than having to wait potentially several decades in a prospective cohort study or an interventional study.

Example 6E: All employees at a nuclear processing facility could be used to form a cohort. The employees could be classified on the amount of radiation exposure during their employment. A cohort study of these employees could determine the short- and long-term effects of the radiation exposures. If a retrospective cohort study began many years after the factory started operation, then the radiation exposure would be based on historical information, but it would be relatively quick to determine the long-term outcome of the radiation exposure.

Finally, a cohort study can be comprehensive. The approach can be used to determine the natural history of the exposure, that is, the spectrum of outcomes occurring following the exposure. In contrast, most interventional studies are focused on a single outcome of primary interest.

Example 6E (continued): Although the cohort study might have been started because of concern about a specific disease (e.g., lung cancer), it would be possible to collect information on a range of outcomes (e.g., the entire medical history after start of exposure). Thus this study could rapidly determine whether there was an association between the radiation exposure and subsequent lung cancer, as well as the association between radiation exposure and other types of cancer, cardiovascular disease, other respiratory diseases, and other diseases.

6.3 Disadvantages of Cohort Studies Compared to Interventional Studies

A cohort study has the same scientific logic as an interventional study: the exposure occurs first, followed by the outcome. There is no question about the temporal sequence of these events. However, even if the temporal sequence is known, this does not ensure that there is a causal relationship.

Example 6B (continued): The investigators compared the outcome (discharge with Crohn's disease resolved) and side effects among those receiving steroids for Crohn's disease to the outcome and side effects among those not receiving steroids. They found that there were significant side effects associated with using steroids, and that the duration of stay was longer.

Such results suggest that steroids do not improve outcome in Crohn's disease. However, this association is only an association. It is not a causal relationship, and may be explained by other factors.

Example 6B (continued): The investigators found that patients receiving steroids generally had much more severe Crohn's disease (e.g., a higher Crohn's disease activity index) when treatment began. This could be just bad luck, of course, but it would raise the concern that the difference between the two groups was due to the worse prognosis among those receiving steroids, rather than an effect of steroid treatment itself. However, this difference might also reflect that patients with higher scores were given steroids because they were sicker, and physicians felt that these patients had more need for steroids – so that more complications and longer hospitalization would be confounded with receiving steroids. This is called confounding by indication.

This illustrates the most important problem with an observational study: exposure is not randomized to participants, but rather is chosen by the participant (or someone else, such as the participant's physician with the patients in Examples 6B and 6C). This can lead to the confounding of participant characteristics with outcome. Confounding variables are variables that are not manipulated by the investigator and are not a focal point of the study, but may affect the relationship between predictors and outcome, and can even cause an apparent reversal of the results. Confounding is discussed extensively in Section 16.2.

Example 6B (continued): Although the investigator found that steroids appeared to lead to more complications and longer hospitalizations than occurred for patients who did not receive steroids, models predicting outcome based on patient characteristics including the severity of the disease at admission found that the patients receiving steroids actually had a better outcome than expected.

Example 6F: In a study of the effect of a chemical exposure, employees volunteered to work in the area with high exposure because the job paid more. One can speculate, therefore, that such employees were of lower socioeconomic status, since they sought out the dirtier but better-paying job. Thus, an increased risk for a variety of health problems might be due to their socioeconomic status rather than the exposure itself. It was also found that there were more minority employees exposed to the chemical than would be expected based on the cohort working in the factory, and minority status is also associated with an increased risk for a variety of health problems.

This confounding can even lead to opposite conclusions from an interventional study.

Example 6G: There is substantial observational data suggesting that hormone replacement therapy reduces cardiovascular disease in women. A systematic review in 1991 found that in 15 of 16 prospective cohort studies, hormone replacement therapy reduced the rate of cardiovascular disease. In contrast, the Women's Health Initiative, a randomized interventional study, found that hormone replacement therapy increased the risk of coronary heart disease in older post-menopausal women. This certainly raises the concern that in these prospective cohort studies women who decided to use hormone replacement therapy had other factors that counteracted the increase in risk from the hormones themselves. Perhaps these women also were more "proactive" with their health, so they had lower levels of other risk factors (e.g., lower smoking rates, better diet, lower body mass index, more exercise, etc.). All of these good behaviors would reduce overall cardiovascular risk.

The other major problem with a cohort study, as with all observational studies, is that the data is generally less reliable than in an interventional study.

Example 6D (continued): Although the data was collected prospectively for the hospital quality improvement program, it may not have been complete for one of the major adverse events. Emergency room visits within 48 hours of the outpatient surgery would only be identified if the patient returned to the hospital doing the study. If the patient went to a different hospital, the event would not be known.

6.4 Prospective versus Retrospective Cohort Studies

There are many trade-offs between a prospective and a retrospective cohort study (Table 6.1). A prospective cohort study compared to a retrospective study:

- generally will take a long time until the outcomes occur;
- generally will have better quality information; and
- generally will be far more expensive.

In contrast a retrospective cohort study compared to a prospective study:

- generally can obtain results quickly;
- potentially has significant data quality issues; and
- is generally less costly.

Table 6.1 Prospective and Retrospective Cohort Studies for Long-Term Outcomes

	Prospective (Concurrent) Cohort Study	Retrospective (Historical) Cohort Study
Duration of study	Duration determined by outcomes of interest: very long term for long-term outcomes	Results potentially available relatively quickly
Data quality: exposure	Exposure information collected specifically for study as it occurs; should be more reliable than retrospective cohort study	Exposure information collected retrospectively. Depending on source of information, can be as reliable as prospective cohort study (if records made concurrent with exposure were systematically kept and can be obtained) but may be very poor
Data quality: outcome	Outcome information collected specifically for study as it occurs; should be more reliable than retrospective cohort study	Outcome information may be collected concurrently specifically for the study and thus be as reliable as prospective cohort study, or may be historical and thus have potentially poorer quality

Table 6.1 (*cont.*)

	Prospective (Concurrent) Cohort Study	Retrospective (Historical) Cohort Study
Potential completeness	Dropouts from the ongoing study limit outcome information. If dropout rate differs between groups based on exposure, this may bias results, but analysis may be able to adjust for this	Potential inability to find all members of the cohort to obtain outcome information may bias study either by missing adverse outcomes or missing healthy outcomes. If exposure information also requires information from all participants, then existence and magnitude of differences not known
Logistics	Sufficient infrastructure to systematically collect information and follow cohort members over time	Less infrastructure than prospective cohort study as cohort members do not have to be systematically followed over time
Costs	May be expensive, particularly for long-term follow-up	Variable: many done "on the cheap"

Example 6E (continued): In the radiation exposure study, a prospective study might require 20–30 years of follow-up to determine the long-term effects of the radiation exposure in the cohort. In contrast, a retrospective cohort study, started 20–30 years after the exposure, could determine the long-term outcomes relatively quickly. However, in a prospective study, investigators can systematically collect individual exposure information (e.g., using individual dosiometers) so that the exposure information would be reliable, while investigators in the retrospective study might have to estimate exposure based on job classification and part of facility in which the participant worked, so that this information would potentially be much less reliable. In addition, in the prospective cohort study participants would have to be systematically followed for a number of years, which is a costly and time-consuming process, while in the retrospective study they would only have to be found and contacted once.

For all these reasons, the first publication for many investigators is a retrospective cohort study based on existing hospital or clinic records, also called a record review (Chapter 9). However, even when the plan is to do such a study, a prospective study may become necessary.

Example 6C (continued): After reviewing the records available at the pain clinic, the investigator realized that only about half the patients had follow-up data, and that most of these patients continued to have significant pain. The investigator speculated that when pain was reduced in patients, they continued the treatment through the physician referring them to the pain clinic. Similarly, if the pain had ceased altogether, they had no further need to attend the clinic. Although the investigator could have contacted the previously treated patients to determine the outcome of their prior treatment, the local Institutional Review Board (IRB) felt that this was an intrusion, since the patients had never consented to the follow-up contact and it was being done only for research purposes. The investigator convinced the clinic to institute a standard follow-up contact for subsequent patients approximately one month after the clinic visit to determine the outcome of treatment as part of the routine clinic procedures, which allowed the investigator to study the outcome of patients attending the clinic.

However, if outcomes are measured short term, then adequate information may be obtained in a short period of time to make the prospective cohort study preferable.

Example 6D (continued): The hospital doing the quality improvement study had approximately 20,000–30,000 outpatient procedures per year. Although the number of adverse events was relatively small (0.2%), even after one year patterns were beginning to emerge that could be used to develop methods to reduce adverse events.

6.5 Ethical Issues

There are several ethical issues relevant to all observational studies. First, if some information becomes known, it can have significant adverse consequences for the participant, possibly impacting access to life insurance, or even leading to legal problems if information involves criminal activities such as recreational drug use or driving while under the influence of alcohol. A major concern in any observational study is whether the procedures to maintain confidentiality of information will be adequate. This issue applies no matter how the information is obtained.

Second, if the study involves direct contact with participants, there is the potential distress to participants. Even asking for information can cause discomfort to the participants by bringing back bad memories or making the participant think about things they would prefer not to think about. This especially applies when a surrogate (for example, a spouse or a friend) is asked for information about the participant after the participant's death or incapacity. When surrogates are contacted, moreover, there is the potential risk to participant's privacy by asking the surrogate for information about the participant of which the surrogate was previously unaware.

Finally, even if the information does not cause distress, often cohort studies collect extensive information, which takes time and effort from the participant. The rationale from the investigators' perspective is that the major costs are in locating and obtaining information, so that the marginal cost of an extra data item is minimal. However, one issue that must be considered is how much information and effort is needed from participants for all the information being collected, and whether all the information will actually be used.

KEY POINTS

- A cohort study follows a group of individuals over time to assess the impact of potential exposures on outcome.
- There are two basic designs:
  - a prospective (concurrent) cohort study in which exposure information is collected as it occurs and outcome determined over time; and
  - a retrospective (historical) cohort study in which exposure information is collected retrospectively and related to current (or previous) outcomes.

- Both designs suffer from the basic problem that since the exposure is not randomly allocated to participants, the effect of the exposure may be confounded by other factors leading participants to choose to be (or not be) exposed.
- Cohort studies have several potential advantages:
  - for exposures that could not ethically be used in an interventional study, they are the only way to determine the outcomes;
  - using a retrospective design allows long-term outcomes to be determined quickly; and
  - a cohort study can provide information on all the outcomes associated with an exposure.
- A major concern in all cohort studies is the quality of the information.
- Because a retrospective cohort study can lead to results relatively quickly, a record review using this design is often the first study an investigator does.

7

Case-Control Studies

A case-control study is a retrospective observational study where the objective is to determine which exposures might be associated with a specific outcome. Exposure is compared between a group of participants who have the outcome of interest and one (or more) groups of participants who do not have the outcome. A case-control study may be used when it is unethical to use a potentially harmful exposure in an interventional study, when a cohort study would have to be impractically large to yield enough participants with the outcome of interest, or when the outcome of interest may take an extended period of time to develop. Case-control studies are often used to screen many different exposures to identify potential risk factors.

7.1 Basic Design

In a case-control study there are at least two groups; cases, who have the outcome of interest (usually disease, disability, or death); and controls, who do not (Figure 7.1). After collecting consents from participants and performing appropriate screening procedures, historical data on exposures is collected and compared between the two groups. The general principle is to have all participants meet the same inclusion and exclusion criteria, with the exception of the outcome of interest. The use of matching to make these groups more similar is described in Chapter 27. In general, controls who are recruited and studied over the same time period as cases (called concurrent controls) are preferable to individuals who were studied at an earlier time (called historical controls).

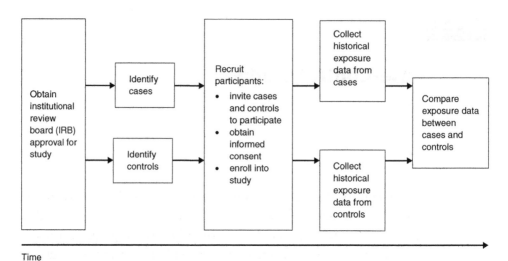

Time

Figure 7.1. Case-Control Study Design.

Example 7A: Investigators propose to do a case-control study to determine if a condition is associated with specific long-term dietary habits. The cases would be individuals newly diagnosed with the condition; the controls would be cases without it; dietary histories would be obtained after the participants are enrolled. Cases and controls will be selected from the same neighborhoods in order to reduce the effects of socioeconomic differences and exposures to local pollutants. To enhance this similarity, both cases and controls will have to have lived in their area for at least 5 years prior to entering the study.

There may be, and often are, multiple exposures of interest. In Example 7A, long-term dietary habits are the exposure of interest. As in many studies, this concept includes several variables, such as fat intake, fiber intake, and salt intake, among many others. Other factors, such as exercise, might be confounding variables. The investigators will often want to see if there is an interaction between multiple factors in predicting the outcome.

It is also possible to have more than one control group for a given group of cases.

Example 7B: In a study to determine if late-onset depression in the elderly was associated with white-matter hyper-intensities (WHI) in the brain, two control groups were selected. The cases were all participants whose first episode of depression occurred after age 50. One control group consisted of participants over age 50 who had never experienced mental illness; the other consisted of participants over age 50 who had recurrent depression, diagnosed using the same criteria as was used to diagnose the participants in the first group, with the first episode before age 35. The first control group tested whether depression might be associated with WHI, while the second group tested whether this was specific to late onset depression.

It is not necessary to have equal numbers of cases and controls in a study. Frequently, only a small number of cases are available, and more controls are used to improve the ability to detect differences between groups (Appendix B, Section B.7).

7.2 Selecting Participants

The identification of participants for each of the groups is a critical part of the study. Care must be taken to avoid introducing bias, which could confound the results. Most investigators prefer to identify cases through health care providers. This can include individual physicians who treat patients with the condition, as well as clinics or hospitals. Potential cases identified in this way are more likely to have the condition of interest. Moreover, these individuals are more likely to have records of medical problems and treatments available. The investigators will have to obtain informed consent as necessary and must protect the privacy of the individual in accordance with government regulations (Section 2.1.2). More details on recruiting participants can be found in Chapter 13.

In many ways the identification of controls is more difficult than the identification of cases, and this topic is discussed in detail in Chapter 26. Ideally, the controls should represent the same population as the cases, and satisfy the same inclusion and exclusion criteria as the cases, with the exception of not having the outcome of interest. Although there may be exceptions in special circumstances, in general you would want as potential controls only people who would be identified as potential cases if they had the condition.

Example 7C: In a study to determine if lack of exercise is associated with the onset of Type II diabetes in adults younger than 40 years, cases were identified and recruited from the diabetes clinic in a public hospital. The investigator initially planned to recruit the controls from individuals who are employed at the hospital and are free of that or related diseases. However, the employees had a higher income, were better educated, and had access to better medical care; they might also have a healthier diet and be more aware of the importance of exercise. A control group that avoided many of these problems could be identified from other clinics in the hospital. However, this means that the controls would have other diseases, which might also be associated with exercise. Parents of children being treated in hospital clinics would likely use the hospital for their own medical care so would be an appropriate control group.

7.3 Matching

A case-control study may be either matched or not matched. A matched case-control study is one in which controls are matched to the cases on important prognostic factors. Controls may be individually matched – that is, each control is matched to a single case on these factors – or the controls may be matched to cases in frequency so that the distributions of these factors are the same in both groups. As an example of the latter, if the cases are 35% female, then the controls would also be 35% female. Matching is described in detail in Chapter 27. We will just give some basic ideas here, because matching is so often used in case-control studies to make the controls as similar as possible to the cases.

For individual matching:

- Control participants must all be matched to specific individual cases, and all cases included in the analysis must have matching controls. Cases without any suitable controls would not be included in any analysis.
- There may be multiple control groups, with control participants in each group matched to a case. Cases are included in the analysis only

when there are matching controls, so some cases may not be compared to all control groups.

- There may be multiple controls in one control group matched to a case, but a control participant may not be matched to multiple cases.
- Cases may have different numbers of matched controls.
- Matching criteria may be exact, such as sex, or within a range, such as age within 5 years.

Example 7D: In a study of a childhood disease, one of the three control groups consisted of children in the same school class as the case. The controls were individually matched to a case, and if no matching child was enrolled into the control group, the case could not be included in the analysis for this specific control group. Using a child from the same classroom controls for a number of factors that are hard to measure, including socioeconomic status of parents, environmental exposures in the neighborhood, community knowledge, behavior, and health care practices.

In a frequency-matched study, there may also be more controls than cases. The goal is to have the control population have the same distribution as the cases on the matching factors. For example, if matching was done on education and one-third of the cases had only a high school degree, one-third had at least some college, and one-third had advanced degrees, then the control group, no matter how large, should consist of one-third high school only, one-third some college, and one-third with advanced degrees.

7.4. Nested Case-Control Studies

In a nested case-control study, both the cases and controls are drawn from a population that has been studied or is being studied as part of a large cohort study. Most large cohort studies, such as the Framingham Heart Study or the Nurses' Health Study mentioned as examples in Chapter 6, include nested case-control studies for studying special topics. This can have several advantages. Because both groups are from the same population (the cohort itself), cases and controls should be similar for many criteria. For example, women in the Nurses' Health Study would have similar levels of education and knowledge of health issues. Other cohorts may be limited by age, income, or ethnicity; for example, in the Framingham Heart Study, the initial cohort only included participants between the ages of 30 and 62 who were resident in a particular city and were considered healthy at the time of enrollment.

Additional advantages of this approach are that the two groups should be comparable with respect to the availability of data, and potentially much of the data needed may have already been obtained as part of the cohort study. The data may even have been obtained before the occurrence of the disease of interest, minimizing differential information biases. The disadvantage of this approach is that you are limited to the population that was selected for the cohort study and to the information collected for the cohort study, unless additional data collection is being done.

Example 7E: Risk factors for syncope were examined in one of the many nested case-control studies using Framingham Heart Study participants. The cases were identified from clinic visits. Controls from the cohort were individually matched to cases on age, sex, and examination period in the ratio of two controls for each case.

Although existing records are being used to identify potential cases and controls, it is often necessary to collect additional information from participants (or, for some diseases, a surrogate respondent after the case's death). Often you must actually confirm that cases do meet the case definition and, equally importantly, that controls do not have the condition being studied.

7.5 Advantages and Disadvantages of Case-Control Studies

A case-control study shares many of the advantages and disadvantages of a cohort study, particularly a retrospective cohort study. Like a cohort study, it may be used when a randomized interventional study is inappropriate. Like a retrospective cohort study, it also has the advantage that all of the relevant events must have occurred, so there is no need to wait for the effect of an exposure to develop. In some cases – particularly in a nested case-control study – most of the information required may already have been recorded and will be readily available. As data on multiple different exposures can be collected on a relatively small number of participants, the case-control study is very useful for generating hypotheses to test in subsequent studies.

As a cohort study might never get enough participants with the outcome of interest, the case-control study is more useful than a cohort study if cases are relatively rare. Also, by focusing on specific outcomes, it may be possible to identify rare exposures related to that outcome. Another advantage is that in a case-control study, matching can be used to diminish the effect of confounding variables.

The same circumstances that give the case-control study these advantages also create some disadvantages. Since participants are not randomized, they choose their own exposures; therefore, their characteristics can be confounded both with exposure and outcome. In many situations the investigators do not control some or all of the data collection, so they are dependent on the efforts of others and often have to depend on someone's recall of events and behaviors far in the past. Therefore, data in a case-control study is generally considered less reliable than data in a prospective cohort study. Another disadvantage is that it may take a relatively long time to locate the cases and verify their eligibility. Moreover, matching, especially individual matching, can further increase the time required to find study participants. Finally, a case-control study may not be as useful as a cohort study, as only one outcome is being studied.

In addition, the logic of the case-control study is different from that of the cohort study. In the cohort study, the investigator is asking whether presence of an exposure is associated with a higher incidence of the subsequent outcome, while in the case-control study, the question is whether the outcome is associated with a higher rate of prior exposure. Although a causative link is not determined in either a case-control or a cohort study, the connection seems clearer in the cohort study because the temporal sequence is clearer.

7.6 Ethical Issues

The ethical issues for observational studies described in Chapter 6 apply equally to case-control studies. Since some information can have significant adverse consequences to the participant if the information becomes known, procedures to maintain confidentiality of information are essential. As cases are often selected because they are sick, you must consider how much information and effort is needed from participants, and whether all the information is actually needed. Causing distress to participants is an even bigger concern in case-control studies, as you are inquiring about potential causes of the disease. If the source of information is a surrogate (for example, a spouse or a friend) who is asked for information about the participant after the participant's death or incapacity, there are concerns both about distress to the surrogate and potentially disclosing information about the deceased participant to the surrogate.

Case-control studies are very susceptible to bias. We assume that the investigators would not let their knowledge of the outcome influence their selection of participants, but there are often problems selecting appropriate controls. The investigator must make sure that cases and controls come from the same population. This problem is discussed further in Chapter 26.

Since case-control studies are retrospective, recall bias (Section 17.1.4) is a particular problem, as is the accuracy and consistency of historical data. Ideally, historical information will be collected by investigators without knowledge of whether the participant is a case or control using appropriate blinding techniques (Chapter 28). Finally, the conditions that define a case may also influence the exposures which the case may have. For example, a case's medical problems may restrict an individual's ability to work, thus reducing his income, thus he may eat a different diet than controls who are healthier and have a larger income.

KEY POINTS

- A case-control study may be done for any of several reasons:
  - when studying a rare outcome;
  - when an interventional study is inappropriate; or
  - when attempting to develop hypotheses for further study.

- A case-control study by definition is retrospective so it can be completed relatively quickly. However, there is a great potential for bias in this type of study.
- The study is based on one outcome, which is known when participants are selected.
- There are at least two groups of participants:
  - those with the outcome of interest – the cases; and
  - one or more groups of individuals who do not have the outcome of interest – the controls.
- Cases and controls should come from the same population so that demographic differences will not influence the analysis. Ideally, anyone used as a control would have been identified as a potential case if they had the outcome of interest at the time of the study.
- The quality of information may be a problem.
- Because the outcome is known, there is a danger of bias when selecting cases and controls and in obtaining information, so steps must be taken to avoid bias.

Cross-Sectional Studies

A cross-sectional study is the clinical research equivalent of a survey in social research. A cross-sectional study can provide a good overview of specific issues, such as the prevalence of a disease in a population. It provides a description of what is and makes no attempt to infer cause-effect relationships.

8.1 Fundamental Features

There are two fundamental features of the cross-sectional study (Figure 8.1). First, each individual's data is considered to apply to a single point in time. Usually, all the data would be physically collected at the same time for a participant, but on occasion data from several different visits may have to be combined. The participants need not all be observed at the same calendar time; usually participants are identified over an interval. More importantly, the data collected is used only to describe results at that point in time.

In some ways, the data collection for a cross-sectional study is very similar to a retrospective cohort study in which all the data collection is done at one point in time, but the objectives are different. In the cohort study the data can be used to infer a cause-effect relationship between historical data (from records or participant recall) and current events (such as disease status). In contrast, in a cross-sectional study you do not attempt to infer cause-effect relationships: you are attempting only to describe what is. As we discussed in Chapter 6, a retrospective (historical) cohort study would be used to infer

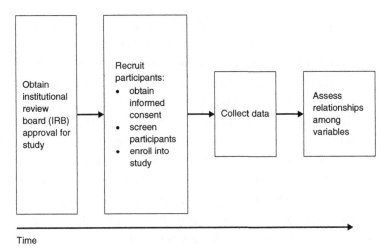

Time

Figure 8.1. Cross-Sectional Study Design.

cause-effect relationships even if all the data is obtained at a single time point.

8.2 Examples of Cross-Sectional Studies

A cross-sectional study can provide a good overview of specific issues, such as the incidence and prevalence of a disease in a population. The data may be abstracted from clinical records or formally collected from questionnaires administered during the observation period or from results of laboratory assays or imaging studies. Although such studies are often thought of as easy, there are many practical issues that can affect the results, which we discuss in Chapter 29. We begin with two large-scale national examples to illustrate how extensive the data collection can be.

Example 8A: The U.S. Centers for Disease Control and Prevention does weekly surveillance of a number of different diseases in the Morbidity and Mortality Weekly Report (MMWR), summarizing data from state public health departments across the country. This weekly data provides the incidence (number of new cases) of various diseases that week.

Although the data collected in Example 8A is from many sources, the objective is fairly simple: to record incidence. Special topics, such as the capacity of state health departments to perform specific diagnostic assays and changes in incidence of a disease over time, may also be studied.

Sometimes cross-sectional studies are done repeatedly over time on different participants, and estimates are compared from one time period to the next to assess time trends. There are, in fact, many national studies that have been done over many years, studying various aspects of health, such as the percentage of patients in hospitals without health insurance coverage, the percentage of patients using emergency rooms because they do not have a primary care provider, risk behaviors (e.g., alcohol, smoking, seatbelt use), and so forth.

Example 8B: The U.S. Department of Health and Human Services has been conducting what is now called the National Health and Nutrition Examination Survey (NHANES) as a series of cross-sectional studies since the early 1960s. It is designed to assess the health and nutritional status of adults and children in the United States. It combines interviews, physical examination, and laboratory tests on a randomly selected population in the United States, which may take one or two years to complete. It provides the prevalence of various health conditions in various populations. The results of a single survey (wave) provide the prevalence of disease at a single point in time, while analysis of results from surveys done over time can identify trends in the data.

The NHANES is a much more complex collection of data than the MMWR is. Data from the NHANES is used not only to estimate prevalence but also to compare demographic subgroups on the prevalence of disorders and to detect associations between health measures and life style and environmental factors. The latter have led to cohort, case-control, or interventional studies to validate a cause-effect relationship. Analyses over time have been used to track recommended changes in behavior, such as a lower cholesterol intake, and to develop growth curves for children. Data from the survey is available to outside investigators for study.

The NHANES and the MMWR are both large surveys covering the entire United States. A more typical example of a cross-sectional study would be the following.

Example 8C: An investigator wants to study the characteristics and particularly the treatments being given to patients admitted to their hospital for Crohn's disease during the past 12 months. All data is collected from the patient's medical record at time of discharge, and might include demographic information about the patient, history of Crohn's disease and other diseases, information about treatments, and even outcome.

This would be a nice descriptive study of the population being treated for Crohn's diseases in that hospital. The results would be information about this specific group of patients – what percentage were female, what the age distribution was, how many other conditions they had, how long they had Crohn's disease, what percentage received various treatments, the distribution of dose received, the distribution of duration of treatment, and so on. The investigator could also summarize hospitalization information, such as how long the patients were in the hospital, and look at the association between demographic and clinical factors such as severity or hospitalization time. Even though the data in Example 8C is collected over time, it is pooled together and treated as a single estimate, for example as the treatment pattern during a specific period.

Example 8D: An investigator collects data on patients arriving with a suspected myocardial infarction (MI) in the emergency room (ER). The data abstracted from the medical record and collected as part of routine care included age, weight, blood pressure, time of day of initial symptoms, among other measurements, with the intent of describing the pattern of these variables over time. In addition to medical record data, the investigator also collects data about some recent activities from the participants using a questionnaire after obtaining informed consent, following the Institutional Review Board (IRB) approved procedures. This includes such information as whether the participant had been driving in a traffic jam or had intercourse during the previous 24 hours and some historical data from the participant, such as prior smoking history and history of a prior MI.

Even though there was an interval between the recent activities and the arrival in the ER, this would still be a cross-sectional study, with the focus again on describing the data for the group of participants arriving at this ER for a suspected MI during this period of time. This data could be used to describe the events prior to coming to the ER, but not to infer a cause-effect relationship, since all the participants have the effect: coming to the ER with a suspected MI.

Example 8D (continued): In addition, the investigator collects data at time of discharge (from the ER or hospital) about whether the suspected MI was, in fact, an acute MI.

Now the question of the study design becomes much more complicated. Although the data is potentially collected over time, the results still apply to a single point in time for the participant, where the point in time is the entire ER and hospitalization history. We would describe this as a cross-sectional study or a cohort study depending on how the study protocol, approved by the IRB prior to collecting data, specified that the data was to be used.

Example 8D (continued): Cross-sectional study: The investigator reports that 20% of the group of participants arriving in the ER with suspected MI had a diagnosis of MI at discharge.
Cohort study: The investigator reports that 20% of the group of participants arriving in the ER with suspected MI had a diagnosis of MI at discharge and that arrival with specific symptoms or physical measurements or prior history were predictive of a diagnosis of MI at discharge.

In the cross-sectional study the data use is descriptive, whereas in the cohort study it is used to explore the relationship between exposures and outcomes. So how the data will be used – and what results will be presented – determines whether the study would be a cross-sectional study or a cohort study.

8.3 Some Common Problems in Cross-Sectional Studies

Cross-sectional studies have many of the same problems as other observational studies. Frequently you may have to find or develop a questionnaire for the study. Sometimes you can find a questionnaire that fits your requirements, but often you find you have to create one or modify an existing one for your study. Like any study based on questionnaires, the results depend on who is asked, what they are asked, and how they are asked, so this is not necessarily a simple project. In Section 29.2.1, we discuss this is some detail.

Cross-sectional studies that use hospital charts or tests as data sources have the problems of all observational studies that rely on data collected outside a formal study protocol. In particular, the data may be incomplete and inconsistent standards used for measuring and reporting data. These data issues are discussed in Chapters 6 and 7 and in detail in Section 25.2.

8.4 Ethical Issues

The same issues that apply to other studies when patient information is being collected apply to these studies, even though they may seem less intrusive, especially if you are only abstracting information from medical records. These issues include IRB approval, informed consent if required by your IRB, and participant confidentiality.

On some occasions, for example if you are asking people in the cafeteria about heartburn, your IRB may allow you to ask questions about a nonsensitive topic without a written informed consent, provided you read a statement at the beginning saying that participants are free not to answer any questions, to stop whenever they would like, and possibly that their medical care will not be affected by participating or not. However, like all studies, your cross-sectional study must be submitted to your IRB and approved by them before you begin the study, and you must follow your IRB's informed consent requirements for your study.

Depending on the nature of the questions being asked, when they are asked, and how they are asked, even asking questions may raise ethical concerns. For example, in Example 8D, asking participants questions when they are concerned that they are having an MI can be quite distressing to the participant – especially if there is an implication that the care they receive is somehow affected by whether they cooperate or not. Moreover, if they are in a crisis situation, they probably do not want to answer questions, and you are adding stress to an already stressful situation.

Even how the questions are being asked can cause stress. Questions should be asked as neutrally as possible, and in as nonthreatening a way as possible. In Example 8D, if the interviewer asks about the participant's behavior before the MI, then this (a) implies that they have had an MI, and (b) raises the concern that somehow their behavior caused the MI. Although asking someone about activities before coming to the emergency room should be less stressful (as there is not an implication that an MI occurred), it is still likely to be stressful.

KEY POINTS

- Cross-sectional studies are the clinical research equivalent of surveys in social research.
- Cross-sectional studies may involve actual questionnaires as well as medical record review, physical examinations, and laboratory tests.
- Cross-sectional studies may be used to determine the prevalence of diseases, to describe the characteristics and behaviors of a population at one point in time, and to examine relationships between variables at that point in time.
- A cross-sectional study should not be designed to use some of the data to predict subsequent data or to identify a cause-effect relationship. If that is the objective, then the study should be considered a cohort study and designed as such.
- Although seemingly simple, the results of a cross-sectional study depend critically on who you study and how you ask your questions or obtain your data.
- Like all observational studies, if data is obtained outside a formal study, there may be problems of completeness and accuracy.

9

Record Reviews

Often, new investigators begin their research with a record review. A record review is not a specific study design, but refers to a study that is based solely on existing data. There is no new data collected for this study. A record review can have a retrospective (historical) cohort study design, a case-control study design, or a cross-sectional study design. Importantly, although as in every study Institutional Review Board (IRB) approval is required, in a record review there is no contact with participants, and the consent requirements are usually waived by your IRB. Here we discuss the conceptual aspects of how record reviews and the different observational study designs are related, as well as the major concerns for all record reviews: data availability and quality.

9.1 Data Availability and Quality

By definition, a record review only uses existing data. No new data is collected as part of the record review, although extensive work may be required to organize the data so that it can be analyzed. Just because the data exists, however, does not mean you have the right to use it without prior IRB permission. When the IRB does approve it, it is normally approved with a waiver of consent, so that you do not have to get informed consent from the participants. This is discussed further in Section 9.3

9.1.1 Data Availability

The existing records may be available in either a single comprehensive electronic medical record with all data easily retrieved and linked together without special assistance, or require work using multiple data sets to obtain the necessary information. Sometimes, even when there is a data warehouse for a health care system, which consolidates information into a single comprehensive record for an individual, retrieval of records is difficult.

Example 9A: The clinic responsible for caring for patients discharged from a hospital on outpatient parenteral antibiotics has maintained a database of all patients treated for several years. In addition to detailed information on all parenteral antibiotics treatment that patients receive, the database includes detailed information on side effects and treatment changes as well as basic patient information including demographics and type of infection. Different fellows have analyzed different aspects of the data, such as the tolerability and efficacy of different antibiotics for the same infection or the outcome of continued treatment following an initial adverse reaction not sufficient to cause a treatment change.

Even then, however, manual data review may be required to assess and confirm some of the data.

In other situations, the records may be pathology log books, which have to be reviewed page by page to identify potential cases for a case-control study. The data may be in patient charts and clinic notes. In fact, many record reviews may require manually reviewing paper records.

Example 9B: Example 6B presents a cohort study involving the use of steroids in patients with Crohn's disease over a 10-year period. Although much of the data was available from online records, the investigators found so many items missing that they eventually did a manual review of the medical record of each of the relevant hospital admissions and then analyzed the re-abstracted data for their publication.

Sometimes data is retrieved from various electronic laboratory data systems, as was done in Example 9A to identify the hospital records needed for the review. Sometimes, the data needed may be found in the text of imaging reports. Enabling automated searches of the various sources of electronic information using natural language processing is a major research focus of some groups. Even then, however, developing and validating an approach to retrieve information may require extensive work and justify a publication solely on the methodology used.

Example 9C: An investigator is interested in identifying foreign-born individuals from a patient data warehouse using natural language processing as one step in a research project. She developed a three stage algorithm using (a) coding as non-English language speaking; (b) searching the electronic medical record for keywords about place of birth and language spoken; and then (c) for the records with keywords, retrieving the text around the keyword and manually confirming the patient as foreign-born. After the algorithm was developed, she did full record reviews of a subset of the data, as well as contacting the patient's primary care provider, to estimate the sensitivity and specificity of the overall algorithm.

9.1.2 Data Quality

Even if retrieving the data is easy, there is always a concern about the quality of the data you are retrieving. Data used in a record review has not been collected for research purposes, usually has not been collected following a specific protocol, and often is incomplete and sometimes even inconsistent. This is particularly true for some material in an online medical record. In part, errors should be expected: the data is entered by each individual caregiver, usually at the time of the encounter, and usually without rigorous data quality control especially of free-text fields. In contrast, in a research study, research staff whose job description includes data entry enter the data. In research studies, the data is normally far more defined and limited, responses are coded rather than free text (or coded shortly after submission as free-text), and data is systematically and rigorously reviewed to ensure data quality.

Example 9D: When patients see their primary care physician (PCP) for medical care, the PCP often enters medical notes for the encounter while meeting with the patient. Certain variables, such as the medication prescribed, would certainly be recorded correctly, since this is part of an electronic prescription. But the symptoms that the patient reported are often recorded as free text during the visit.

9.1.3 What Can Be Done about Data Problems?

Given that the data has often been collected over an extended period by multiple individuals, it is not clear whether or not the data can be corrected. Thus, after doing a preliminary review of the data available, decisions are needed about how missing and inconsistent data items will be handled. Importantly, decisions about handling missing and inconsistent data should be made before attempting to answer the research questions driving the study, and done independently of information about the primary exposures and outcomes of the study.

Example 9B (continued): After checking the entire medical record, there were still some patients who had no information, either positive or negative, about prior attacks of Crohn's disease. For patients who had had encounters with the medical system from before the hospitalization without information about prior attacks of Crohn's disease, it was decided that this would be interpreted as if they had not had a history of prior attacks. For several patients who had not previously been seen in the medical system, however, it was not clear whether this was their first attack or their first admission to the specific hospital. For these patients, the prior medical history was treated as missing and they were excluded from analyses using this variable. All these decisions were made as policy decisions, without knowledge of the exposure variable (steroid use).

Generally, the approach we would recommend is going back to original records, if they exist or can be accessed, to resolve data issues. Sometimes this can lead to unexpected corrections and changes to the data.

Ultimately, however, you need to decide what to do about the data problems, without biasing the results of any subsequent analyses. To do this, the decisions should be made without knowledge of how they will affect the outcomes. This means, in particular, that in a cohort study (like Example 9A), decisions about the exposure (for example, whether there was an adverse reaction to a drug or not) are made without knowledge of the outcome (subsequent adverse reactions, treatment changes, and outcome on treatment). Similarly, when decisions about whether a patient is a case or a control are being made for a case-control study, the decisions should be made without any knowledge of the exposure variables (Section 28.2). The issue of validating data and correcting errors is discussed further in Section 30.5.

9.2 Examples of Record Reviews

Examples of record reviews are scattered throughout the chapters on cohort studies, case-control studies, and cross-sectional studies. In a record review, the conventional designs shown in the previous chapters are modified to reflect that only historical data is collected, without any patient contact. These modifications are shown in Figure 9.1 for the retrospective cohort study, Figure 9.2 for a case-control study, and Figure 9.3 for a cross-sectional study. Comparing these to the original figures, there are two major changes: the IRB approves the study with a waiver of consent, and the participant consent, screening, and enrollment procedures are not needed.

We show here how a record review can be used for a range of study designs.

Example 9E: An investigator wants to investigate the use of antidepressants for the control of pain. He works in a pain clinic that has treated approximately 5,000 patients in the previous 5 years. Data collected during the initial clinic visit include primary and secondary diagnoses

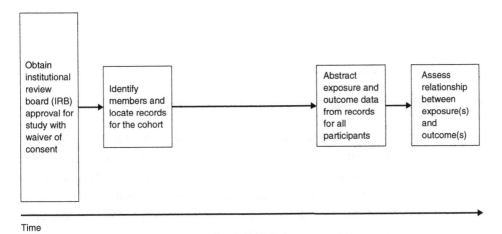

Figure 9.1. Record Review Using Retrospective Cohort Study Design.

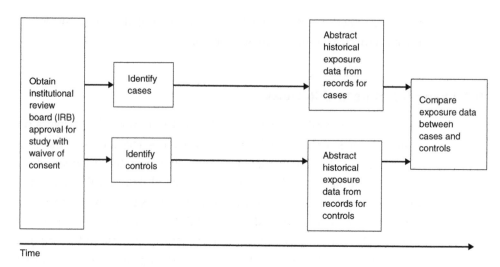

Figure 9.2. Record Review Using Case-Control Study Design.

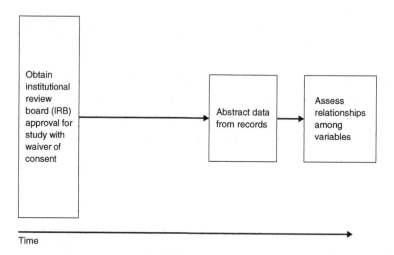

Figure 9.3. Record Review Using Cross-Sectional Study Design.

for the cause of pain, duration of pain, and prior treatment history for pain. At each visit, a current medication history, the current pain level, and any treatments prescribed are recorded. Thus, patients returning to the clinic provide serial measurements of pain control and effectiveness of treatments given at the clinic. There was no systematic follow-up of patients who do not return to the clinic.

There are several possible ways the data could be used to answer different questions about the use of antidepressants for the control of pain.

1. The investigator could do a cross-sectional study of the current medication history to answer the question: "How common is antidepressant usage in patients coming to the clinic?"

2. The investigator could do a cross-sectional study of the treatments assigned at the initial visit of a patient, to answer the question: "How often are antidepressants prescribed to patients at their initial visit coming to the clinic?"

3. The investigator could do a cohort study that can answer the question: "How often are antidepressants prescribed to patients attending the clinic?"

4. The investigator could do a study that can answer the question: "What factors predict which patients coming to the clinic are prescribed anti-depressants?" We consider this a cohort study because it is using existing factors (patient history characteristics) to predict a future outcome (prescription of antidepressants), but others might argue that it is a cross-sectional study because it is using concurrently collected data to examine an association.

5. The investigator could do a case-control study, comparing a sample of records for patients prescribed antidepressants at their initial visit (which may include continuing an existing prescription) to a sample of other patients to answer the question: "What factors are associated with prescribing antidepressants when patients enter the clinic?"

These different possibilities illustrate how important it is to be clear about the purpose of the record review before starting. All of the questions are legitimate, and all "investigate the use of antidepressants for the control of pain," the investigator's stated goal. Any one of these studies could be done entirely using existing records, with no additional data being collected from participants. Thus, a record review can be done using different study designs to answer all these different questions.

Precisely what can be done in the record review depends on what data is already collected, how reliable the data is, and how easy it would be to abstract and use for a project. These practical aspects, which make record reviews complicated, are discussed in detail in Section 25.2.

9.3 Ethical Issues

The primary ethical issues in a record review relate to confidentiality (Section 2.1.2) of individual patient data and the ethical aspects of accessing this data. Even though a record review might appear to be exempt research, an IRB application should always be submitted unless your institution has specific exemption pathways for a record review, in which case you should follow the specified procedures. In our experience, it is usually necessary to be able to link data used in the analysis to actual individuals, at least until the analysis is complete, to check that the data abstraction and data management were correctly done (Chapter 30), and thus such research is not exempt from IRB review. The IRB can, however, waive any requirement for participant consent so that informed consent for the record review is not required from participants. Without such a waiver of the informed consent requirement, you cannot do a record review.

KEY POINTS

- A record review is not a study design: it is an approach to using existing data from records for an observational study.
- A record review can use a retrospective (historical) cohort study design, a case-control study design, or a cross-sectional study design.
- It is critical to be clear about what question you are attempting to answer with the record review before starting it.
- It is essential to have IRB approval (or waiver) for the project before beginning the data abstraction.

Selecting a Design

Now that you know something about study designs, which one should you choose? In this chapter we provide a systematic framework for selecting a reasonable design for your study. Often multiple designs may be possible for similar questions – or even the same question – but all designs have their own strengths and weaknesses.

10.1 A Range of Designs

Sometimes, you could use almost any design for a study.

Example 10A: You are interested in how c-reactive protein (CRP) levels relate to the risk of heart disease. This could be studied in several different ways:

- a cohort study, in which a large group of participants with CRP measurements are followed (either prospectively or retrospectively) to determine the occurrence of heart disease;
- a case-control study, in which a group of cases with heart disease and controls without heart disease are identified and prior CRP measurements obtained from medical records; or
- a randomized interventional study to assess whether treatment with a therapy which affects CRP reduces the occurrence of subsequent heart disease.

Any one of these three designs could potentially answer your underlying question. The three designs involve trade-offs of feasibility, practicality, and timeliness among other issues, so this question, like many questions, does not uniquely determine a particular study design.

Unfortunately, these studies can give different answers. For example, there is extensive evidence from observational studies that a high HDL level reduces the risk of coronary heart disease. However, in randomized interventional studies, drugs developed to raise HDL were successful in raising participants HDL level but had no effect on the rate of coronary heart disease. Similarly, as discussed in Example 6G of the relationship of hormonal replacement therapy and the risk of coronary heart disease in women, the observational studies and randomized studies gave different results.

There are occasions in which the question does determine a specific study design, however. One such type of question is when you are trying to describe something in a particular time frame, such as a description of the patient characteristics and treatments used in your clinic during a specific time period, or how current patients in your clinic describe certain complaints, both of which would be studied using a cross-sectional design. However, such questions are relatively rare.

10.2 Interventional or Observational Study?

10.2.1 Is an Interventional Study Ethical?

Although interventional studies provide the strongest evidence for a causal association between the intervention and the outcome, there is a fundamental issue that must always be considered before starting to consider various interventional designs: Is an interventional study using this intervention ethical?

We wish there was a single standard that gave a YES or NO answer to this question, but such absolute answers are extremely rare.

Example10B: An investigator proposes to study whether a medical procedure – not needed by the population being studied – poses any risks. This is clearly unethical: there is no potential benefit, and there is at least some potential risk. Such a study would never be ethical.

In this example it is clearly not ethical to do an interventional study. However, various observational designs can be used to answer this question. In fact, observational studies are the only way to assess exposures that could not be used in an interventional study.

Rarely is the answer so clear-cut. If the study involves comparison of two interventions for the treatment of disease, then there is a requirement for clinical equipoise, meaning that there is a real question in the minds of the medical community about which of the two treatments are better. Usually this is a far more difficult question to answer and the answer may even vary depending on where you practice.

Example 10C: A group of investigators proposed studying whether patients presenting with an initial AIDS defining illness should be immediately treated with antiretroviral agents as well as treatment for the presenting illness, or whether antiretroviral treatment should be deferred until the presenting illness was treated. Among the over 30 clinics asked to participate, two refused because they already "knew" as a group which approach was better. In the two centers that "knew" which treatment was better, the clinical trial would be considered unethical. In all the other clinical centers, the trial was considered ethical.

In Example 10C, the investigators were not surprised when they learned that at one clinic immediate treatment was always instituted, while at the other clinic treatment was always deferred. Given that there was not even a consensus among those who "knew" the best treatment, there clearly was clinical equipoise on the question.

The decision becomes far more difficult when one is questioning accepted practice.

Example 10D: A group of investigators proposed studying whether drugs used to suppress ventricular arrhythmia actually reduced mortality. When the study was initially proposed, arguments were made that such a study was unethical, because everyone "knew" that treatment with anti-arrhythmia drugs improves survival. Some years later, as more and more questions arose about whether the active treatments actually had benefit, a randomized trial was finally started comparing three standard drugs to placebo. Two of the standard drugs were stopped early in the study because of excessive mortality, and the third drug was later stopped for futility, as it increased early mortality and had little chance of actually reducing overall mortality compared to placebo.

Ultimately, the decision about whether a study is ethical depends on the perceived risk-benefit relationship for the proposed intervention.

Example 10E: A group of investigators proposed using sham surgery to determine whether a surgical procedure actually benefited patients receiving the surgery or whether the benefits reported in multiple independent cases series of the surgery only reflected the patients' belief in the efficacy of the procedure.

The decision on whether such a study is ethical is hardly simple. There is clear potential risk to participants receiving the sham surgery related to the procedures involved in the surgery itself. There are also potential complications arising from the surgery. There would appear to be no potential benefit to the participant from the procedure itself unless one assumes that there could be potential benefit to the participant from the placebo effect. Several such studies have been done in the last few years, one involving a low-risk athroscopic procedure and another higher-risk neurosurgery, both showing that the surgical procedure offered little benefit to participants.

Example 10F: An investigator has observed that despite receiving an adenotonsillectomy (the standard of care), many children continue to have breathing and sleep disturbances with potential long-term adverse cognitive and behavioral outcomes. The investigator proposes to study the effect of continuous positive airway pressure (CPAP) in children with sleep disturbances following adenotonsillectomy in a randomized study to determine the effect on cognitive outcomes. Preliminary studies have already demonstrated that CPAP appears to be safe and tolerable to these children, and appears to have benefit in reducing sleep disturbances. The investigator designed a randomized, open-label study to compare the effect of CPAP on both sleep disturbance and neurocognitive outcomes before and following 6 months of treatment in children continuing to have sleep disturbances after surgery.

Given the prior experience showing that the procedures appeared to be safe and tolerable, and the potential benefit to the children participating, no ethical concerns were raised by any of the groups reviewing the study prior to its starting.

10.2.2 Is an Interventional Study Practical?

Assuming that a potential interventional study is ethical, one then needs to consider the practical aspects of an interventional study compared to an observational study. There are many different practical considerations, but we discuss only three factors that always need to be considered: time, resources, and feasibility. These three factors are usually interrelated.

Interventional studies always take longer than the investigator imagines they will. Depending on the particular intervention being considered, there may be substantial delays in getting the necessary approvals to even begin the research. We are aware of funded studies that have waited for years for various approvals, although most studies take only a few weeks to several months to be approved. Once approval is obtained from your Institutional Review Board (IRB) (and others, if necessary), you then have to identify and screen potential participants, recruit them into the study, do the intervention, and then follow them for the outcome. This follow-up may range from a few days to decades, depending on your question.

Observational studies can, under the right circumstances, be done much more quickly. First, if you do not require collection of data from participants, it may be possible to get a waiver from the IRB for both informed consent and an authorization for data use. This would allow you to retrieve records without individual consent, which will ensure that you can obtain available information on all the participants in whom you are interested. If your institution has extensive electronic medical records, it may be possible to actually extract the data you need for the project in a matter of days or weeks. This assumes, of course, that the data you need is available in the electronic records. Even if it is not, however, you might be able to use the available electronic records to identify the patients needed for your study. Then you can retrieve and extract the data from paper records for the retrospective study. If data needs to be collected prospectively, then there may well be no time advantage compared to an interventional study.

Resources are another practical consideration that may affect design decisions. Generally, an interventional study will be the most resource intensive for a given number of participants. This occurs for several reasons, including the greater difficulty in recruiting a participant into an interventional study compared to recruiting a participant into a prospective cohort study, the greater costs for measuring and trying to encourage adherence to the assigned intervention, including safety monitoring, and the requirement for continued follow-up for outcome. In contrast, in a prospective cohort study there needs to be continuing contact with participants and data collection (potentially including visits and study measurements), but the intensity and frequency of visits or contacts is usually less. For retrospective cohort studies and case-control studies, there are data acquisition costs plus potential costs for locating participants and collection of new data, but this is usually only a single study contact.

Finally, there is the underlying feasibility issue of the study. Although in principal a retrospective cohort study or a case-control study could be done very easily, this assumes that the data needed is readily available and of adequate quality for the study. Often, however, even if the data is supposed to be available, review of the data finds that much information is missing and that the quality is not as high as one would hope. In fact, on occasion, the quality of the existing data was so poor that we recommended that investigators start collecting new data rather than trying to salvage the old information. For both the interventional and prospective cohort studies, a major feasibility issue is the availability of an adequate number of potential participants. An old rule of thumb – which some feel is optimistic – is that the number of potential participants for an interventional study drops by 90% on the day recruitment opens.

10.3 Selecting an Interventional Study Design

10.3.1 Randomized or Non-Randomized Study?

There are four basic designs for interventional studies:

- single arm study (also called a case series);
- parallel group study;
- crossover study; and
- pre-post study.

We believe that two of these designs, the single arm study and the pre-post study should only rarely be used, and then only in specific circumstances outlined below. Except in those circumstances, the decision is between a parallel group and a crossover study, discussed in the next section.

For the single arm study to be the optimal design, both of the following conditions are needed:

- the outcome of the condition is (virtually) uniform; and
- the outcome is significant mortality or morbidity, so that a true control group would be unethical.

Example 10G: An investigator wants to study a new intervention in a disease where patients have a uniform course leading to death. Here a single arm study is appropriate, since any survival would be unexpected and evidence of an effect.

A pre-post study is actually a single arm study with a baseline measurement, focusing on the change in the measurement over time. For this design to be optimal, both of the following conditions are needed:

- strong evidence that no change would be expected in the measurement in the absence of the intervention, so that any changes in the measurement can be attributed to the intervention; and
- strong arguments against doing this as a parallel group study with even a small control group.

In Example 5L a pre-post study is appropriate. In that example, involving measurements of metabolic pathways assessed in muscle biopsies both before and after an extended exercise program, there were several reasons why a pre-post design was the only feasible design. The primary reason that a control group would not be appropriate in this study was that taking two muscle biopsies is both painful and invasive. Thus, including control participants having two such biopsies to rule out potential temporal effects would raise both ethical and logistic issues, making a control group infeasible at best and potentially unethical. The study could not feasibly be done as a crossover with the order of the biopsies randomized. Taking an initial muscle biopsy after an extended exercise program, and then taking a second biopsy some months later after the effect of the exercise program had dissipated, would substantially increase the duration of the study. In addition, some participants might like exercising and not stop as required by the crossover design.

10.3.2 Parallel Group or Crossover Study?

A crossover study is feasible only if both the following conditions are met:

- the interventions are unlikely to have a permanent impact on the underlying condition; and
- the underlying condition is basically stable over time.

Example 10H: An investigator wants to determine whether a treatment for rheumatoid arthritis reduces symptoms. Although rheumatoid arthritis is a progressive disease, over short periods of time it is (on average) stable symptomatically, so a crossover design could be used.

Example 10I: An investigator wants to determine whether a treatment for amyotrophic lateral sclerosis delays progression of the disease. Because the endpoint requires a change in the underlying disease, which requires extended observation, a crossover design could not be used for this study.

Assuming that a crossover design could be used, then deciding between a parallel group and a crossover study involves a number of factors that affect the feasibility of the two designs.

A crossover study is appealing because it reduces the impact of variability between individuals so should require fewer participants. This is important if the pool of potential participants is small or it is difficult to recruit participants, but time and resources are wasted if the participant does not complete the crossover study. This can be a major problem if the protocol is demanding, as such a study requires strong commitment from the participants. If the number of potential participants is large and they are relatively easy to recruit, then a parallel group study is generally preferable. In addition, it will likely not be as demanding as a crossover study for the participant. Often a parallel group study can be completed more rapidly as well. We cannot categorically recommend one over the other, but most of the time the study details and participant availability will indicate which would be the better design. In our experience, most studies use a parallel group design.

10.4 Observational Studies

Observational studies are optimal in many circumstances. For some research questions, when there would be ethical issues in deliberately exposing participants to the intervention, observational studies are the only possible research design. Even if an interventional study is possible, there may often be logistical and practical reasons making an observational study preferable.

10.4.1 Case-Control or Cohort Study?

The first major decision you face when deciding to do an observational study is whether to design it as a case-control study or a cohort study.

The major difference between the two designs is in the type of question you are attempting to answer. If you are trying to find exposures related to a specific outcome, then the obvious choice would be a case-control study. If instead you are interested in a range of different outcomes from one (or more) exposures, then the obvious choice would be a cohort study. However, studies sometimes mutate from a relatively focused case-control study to a much broader cohort study just because one is collecting data. Broad large-scale cohort studies often lend themselves to multiple nested case-control studies as well.

Example 10J: An investigator is attempting to assess the effect of prenatal medication on a range of birth defects. This would suggest that a cohort study should be done. However, the number of different medications prescribed would likely be very large with relatively few women given any specific medication, so that only a small fraction of the entire cohort would be providing information about any specific medication. Thus, a case-control study would likely be a far more effective approach than a cohort study. The cases would be women who have infants who have a range of birth defects. The cases could be compared to a specific control population of women who have infants without these birth defects, women who have infants with no birth defects, or the general population of all pregnant women in the medical system (technically called a "case-cohort" study). No matter which control group is used, however, this study would not identify all adverse events of the medications – only those adverse events specifically used to identify the cases in the study.

The decision between a case-control study and a cohort study also impacts how you recruit participants. In a case-control study, you need to recruit both cases (with the outcome of interest) and appropriate controls (without the outcome of interest). In a cohort study, depending on the type of exposure you are interested in, you might need to recruit either a single group that would be expected to have a range of exposures to provide both exposed and unexposed individuals from within this single group, or two separate cohorts – one with the exposure of interest and one known not to have the exposure of interest – and form a single cohort study from the two cohorts.

Example 10K: An investigator wants to study the range of potential effects of exposure to an industrial chemical, so a cohort design would be appropriate. There is a factory where the chemical has been used, but only a small subset of the factory workers would have any exposure. This would argue for defining all the individuals who have been exposed to the chemical in the factory and a random subset of the much larger factory population with no exposure to the chemical as the cohort for the study.

Practical issues may also impact the choice between a case-control study and a cohort study. If there is no reasonable method to identify the cases you are interested in, then this would make a case-control study impractical. One might imagine that with the expansion of electronic medical records this should become less of a problem over time. Depending on how privacy regulations are interpreted, however, it may become increasingly difficult to do case-control studies, as one may not be able to contact cases to collect the detailed exposure information needed.

Another practical issue is the length of time it will take to do the study. Both the case-control study and a retrospective cohort study are likely to take similar amounts of time, but a prospective cohort study is likely to take substantially longer to complete. Thus, if speed is important, then a prospective cohort study is unlikely to be an optimal design.

Finally, there are data quality issues – both in terms of the existing data and the data to be collected. The prospective cohort study is likely to have the best data, while the choice between the case-control study and the retrospective cohort study depends on the quality of the data already available and to be collected. If the exposure data used to form the cohort is relatively poor, for example, then the case-control study, despite its potential for recall bias, may actually have the more reliable data.

10.4.2 Cohort Study: Retrospective or Prospective?

In a retrospective cohort, the cohort is identified based on historical records and the outcome may be determined either by locating cohort members and then obtaining new information or by using historical records. In a prospective cohort study, the cohort is identified prospectively and then followed over time for the outcome of interest.

Sometimes, this decision is very simple. If there are no records that allow for the historical cohort to be identified, then you must do a prospective cohort study. In that situation, we would suggest you reconsider whether a case-control study might be almost as good and far faster to complete.

The decision on whether to use a retrospective or a prospective cohort study involves a number of feasibility and practical issues, including concerns about data quality and reliability and completeness of records. In general, if the information for the cohort is available in existing records, the quality of the information is reasonable, and these records are easy to access, then a retrospective cohort will usually use fewer resources and be completed far more rapidly than a prospective cohort study. If the data quality is unacceptable or the data are not accessible, then a prospective study would be required. Sometimes a small but essential part of the information needed for the study, such as family history, has not been collected. In this case, if existing members of the cohort can be contacted for this information, then you can still do a retrospective study, but if you cannot get this information, a prospective cohort study would be necessary. We cannot categorically recommend one design over the other, but most of the time the study details and the resources available, particularly the historical data available, will indicate which would be the better design. Speed would favor the retrospective cohort study when it is feasible.

10.5 Example of Developing a Design

This example, based on an actual study, illustrates some of the decisions involved in developing a design for a record review.

Example 10L: An investigator wants to determine whether one of two different surgical placements of inferior vena cava (IVC) filters used for the treatment of potential pulmonary embolisms has a better outcome. There is an available cohort in the hospital records of several thousand patients receiving the different placements over a period of time. The investigator is particularly concerned about which placement has a lower thrombotic rate, so he decides to do a case-control study.

Here the interest is in a single outcome, so that the decision is clear: the case-control study would be preferred. Cases would be those with a thrombosis following an IVC filter placement while controls would be individuals without a thrombosis following the procedure.

Example 10L (continued): Given the hospital record system, it is easy for the investigator to identify patients with an IVC filter placed, or to identify patients with a thrombosis, but not to identify patients with a thrombosis after an IVC filter has been placed.

Now practical issues seem to override the obvious choice. As the investigator did not have a simple method to identify cases, the investigator decides he has to do a cohort study.

Example 10L (continued): Since the investigator has to do a cohort study, the investigator decides that he might as well determine the full range of outcomes among patients having the procedure. This includes both short-term complications from the procedure and longer term (6–12 months) outcomes following the procedure. After all, this only involves a bit more data abstraction, and because charts need to be reviewed anyway, it will not be a lot more work.

This shows the creep that develops in many projects.

Example 10L (continued): The investigator realizes that for many of the outcomes of interest the medical records are unlikely to be very comprehensive. Thus, it would be necessary to contact participants to collect much of the data needed for the review. Because of concerns about the reliability of collecting results retrospectively, and the ease of forming a new cohort – several hundred patients have the procedure each year at his institution – the investigator decided that a prospective cohort study would allow the information to be collected systematically and could be done in a feasible amount of time.

So the investigator has now moved from what started as a relatively quick case-control study, through a retrospective cohort study, to a prospective cohort study to collect reliable information on all the different outcomes, even though the project started out as one focused on a single – and reliably collected – significant adverse outcome.

Example 10L (continued): The investigator discusses his proposal with a colleague. The colleague asks a pointed question: Why are the relatively minor complications of any interest? Didn't you start out being concerned only about the major complication? The investigator reconsiders what, precisely, he is trying to assess and decides that a retrospective cohort study focusing solely on the outcome of interest, which would be expected to be reliably recorded if the patient returns to the institution, will be more practical and will answer the question far sooner than the expanded project will.

The investigator has gone back to the retrospective cohort study.

Example 10L (concluded): Finally, since the investigator has access to a statistician, he discusses his proposal with the statistician. The statistician asks why the investigator could not get both lists from the hospital record system (those with the procedure and those with a thrombosis) and then manually identify the cases. Then the controls would be a random sample of individuals with the procedure who did not have a thrombosis.

So the investigator ends up back where he started – doing a case-control study using only historical records.

10.6 Ethical Issues

There is a fundamental ethical issue in selecting an appropriate study design. Deciding whether an interventional study is even possible is strictly an ethical issue: Is it ethical to test the intervention in a population? If the answer to this is yes, then you can decide among the different interventional designs, or perhaps decide that even though an interventional study might be acceptable, an alternate design, such as a retrospective cohort study, might be more practical and feasible. If the answer is no, you need to choose among the different observational designs to study the question.

Once you have answered this question, however, there are other considerations. The most important, in our opinion, is the practicality and feasibility of the proposed design. Although some do not feel that this is an ethical issue, we believe that there is an ethical component in selecting a design. No matter what design you are selecting, you are using participant information. Sometimes this extends to contacting them and using the participant's time and assistance to help in your research. When this happens, you have an obligation to ensure that the information will be used and is being used efficiently, and that you trouble as few participants as possible. Choosing the right design can reduce the number of participants dramatically. Example 10L, for example, discussed a range of studies, from a case-control study of a single outcome, to a retrospective cohort study involving a record review of thousands of individuals, to a prospective cohort study, back to the case-control study design. The final case-control study, which was by far the smallest of the studies considered, would provide as much or more information about the most severe outcome as would the historical cohort study with thousands of individuals. Being smaller, it is also easier and faster to do, and none of the participants need to be contacted for it.

KEY POINTS

- The first step in selecting a design is to determine whether an interventional study is ethical. Unless it is ethical, you cannot do an interventional study.
- If a study can be done either as an interventional study or an observational study, the decision between the two revolves around a number of practical issues including time, resources, and feasibility.
- The major decision in planning an interventional study is between a parallel group study and a crossover study. This decision is based on issues including the number of potential participants, the ease of recruiting participants, and their likely commitment to the study.
- The major decision in planning an observational study is between a case-control study and a cohort study. This is determined by the nature of the question being asked and, to an extent, by whether the condition of interest is rare.
- When deciding between a historical (retrospective) cohort and a prospective cohort study, the decision is based on issues including availability, completeness, and reliability of data for a retrospective study, whether members of this cohort can be contacted, and the time pressure for generating results of the study.

Part III

CORE CONCEPTS APPLICABLE TO ALL STUDY DESIGNS

11

Generalizability and Validity

Generalizability is the ability to draw widely or even universally applicable conclusions from a study. Generalizability is an important goal, because if the conclusions of the study cannot be applied to a broader population, then the results have little or no value to the larger community. Ideally, a study would be generalizable to a large population, but often practical limitations such as time, money, and the population available mean that the study's generalizability must be reduced to preserve its validity. Validity means that the results of the study are true for the population studied. Every effort must be made to maintain study validity.

11.1 The Population

The participants in a clinical study are assumed to be representative of some population, and when you specify what individuals you will select, you determine which population they represent. For maximum generalizability, the population should be all people who could benefit from the study's results. However, the more varied the population is, the more individuals you must study to ensure that the effect of interest can be detected despite the variation within the study population. If you limit a study to a specific, narrowly defined group, interpersonal variation is reduced so you can do a smaller study and still be able to detect the effect of interest; however, you then have no information about the effect in other groups. As a rule, the individuals studied will represent a compromise between generalizability and feasibility.

Example 11A: Many patients with major depression also suffer from other related disorders, such as anxiety disorder, which may add more variability to a study's results. Restricting the target population to patients with no other disorders will reduce the variability among participants and thus improve the ability to detect an effect, but it will exclude a large proportion of patients and thus severely reduce generalizability. If resources are sufficient to study a larger population, investigators may allow the inclusion of participants with other disorders that do not interact with the pharmacological effect of the therapy, thereby increasing the generalizability without adversely affecting validity.

There are practical advantages to either approach. Fewer patients would be required if only participants with no other disorders were included, but because so many patients will have multiple disorders, it may be more difficult to recruit even this smaller number of patients.

Often it can be very difficult to decide what the study population should be, and validity needs to be protected at the cost of generalizability.

Example 11B: Many nephrologists are interested in whether dietary supplements improve nutritional status in individuals who are undergoing renal dialysis. To reduce variability among the participants, such a study might include only individuals who are stable on dialysis. The investigators may also want to exclude individuals with Non-Insulin Dependent Diabetes Mellitus (NIDDM), which may affect nutritional parameters independent of the dialysis. Alternatively, the investigator might want to include only individuals with NIDDM, since they constitute a large fraction of the population on dialysis. In either case, such a study would have validity for the population studied, but not necessarily have generalizability to the total population of individuals on dialysis.

For a study of a rare outcome, a population with a high prevalence of the outcome is necessary so that there will be enough participants with the condition to make conclusions about the effect of therapies or exposures (see Appendix B on sample size). Sometimes it is possible to use a restricted study sample without losing generalizability.

Example 11C: An investigator wants to study whether a high dose of a nutritional supplement during pregnancy reduces the risk of early delivery. The inexpensive supplement has been in general use for many years and has been shown to be nontoxic to the mother and the fetus at the dosage specified. The true target population for this drug would be all pregnant women, since early delivery cannot be ruled out in any pregnancy. Because the rate of early delivery in the general population is low, an impractically large number of participants would have to be studied to detect a reduction. Restricting the study to women at high risk for early delivery makes the study feasible. Positive results in this group would still allow the investigator to recommend use of the supplement for all pregnant women, since the supplement is known to be safe and potentially would reduce the risk of early delivery in low risk women as well. Thus, the investigator's choice to improve feasibility should not compromise generalizability or validity.

But sometimes generalizability must be sacrificed for feasibility, although validity can never be sacrificed.

Example 11D: Several studies of gestational diabetes and the incidence and timing of metabolic disorders after pregnancy have been conducted in a hospital serving a largely Hispanic population. Hispanics have higher rates of gestational diabetes than do other ethnic groups, as well as higher rates of metabolic diabetes, so fewer participants would need to be enrolled and followed to obtain the needed number of cases. Therefore, these studies were limited to women of Hispanic background. However, the results from these studies may not be applicable to women of other ethnic groups.

Sometimes it is reasonable to apply results in a subgroup to the general population, as in the interventional study in Example 11C. In other circumstances, such as in Example 11D, studies involving other groups are required to confirm that the findings in one specific population are generalizable.

Even if the sample is representative of the total population with the disease, generalizability may be diminished if enrollment is limited only to highly motivated individuals who are very likely to remain in the study and adhere to the protocol. This helps the study progress well and maximizes the chance of detecting an effect, but the results may not apply to the general population, which includes many less motivated individuals.

Example 11E: The Diabetes Control and Complications Trial (DCCT) demonstrated convincingly that intensive monitoring and treatment of Type I diabetes was extremely effective in reducing the risks of diabetic sequelae. But the results are only directly generalizable to Type I diabetics willing to follow the intensive monitoring and treatment plan, requiring participants to test blood glucose levels four or more times a day, adjust their insulin dose based on those measurements, and follow a diet and exercise plan. Therefore, these results may not be generalizable to Type I diabetics who will not or cannot follow such a strict regimen.

Example 11E illustrates the trade-off between efficacy and effectiveness (see Section 24.1). The intensive monitoring and treatment was clearly efficacious: it definitely improved outcomes in participants willing to be in a study with such rigorous monitoring and treatment. It does not show that the program would be effective in the general population of Type I diabetics, who might not be able to comply with the strict requirements for monitoring and treatment. Only after efficacy has been demonstrated for a treatment does the question of whether the treatment is effective in the general population of patients become important.

Characteristics of study populations are discussed in more detail in Chapter 12.

11.2 Study Methods

Generalizability includes not only the question of whether the results apply to the general population but also whether the intervention is practical; that is, is it feasible and acceptable in the general population? This is very dependent on the complexity and cost of the methods for treatment and monitoring of treatment.

11.2.1 Treatment and Treatment Monitoring

In many studies the protocol specifies a very rigorously defined, complex, and closely monitored treatment. Sometimes special staff are used to provide additional or specialized participant care not generally available as part of standard care. Often the treatment monitoring involves frequent evaluations to ensure that participants are adhering to the treatment and that the treatment is properly delivered. This is particularly important in initial studies of a new therapy, where little is known about the treatment and you need detailed information to detect not only efficacy but also possible adverse effects. This level of attention may be difficult to achieve outside the study setting, however, so unless the procedures can be simplified for application in the field without affecting the efficacy of the treatment, the generalizability of the study results may be limited.

Example 11F: In a study of a drug therapy, the investigators believe that the maximum benefit of the therapy is obtained only when the serum blood levels reach a specified amount. During the study, investigators test the blood on a weekly basis to adjust dosages to ensure that this level is reached as soon as possible. If the drug were used in general practice, however, blood levels would probably be tested only monthly because of the test cost, so that patients might become discouraged or even develop complications before the optimum dose is reached. Although frequent monitoring during the study increases the chance that the new therapy will succeed, its use may limit the generalizability of the results.

Example 11G: An intensive intervention study for weight reduction provided special counselors in three areas; psychological, exercise planning, and nutrition. The participants met with the study coordinator and the counselors weekly for the first month, and after the first month they met biweekly with the coordinator and could schedule visits with the counselors at their own request. The investigators found that, although the program resulted in significant weight loss during the first six months of the study, the participants who continued to meet with the counselors had a better than average maintenance record during the remaining 6 months of the study. Thus, the intervention might not be successful in an individual who, even though interested in success, did not have access to as much personal support.

Example 11E (continued): The intensive diabetes control in the DCCT study required a highly motivated population because of the demanding procedures. But the success of the DCCT led to many studies of methods to simplify implementing intensive diabetes control, mainly by use of a wearable instrument that automatically monitors glucose level and releases the correct amount of insulin as required without intervention by the individual. Such devices allow intensive diabetes control in a much larger population.

A treatment that is effective may not be useful in particular environments because of economic, structural, and political limitations.

Example 11H: Neonatal conjunctivitis is a serious cause of blindness in newborns, particularly in the developing world. Agents such as silver nitrate and erythromycin in eyes immediately after birth are effective but they are expensive, require special storage, and are not widely available. In a randomized clinical trial conducted in Kenya, investigators showed that povidone-iodine was as effective in reducing infection as the other agents. Moreover, it was much less expensive, did not require refrigeration, and, because it had a color that showed up in the infant's eye when it was applied, it was easy for even minimally trained personnel to verify that the child had received the treatment. Thus, it was recommended for use in this type of environment.

11.2.2 Assessment Methods

A treatment may use very sophisticated and frequent assessment measures that are expensive to perform or require specially trained personnel. These procedures may be too expensive and demanding for general use outside the study. If the assessment methods used are critical to the treatment, then unless they, as well as the treatment methods, are available and easily usable in the general practice setting, the generalizability of the study will be compromised.

Example 11I: There are currently several approved drugs for treating major depression. They differ in the neurological systems they act on and on the response of the patient. Research protocols to study which participants are most likely to respond to a treatment typically use a battery of instruments twice weekly in the early treatment period to assess aspects of the disease. Specific algorithms are used to predict response, and participants unlikely to respond are switched to another drug. This method will not be generalizable to private practice unless the assessment method is simplified and practitioners are given easy ways to apply the algorithms.

It is important to distinguish between assessment methods that are used during the study only to evaluate whether the therapy is effective and those that are necessary to implement the treatment. In the former case, there is no need to use these methods in practice, so they do not affect generalizability, but in the latter case they do.

Example 11J: A study involving exercise as a therapy for fibromyalgia will be done in a special exercise clinic. The investigators develop an individualized exercise plan for each participant and will use special equipment to monitor pulmonary and cardiac function. The exercise plan is based on the participant's age, weight, and results of a standard physical and can be implemented by varying speed and resistance on a standard exercise bicycle. The cardiac and pulmonary function measures are only used to evaluate the effectiveness of the program. Therefore, the results are generalizable to any population that has access to a standard exercise bicycle.

Example 11K: This study is similar to that in Example 11J, but the investigators feel that the cardiac and pulmonary measures are necessary to modify the exercise plan for a participant. In this case, the results cannot be used in general practice.

11.3 Validity

Most of this book is concerned with providing you techniques to ensure that your study is valid. Validity is separate from generalizability. It means that the results of the study are in fact true for the population studied. This is essential for any study. Without validity it does not matter whether the study is generalizable or not, as it is not clear what the true results of the study are. Therefore, in developing your study design and procedures, each decision should preserve the validity of the study.

Appropriately selected participants, with clear-cut inclusion and exclusion criteria (Chapter 12) are critical, especially when more than one group of participants are being recruited (Chapters 26 and 27). Clearly defined data and data collection procedures (Chapters 14, 15, 16, and 29) are essential for a valid study. Avoiding bias in general is critical (Chapters 17 and 18). For interventional studies, the key techniques are randomization (Chapters 20 and 21) and blinding (also called masking; Chapters 22 and 23). Blinding should also be used whenever possible in observational studies (Chapter 28). Although you may not have the expertise to define the statistical methods for your study, you should consult with a qualified statistician, if possible, to ensure that your hypotheses directly address the objectives of the study, the statistical methods to be used are appropriate for the data, and the question and your study are adequate to provide confidence in your results (Appendixes A and B).

You must always ensure validity, even if this means limiting the generalizability of the study.

11.4 Ethical Issues

Ideally, the results of a study would be generalizable to all individuals who might benefit from them. In reality, generalizability usually is limited because of practical considerations. A major ethical concern is the exclusion of subgroups of individuals, especially when this is done deliberately. This may result in the excluded groups not being properly diagnosed, not being considered for new and better treatments, or being given dosages that may not be optimal for them. For example, in early studies of AIDS, the exclusion of women meant that certain disorders in the female reproductive system were not recognized as early manifestations of AIDS. Another example is that the risk of adverse effects in fragile populations, such as elderly individuals or those with rare disorders, may be underestimated because they are not represented in the study population. Elderly individuals tend both to be taking more medications than the general population, which may interact with the study medication, and to be more susceptible to adverse effects from a study medication.

Another ethical concern is the effort that may be spent on studies that have no practical application because of the demanding methods used. This may be because of extensive requirements for using medical personnel or facilities, painful procedures, or demands on the participant or caretaker involving time, effort, and resources. This is true of almost all diet or exercise programs. Sometimes a difficult protocol may have benefit for the insights it provides on the disease process and has the possibility of leading to less difficult regimes. If the probability is high that an intervention cannot or will not be followed in the population of interest and will not provide information that could help inform future studies, then the investigator should consider whether a less demanding and more acceptable alternative, even if it is less effective than the more difficult method, would be more useful.

Finally, we point out the obvious: deliberately doing a study that will not provide valid results is not only unethical but a waste of time, effort, and energy for everyone involved.

KEY POINTS

- Although generalizability to all individuals with the condition of interest is desirable for a study, it is usually limited by what is feasible to do. No matter what is done, the validity (scientific integrity) of the study cannot be sacrificed.
- An expansive population definition with few restrictions will enhance generalizability, but in practice, the population studied is usually limited
  - to reduce interpersonal variability;
  - to have a high enough rate of a rare outcome in the study population; and
  - to eliminate the effect of concomitant conditions on the outcome.
- Narrowly defined treatment plans with many visits and extensive staff time to ensure participant adherence may be necessary to ensure that the study assesses the proposed treatment under optimal circumstances, enhancing the validity of the study. If these methods are not feasible in a non-research setting, then generalizability will be limited.
- For generalizability, monitoring procedures that affect treatment decisions should be able to be done by health care providers in local facilities using laboratory and evaluation methods in general use. If a treatment requires specialized laboratory tests or assessment by

specially trained personnel for treatment monitoring, then the results of the study may not be generalizable.

- Using specialized tests, centralized laboratories, and specialized staff to perform outcome assessments increases the validity of the study.
- You must take steps to ensure validity of your study from the original planning to the final analysis and interpretation.

12

Study Population

A key factor in generalizability is the target population, the people who are the object of the study. In this chapter we discuss the target population versus the actual study pool of available individuals. We focus on the eligibility criteria, since this is critical to the validity (scientific integrity) of the study. The actual individuals who participate in the study, the study group, are recruited from the group of eligible individuals. The study design must specify in detail which individuals within the study pool are eligible for the study to ensure the validity of the study.

12.1 The Target Population and the Study Pool

The target population is the largest group of people to whom the results of your study may apply. It may be very general, for example simply "being human" for studies of basic physiological mechanisms, or very narrow, such as a group with a carefully defined and very homogeneous disease. Within the target population we define the study pool, which is the group of individuals who could actually be observed in the study. The study pool could be the same as the target population but is usually a subset of the target population observed in one or more specific locations while the study is being done. Sometimes the study pool is not representative of the target population, or you may not have access to enough individuals in the target population in your area to test your hypothesis. The study pool may be expanded to resemble the target population more closely by designing a multi-center study, in which several centers or hospitals all follow the same protocol and use the same techniques.

Example 12A: In the study described in Example 11C on the use of a nutritional supplement during pregnancy, the treatment was to be started in the fifth month of pregnancy. Thus, the study pool would be limited to women in prenatal care by the fifth month of their pregnancy. This means that the study pool may underrepresent certain groups of women who are at risk for early delivery, such as intravenous drug users, because they are less likely to have prenatal care. The investigators plan to take extra steps, such as working with community outreach programs, to try to recruit more of these women.

Example 12B: In a physiological study of the impact of an insulin clamp, the goal was to determine what was abnormal in the response of Type 1 diabetics compared to a normal physiological response. This requires a group of "normal healthy individuals." Although it is straightforward to define Type 1 diabetics, it is much harder to define a "normal healthy individual."

12.2 The Eligible Group

Within the study pool, specific criteria for inclusion and exclusion will identify a subset of individuals who are eligible for the study. The eligibility standards defined in the study protocol are a set of physical, demographic, and medical standards that the individual must meet to be included (inclusion criteria) and another set of standards that they must not meet or else they are excluded (exclusion criteria). The specification and implementation of these criteria are critical to the success of the study. They must be spelled out precisely and without ambiguity, or the results of the study may not be interpretable or credible.

The first and most important inclusion criterion is that a participant be able to understand and give informed consent, usually a signed document. Chapter 3 describes the details of creating an informed consent document, presenting it, and discussing the details with a participant in an interview. Most of the time this process is straightforward, but if your study involves special populations (such as pregnant women, children, and individuals with impairments), then special procedures apply (Section 3.4). Your Institutional Review Board (IRB) will be able to provide advice and assistance for these special populations. Sometimes informed consent is waived (Section 3.6), most usually for record reviews (Chapter 9). Your IRB can provide information about waivers of consent as well, and will have to authorize it, if appropriate for your study, before your study begins.

Table 12.1 is a list of some participant characteristics in addition to informed consent that are often specified in inclusion or exclusion criteria. This list cannot be exhaustive, as each study will have specific requirements. Also, not all categories on the list will be important for every study. Items in most categories can be either inclusion or exclusion criteria. Usually it is easier to understand a requirement when it is presented positively, so that the exclusion criterion "allergic to drug" is easier to understand than the inclusion criterion "not allergic to drug," but the investigator decides which way to present it.

The protocol must specify methods for assessing the variables that comprise the inclusion and exclusion criteria. Many criteria include lists of items, such as other diagnoses or medications. In general, if a list in

Table 12.1 Common Categories of Inclusion and Exclusion Criteria

- Diagnosis
- Demographic factors
  - Sex
  - Age
  - Ethnicity
- Current physical condition from a recent examination or laboratory tests (possibly from history; possibly done as part of the study)
- Medical history
- Family history
- Current treatments or medications, including contraceptives
- Over-the-counter medications
- Lifestyle factors
  - Diet
  - Alcohol
  - Recreational drug use
- Expected to complete the study
- Ability to communicate with study staff

the inclusion criteria is all wanted items, others are not of interest unless they are in the exclusion criteria. If a list is in the exclusion criteria, then it is assumed that items not on this list are allowed.

Example 12C: In the study in Example 10C to assess whether patients presenting with an AIDS-defining opportunistic infection (OI) should be treated first for the OI and defer antiretroviral treatment (ART) until the OI was resolved, or should be treated concurrently with ART, detailed criterion for each specific OI was needed. For some OIs the specific criteria for diagnosis varied by site, as in some parts of the United States certain OIs are frequently seen and thus are treated empirically without definitive diagnosis, while at other sites the specific OI is sufficiently uncommon that physicians routinely do a definitive workup prior to initiating treatment for the OI.

Diagnosis is probably the most common criteria, and frequently the focus of the study. A study protocol might specify what diagnosis the participant must have and what diagnoses would make the participant ineligible for the study. The method of ascertaining the diagnosis must be spelled out in detail. If laboratory tests are used, what are the ranges for pathology? May prior or current results from the participant's usual laboratory tests be used, or must the participant be tested at a central laboratory? If it is a physical limitation, how will it be tested and what range of results is considered diagnostic? If the diagnosis is derived according to a manual of diagnosis such as the Diagnostic and Statistical Manual of Mental Disorders (DSM), how is the information required for the diagnosis obtained? Similarly, if information is from a current history, what sources are considered reliable?

Example 12D: In a study of treatment for depression in an outpatient population, the primary inclusion criteria were that participants be diagnosed with major depression. This was defined according to the current DSM, using data from the Structural Clinical Interview for the DSM (SCID). The SCID includes criteria for deriving DSM diagnoses, and the two together are accepted standards of diagnosis in the field of depression. Patients with major depression frequently have other psychiatric disorders. In this study the investigators decided to allow the presence of comorbid generalized anxiety disorder if major depression was also present. This was stated specifically in the inclusion criteria. All other DSM comorbid disorders, such as obsessive-compulsive disorder or posttraumatic stress disorder, were exclusion criteria, since there was evidence that these disorders affected the response to one of the drugs being studied.

Example 12E: Diabetes mellitus is included in the eligibility criteria in many studies, either as an inclusion requirement, when it is being studied, or as an exclusion criterion. In some cases the medical record may be sufficient to ascertain the presence or absence of diabetes. If not, the criteria for diagnosing Type 1 diabetes are well defined, but different methods may be used for diagnosing Type 2. For some studies a fasting blood glucose measurement is sufficient, while others may require that the participant undergo an oral glucose tolerance test.

Example 12A (continued): The primary inclusion criteria for this study was that the woman be at high risk for early delivery, therefore the criteria for "high risk" must be spelled out clearly and unambiguously, and only women who meet those criteria would be eligible. It might include several separate conditions, such as age under 16, age above 40, a previous history of early delivery or other related problems, or physiological problems that would make it difficult to carry a child to term, any one of which would qualify the woman for the study.

Even using the best current standard for diagnosis, problems can occur during the study as standards for diagnosis or treatment can change over time. The American Diabetes Association criteria for Type II diabetes were modified in 1997 to simplify methods of diagnosis. The guidelines for treating elevated cholesterol levels for individuals at increased risk of cardiovascular disease was changed in 2013. If standards for diagnosis or treatment change but all participants are selected according to the same criteria, then the results will be valid but may be less generalizable than originally hoped.

On some occasions a diagnostic result in an individual may change during the study. For example, a patient may be admitted to a psychiatric study as a unipolar depressive, but the participant may have his first manic episode during the course of the study, so that the unipolar depression diagnosis is no longer valid. You cannot be expected to foresee the future, but possible changes should be considered when you are developing your inclusion and exclusion criteria.

Demographic variables are generally less complicated to describe, but they still require definition. Sex is usually clear, although in some studies the protocol must specify how to deal with adults who have had sex change operations or newborns who have characteristics of both sexes. Age can be more complicated. Although age is usually calculated as current age at time of screening, in the study of premature neonates, age is usually based on known or estimated gestational age at birth rather than time since birth. In multinational trials, it is even necessary to specify how age is calculated – from conception or from birth, as different countries calculate age differently. In addition to age, menopausal status may be a criterion in women, and Turner stage or pubertal status may be important in children. A "full-term infant" may be defined by gestational age, birth weight, or a combination of the two. If ethnicity is a criterion, then the protocol must define ethnicity and specify how it is determined.

Example 12A (continued): In this study, the woman's age was her age at time of conception, estimated from the last menstrual period. Extreme age, young or old for pregnancy, would be one of the risk factors and therefore was an inclusion criterion, but normal age for maternity was not an exclusion criterion if other risk factors were present.

Example 12F: In a study of the genetics of response to psychotropic drugs, the association between genotype and enzymatic action was compared between Caucasians, African Americans, and Mexicans. Potential participants were required to verify that all four grandparents were of the same ethnic group to be included. Their response was considered adequate.

If the eligibility criteria are to be verified by a physical examination, will this be done by the investigator's staff, as part of the screening process, or will information from medical records be sufficient? Most interventional studies require a physical examination to verify eligibility.

Example 12G: As part of the screening process in a study of testosterone replacement in hypogonadal men, all potential participants had a complete physical examination by the investigators staff, including a prostate examination and measurement of prostate-specific androgen (PSA). Since testosterone may exacerbate certain prostate problems, individuals with elevated PSA or any abnormalities on the prostate examination were excluded.

Example 12B (continued). For the group of "healthy normal controls," diabetes was ruled out using a 2-hour oral glucose tolerance test.

Sometimes information about the individual must be obtained from records (with the individual's permission) or from an interview. An interview is only as good as the person's recall, so it may not be possible to obtain very specific or detailed information. If the accuracy of the historical information is very important, then sometimes individuals may be excluded if the information cannot be verified from records.

Example 12A (continued): The occurrence of prior gestational diabetes was an exclusion criterion for this study because of the possibility of metabolic abnormalities. In the center doing this study, many of the participants were immigrants from rural areas, and may not have been tested in previous pregnancies. However, since the gravida would be tested for diabetes at least once in the pregnancy, it was decided that the investigators would accept a no response, even though it might be erroneous. Women who reported very large babies or other symptoms associated with gestational diabetes would be tested a second time. This problem may not occur in another institution, and this difference should be noted if results are compared.

Example 12B (continued): In this study, the inclusion criterion for "normal healthy volunteers" was quite lengthy, as it usually needs to be. In addition to the control group not having diabetes (based on an actual test performed by the investigators), the investigators decided to rule out a family history of diabetes, since this might have genetic consequences that would compromise the physiological pathways being studied. The investigators asked about a history of diabetes in grandparents, parents, uncles, aunts, and siblings. Any history of diabetes excluded the participant from the study.

Example 12D (continued): In addition to describing their current mental state, participants were questioned about their medical history, including the number of previous episodes of depression, the duration of these episodes, and the number of previous hospitalizations for depression. They were asked to allow examination of earlier medical records, if available. The focus of the study was the results of the current treatment, so that individuals were not excluded if this information was missing, but they were excluded from secondary analyses that examined the impact of prior history on the current results.

If family information is critical to the study, then the inclusion criteria may specify that all relatives up to a certain level must also agree to participate for the family to be included. This may lead to an ethical problem, if relatives feel compelled to participate (Section 12.4). In general, any requirements for the participation of family members should be kept to a minimum (e.g., limiting the requirement to first-degree relatives only), and minimizing the procedures requested from family members (e.g., minimally invasive procedures or questions that violate privacy). If possible, alternatives that would allow an individual to participate without the inclusion of family members should be specified.

Frequently participants are on some kind of treatment when they enter the study. The protocol must specify what current treatments are acceptable, whether a washout period is required, and if so, how long the washout period must be.

Example 12G (continued): Men were diagnosed as hypogonadal based on a single morning testosterone level below an established limit for normal. Men who were already receiving testosterone replacement therapy were asked to stop treatment for 4 to 6 weeks, depending on the treatment, before the screening test was done and potentially entering the study.

Example 12D (continued): Most participants were taking medications for depression when they entered the study. Most of these were not considered cause for exclusion if the participant was willing and able to undergo a washout period of 10 days. However, one class of medications had a half-life that would have required a much longer washout period. Since the investigators did not feel it was ethical to ask a participant to go for such a long period untreated, patients currently using those medications were excluded.

Sometimes the intervention is to be used as a supplement to a treatment currently in use. In these studies, use of the treatment would be an inclusion rather than an exclusion criterion.

Example 12H: Sulfonylureas are drugs used for treatment of type 2 diabetes by increasing the amount of insulin released from the beta cells. Biguanides have a different action, enhancing the response to insulin. Although biguanides were tested as monotherapy, there was interest in their added benefit when used in combination with sulfonylureas or insulin. Therefore, some clinical trials of biguanides specified current use of a sulfonylurea as an inclusion criteria.

The effect of a pharmaceutical intervention, particularly an experimental one, on pregnancy and outcome is of particular concern. Therefore, it is a common requirement that women of childbearing age be practicing a proven method of birth control. Frequently the exact method of birth control may be specified, particularly if pharmaceutical methods might interact with the intervention.

Example 12I: In a study of a proposed method of male contraception, the participants were males with normal sperm counts, in general good health according to a physical examination, and known to have fathered at least one child. They also had to have a current female partner who was not pregnant at the time of the study, and have no plans to initiate a pregnancy during the study period. The study was to determine the effect of the method on spermatogenesis and also do safety evaluations, but not to determine its efficacy as a method of birth control. Therefore, the participants were required to agree to use a barrier method of birth control, which was considered more reliable than hormonal methods, during the study.

In Example 12I, the participants were required to be in "general good health based on a health examination." This is a very loose criterion, and should be specified in some detail to be clear. How extensive is the physical examination? Does it include a prostate exam? If it does, the number of potential participants agreeing to screening would likely drop substantially; for this example, however, it would seem to be needed. What about vision and hearing? Is someone requiring very strong glasses to see in "general good health"? This becomes even more important in a study where one group is specifically recruited to be "healthy normal volunteers."

Example 12B (continued): In this study, the "healthy normal volunteers" had a complete physical examination (which did not include either a prostate exam for males or a pelvic exam for females) and standard laboratory tests, all required to be in the laboratory normal range, to ensure that they were healthy. They were excluded for any medical history suggesting a metabolic disorder and were required to have a normal BMI (defined as 18–25 for the study). The investigators had limits on physical activity in both groups as they anticipated that competitive athletes would have an altered physiological response. Initially, the investigators had intended to exclude both diabetics and controls who were taking any medication (except for insulin for diabetes), but found that many of the women being recruited in the study were using hormonal contraceptives, so they amended the inclusion criteria to allow this specific medication.

Because "normal healthy controls" are often used in case-control studies, this topic is discussed further in Section 26.2.

Lifestyle factors may also be inclusion or exclusion criteria. These factors include such things as usual diet, exercise, smoking, and alcohol use. They are particularly important when an intervention is designed to modify behavior, but may also affect both physiological and behavioral results in a study. Methods of assessing these factors must be clearly defined in the protocol. Individuals are often asked to agree to a drug screening, and positive results on the test or reported heavy alcohol consumption would be exclusion criteria for a study.

Example 12J: Before entry into a study of the effects of a low-fat, high-fiber diet on reproductive factors in men who were normally on a high-fat, low-fiber diet, all potential participants were screened by a dietitian and completed a four-day food record to ensure that they were consuming a high-fat, low-fiber diet, defined as more than 30% calories from fat and less than 20g of fiber a day, for enrollment in the study. Participants were allowed limited use of alcohol (as defined in the protocol), but were excluded if they tested positive for recreational drugs.

In studies where lifestyle factors are inclusion criteria, it is often the less desirable ones that are of interest. For example, studies of weight loss regimens will list obesity as an inclusion criterion, usually defined by the body mass index. Studies of the effect of exercise may exclude individuals who are already physically active and require that participants fit the study's definition of inactive. Lean or physically active individuals may be recruited as controls in some studies.

The investigator's assessment that the participant is likely to complete the study is a necessary condition. Will the individual be able to attend visits as required? Is this person planning to move from the area, take a long vacation, or have other problems returning for study visits? Recruiting a participant who is likely to drop out of the study soon after enrolling is a waste of effort. This can be a very subjective evaluation, and procedures for ascertaining this should be specified to avoid the potential for bias.

12.3 The Study Group

Finally, there is the study group, which is the group of individuals that are actually studied. This is almost always a subset of the eligible individuals. Not all eligible individuals will be willing or able to participate; their personal physicians may not want them to participate; or the study requires fewer participants than there are eligible individuals. To maintain the generalizability of the results, the individuals in the study group would be selected at random from the eligible individuals and have no special reason, related to the condition being studied, for being in the study. In practice, this ideal can never be truly achieved, but by strict adherence to the eligibility criteria you can minimize problems of generalizability in the study group. Participants should not be selected because they are more likely to benefit from the intervention than other eligible individuals. It is important that the participants are independent – that is, inclusion of one individual does not affect the chances of another being included. If some participants have a closer relationship between them than other individuals (e.g., brothers), then standard statistical tests may not be valid. Occasionally a relationship between participants may be built into the study design, but that is relatively rare in clinical studies (see Chapter 27 on matching in observational studies), and then all participants are enrolled based on such relationships.

Example 12K: In all of the above examples, the study group consists of all individuals, up to the number defined in the protocol, who are able to understand and sign an informed consent, meet all of the inclusion criteria, and do not meet any of the exclusion criteria.

12.4 Ethical Issues

This chapter deals with the people you will be studying; therefore, there are many ethical issues. Chapter 2 presented a detailed discussion of these issues; we discuss them only briefly in this section. First and foremost, the study must be ethical in itself. The risk-benefit ratio must be such that the benefits outweigh the risk to the participants. The IRB grapples with this question on a regular basis.

All participants must understand and give informed consent. Some populations may require special documents or techniques for interviewing these potential participants. The IRB must approve the use of these populations and the special procedures involved in obtaining consent. We discuss this issue extensively in Section 3.4.

The exclusion of subgroups, either deliberately or because of problems with recruiting such individuals, is another ethical concern. This may result in the excluded groups not being considered for new and better treatments, or being given dosages that may not be best for them. This issue has been demonstrated to have serious consequences. Previously studies of cardiovascular disease were often restricted to males because it was felt that women were not at sufficiently high risk for cardiovascular disease. This meant that the results of the studies were based only on males, without consideration of different dosing requirements, hormone interactions, or lifestyle differences that made the recommendations of these studies inappropriate for women. Similarly, studies of pharmacological therapies routinely exclude children, but the results were often applied to children on the basis that they were simply smaller adults.

But children are physiologically different from adults, and the therapies could be ineffective or sometimes dangerous in children.

Another issue is the extent of the screening procedures, the order in which they are applied, and when an individual would be excluded. Ideally, the least invasive screening should be done first, and only if the person is acceptable on these criteria should more invasive tests be done. It is not ethical to make someone have a blood draw or spend his time doing a long and perhaps disconcerting interview if he is going to be excluded because of his age.

Some studies require that individuals be able to provide information on their family history or current status of some family members to participate in the study. This raises additional ethical problems. What information can a participant report without the consent of the family member or an authorized surrogate? Death certificates are public information, but if the information has to be verified through medical records, then there must be some mechanism to obtain consent from the decedent's personal representative. Similarly, the family member must consent to be interviewed or undergo any testing that is required. This raises the issue of coercion, because the family member may be reluctant to participate, but feel they must help their relative, particularly if the person is "sick."

It is important that whatever population is studied, any publications clearly describe who was studied and any limitations in having a representative sample of the population in your study.

KEY POINTS

- The target population is the group to whom you want the results of your study to apply.
- The study pool is the group within the target population that are available for study.
- The eligible participants are those who meet the specific list of eligibility criteria, meeting all inclusion criteria and not meeting any exclusion criterion.

- The most important inclusion criterion is that the participant (or an appropriate surrogate) understand the study and provide informed consent for participation, unless informed consent was waived by the IRB for exceptional circumstances.
- The inclusion and exclusion criteria must be clear, comprehensive, and unambiguous. Standards for assessing the criteria must be explicitly defined.
- The study group is the group actually enrolled in the study.

13

Getting and Keeping Participants

You have determined the study design and the target population, defined the criteria for eligible participants, and determined how many participants you will need to complete the study. The next issue to consider is how you will identify potential participants, how you will interest them in volunteering for the study, and how you will keep those who are enrolled in the study actively participating. In this chapter we discuss recruiting and retaining participants. It may be tempting to think that you will worry about this when the time comes, but by then it is too late: your design may not even be feasible.

13.1 Recruiting the Right Number of Participants

In any protocol you must specify the number of participants you plan to have complete the study as part of the study design. Appendix B discusses issues involved in determining a sample size. Some studies require either a number of events or a specific duration of follow-up rather than a fixed number of participants completing the study (which we term "completers,") but for simplicity we will word this discussion in terms of completers. Achieving the specified number involves three steps. First, you must determine what sources are available to reach possible volunteers for the study and develop methods to engage their interest. If participants express an interest in participating in the study, then you must see whether they meet the eligibility criteria (Chapter 12). The most important criterion is the ability and willingness to give informed consent, usually including signing a consent form (Chapter 3). Once participants are enrolled, you must initiate procedures to encourage them to stay in the study until they complete it. Often investigators work backwards from the number of participants they need to complete the study and adjust this number to allow for dropouts during the study, and finally further adjust this for participants consenting to the study but then found to be ineligible.

Example 13A: An investigator wants to conduct a study of 5-weeks duration and has determined he must have 60 participants complete the study. The flow of participants is shown in Figure 13.1. Working backwards from the final number, he assumes that 20% of the participants enrolled will not complete the study, therefore the investigator needs to enroll 75 participants. He will advertise for participants in the hospital clinic. He expects that only about 50% of the respondents will be eligible for the study, therefore he has to recruit at least 150 participants into screening for the study. There are about 50 cases a month seen in the clinic. Assuming that about one-quarter of them would agree to be screened for the study, there would be about 12 screened and 6 enrolling

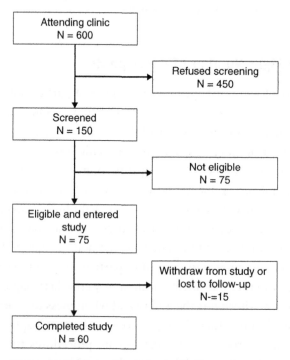

Figure 13.1. Flow of Participants for Example 13A.

each month. At this rate, he would need at least 1 year to recruit the 75 participants needed to have 60 participants complete the study.

Note that although there are about 50 patients attending the clinic, the investigator estimates that only about 5 per month will be willing to participate, eligible, and complete the study. This reflects the reality that only a small proportion of potentially eligible individuals may be interested in your study.

13.2 Recruitment and Retention Is Part of Planning

In addition to determining if the study is feasible, there are many other reasons that methods of recruiting and retaining participants must be part of your planning. If you are writing a proposal, then you must convince the potential sponsor that you can find and retain the number of participants you specified and budgeted for this activity. If the study has any longitudinal component, you must have a realistic estimate of the proportion that can be expected to complete the study to determine the number of participants that must be enrolled to achieve the specified number of participants completing the study. This may also impact the feasibility of the design.

Example 13B: You have designed a crossover study with 3 treatment periods of 8 weeks each and a 2-week washout period between each treatment period. This is a very demanding study for the participants, who would need to participate for a total of 28 weeks. Is it likely that you can find enough participants in the population at your center that will agree to this, and will stay in the study? If the study only requires a small number of participants to complete the 3 treatment periods, or if the participants are people with whom you interact on a regular basis, such as patients in a diabetes clinic, then this study may be feasible. Recruiting your own patients, however, raises the potential for coercion, discussed in Section 3.3. Otherwise, since it is likely that there will be a lot of dropouts, it may be better to do this study using a parallel group design with each participant receiving one treatment.

Recruitment and retention are costly, time-consuming tasks, and you must allow for adequate personnel time and financial support. The personnel who interact with the participants are the key to successful recruitment and retention. They must be readily accessible to answer questions, be nonjudgmental, and show respect for the participant at all times. Most importantly, the staff members must be problem solvers. If study staff are evaluating participants, filling out forms for the study, entering data, and performing all the other duties necessary to keep a study running, will they have the time needed to communicate with participants and to address their concerns? Your staffing plan must allow sufficient time for nonspecific interaction with participants.

13.3 Locating and Recruiting Participants

Locating and recruiting participants can be done in many ways, listed in Table 13.1. The approaches range from a targeted appeal to a limited group (e.g., clinic patients, referrals from specialists in the disease), to broad, "shotgun" approaches (e.g., Internet and media advertising). In between these extremes are more general but still targeted approaches (presentations to support groups and posting to Internet groups focusing on the groups of interest, etc.).

Example 13C: You intend to recruit participants with a specific condition from clinics in your institution. You must review the clinic reports to ensure that there are enough participants available who will meet your inclusion and exclusion criteria, assuming that most will refuse to participate. If there are not enough patients in your clinic, you may need to expand the eligible population by making arrangements with other institutions. This may be an informal agreement with a neighboring institution or with specialists in the community to refer patients, or formal arrangements with institutions in other locations.

Recruiting from a clinic might require placing posters or pamphlets written in layman's language, often in multiple languages, in the clinic's waiting area with information on the study, or arranging for clinic personnel to describe the study briefly and ask prospective participants if they would be willing to be contacted about participating. Sometimes a recruiter for the study, with the approval of the Institutional Review

Table 13.1 Possible Recruitment Methods

Source of Participants	Advantages	Disadvantages
Hospital Clinic	• Known participant characteristics • Number of participants with specific characteristics may be high • Existing relationship helps recruitment	• Limited population • Possibility that patients feel pressured to participate
Physician Referrals	• Inexpensive • Likely to understand research requirements	• Often not much variation in population • Recruitment by primary physician may seem coercive • May not be committed to long-term involvement • Usually referring physicians are overcommitted, and so have minimal time to refer potential participants
Disease Specific Support Groups	• Inexpensive	• May attract a sicker population
Word of Mouth	• Cheap	• Usually not very effective • Potentially few volunteers screened for study actually have the disease of interest
Internet Bulletin Boards and News Groups	• Probably widest audience • Not expensive (so far)	• Completely unselected audience will give low proportion of contacts who are eligible.
Paid Recruiters	• Experienced recruiter who is knowledgeable about recruiting methods • Links to the community • May select for specific characteristics • May help with retention and compliance	• Expensive • Payment depending on success may result in coercive methods to enroll participants • Payment depending on success may result in participants being recruited who do not fully meet the inclusion and exclusion criteria • Payment depending on success may result in persuasion of participants to enlist in the study who are not likely to stay in the study

(continued)

Table 13.1 (*cont.*)

Source of Participants	Advantages	Disadvantages
Institutional Recruiting Support	• Experienced recruiter • May have same advantages as paid recruiter • May not require funds from the study budget • For advertising, may be able to include your study with others to reduce cost	• May be recruiting for several similar protocols • Limited time for your study • An advertisement with multiple studies has less focus on your study
Community Groups and Community Bulletin Boards	• Less expensive than media • Good community relations • May be directed at a particular audience	• Proportion of contacts who are eligible is usually low
Mass Mailing	• Reaches many potential participants	• Expensive • Proportion of contacts who are eligible is usually low • May attract participants with a different agenda (e.g., suspected problems)
Media Advertising (Radio, Newspapers, TV)	• Reaches a wide audience • May be directed at a particular audience or the general population	• Expensive • Proportion of eligible contacts is usually low • May attract participants with a different agenda (e.g., suspected problems)

Board (IRB), will attend the clinic to ask patients if they would be willing to talk about the study while waiting, and to answer questions about it.

If participants are to be recruited from the general population, methods to advertise the study include word of mouth (usually not sufficient), advertising on local bulletin boards, newspaper and radio advertising, the Internet, presentations at community groups, and the like. Occasionally mass mailings are used to locate study participants, but this is not very efficient and is only done for very large studies. Mailing lists based on basic characteristics such as age and sex can be purchased from marketing firms, but this is expensive. Frequently, a brochure and a website describing the study will be prepared. Some studies use professional recruiters, although this is also expensive. Many institutions have staff members who aid investigators in developing and implementing plans for recruiting and who can be reached in the evenings or weekends.

Example 13D: The study in high-risk mothers cited in Examples 11C and 12A requires a large number of participants. To recruit them, the study would be announced in local newspapers and radio stations and presented at local meetings of obstetricians. Participants would be recruited from hospital clinics, outlying clinics, and private physicians. A letter describing the study would be sent to care providers. Care providers would be asked to identify potential high-risk participants and give them a pamphlet, but not ask them to participate. A special phone number would be set up for questions about the study.

Sometimes institutions or government organizations will post information on their websites about clinical studies that are recruiting participants. You may be able to use this resource as a way for patients to find out about your study and for potential participants to contact you about the study. Unless appropriate security measures have been taken, however, only very limited information can be collected using e-mail or the Internet (Section 13.5). For example, someone can contact you about a particular study and provide their contact information, but you should not be receiving any detailed medical information.

Random digit dialing is a method sometimes used for recruiting controls for case-control studies or for surveys from the general public. Telephone numbers are randomly generated, usually by a computer, which will also dial them. The possible telephone numbers can be restricted by area code and sometimes by exchange to sample from a restricted geographical area. It has the advantage that it would include unlisted numbers that would be missed if the numbers were selected from a telephone book. However, it has the disadvantage that it may create a biased sample. Calling would be limited to daytime or early evening hours, and people who are not available at that time because they work late, have a long commute, or have multiple jobs would be excluded. Leaving messages is one option, but people may be reluctant to call back an unknown person, and people with lower incomes may not have answering machines. Another potential bias occurs when individuals have multiple phones, such as home and business landlines and cell phones, which makes them more likely to be called. In addition, individuals often retain mobile numbers when moving, so that over time they are no longer representative of a geographic area.

For studies in special populations, you must tailor your recruitment methods to that population. If you are studying the elderly, you may need an alternative to telephone contact for those who are hard of hearing. If the participants have limited mobility, you may want to have a staff member go to their homes or other sites. You must devise special ways to protect participants' privacy when you are discussing the study in assisted living or nursing homes. In an area where many of your participants may not be English speaking, you must find staff members fluent in the languages used in the area.

Example 13E: In the study of gestational diabetes in Hispanic women in Example 11D, the Hispanic women were recruited from the postnatal clinic at the institution. The investigators realized that this population might have particular concerns about such a study and therefore conducted a series of focus groups to define these issues and develop ways to address them in recruiting material and interviews. All printed material was available in English and Spanish and all the staff involved in recruitment and interactions with participants were bilingual.

If you plan to do a series of studies, then it may turn out that a participant who was not eligible for the current study may be eligible for the next, or may be eligible for another study in your research group. You may ask if the participant would be interested in the other studies or could be contacted in the future for new studies.

13.4 Retention and Adherence

Many clinical studies involve observations over time to assess the effect of an intervention. You must plan how to retain the participants in these studies and how to measure and enhance the participant's adherence with the study protocol. Adherence means that the participant is choosing to comply with the study requirements. Although an investigator wants all participants to comply with the study protocol, it is up to the participant whether to adhere to the investigator's requests. Adherence is a choice that the participant makes. A participant can decide to only do certain parts of the study, such as to attend clinic visits but not to keep a daily activity log. A participant has the right to decide at any time not to continue in the study without penalty and does not have to give you a reason for this or even have to tell you about leaving the study. However, if the participant's leaving would pose a potential danger to himself or others, then you have a responsibility to see that this danger is minimized, as discussed in Example 3D, which involved a study requiring alcohol consumption. It is allowable to try to determine the participants' reasons for leaving and, if possible, resolve the issues so that they are willing to continue.

Although adherence is sometimes thought to be a problem only in interventional studies, anytime you need participants to do anything, such as responding to questions in an interview, you need their cooperation. When more than one contact is required, this problem becomes even more critical to the successful completion of the study. We discuss the special issues involved in adherence in interventional studies and ways to improve this in Chapter 24.

Probably the most important factor affecting retention, whether for an interventional study or an observational study, is the study staff who interact with the participants. Although it should go without saying, they need to treat participants with respect at all times. They should try to be helpful and resolve participant problems whenever they can. They should be warm and friendly to the participants. If acceptable to the participant, an occasional call just to keep in touch and see how the participant is doing is a good way to keep a participant involved in a study. We talk more about how this factor affects adherence and retention in Section 24.3.

One way to improve retention and adherence is to exclude participants who are planning to leave the area for an extended period of time during the study period. You may also try to select participants who are highly motivated and likely to stay in the study and exclude participants who might not. This is often an appropriate choice, but it reduces generalizability in favor of feasibility. If the participant is receiving financial compensation, then you may institute a system of graduated payments, with small amounts being paid at each visit and a larger sum after the study is completed, provided your IRB approves this strategy.

If there are long periods between study visits, you should find other reasons to contact the participants during the interval if acceptable to the participant. If your group has a newsletter about the study written for the general public, then sending this to study participants will not only remind them to stick to the study protocol but also make them feel they are part of something important. Birthday, anniversary, and holiday cards are extremely useful. In studies where information is being collected periodically, you may call to do periodic reminders of some sort to maintain contact.

Example 13F: An investigator wants to study factors affecting long-term adherence to exercise programs in patients enrolled in a cardiac rehabilitation program after a myocardial infarction. The investigator plans to record information about exercise participation during the rehabilitation program, along with various measures of physical condition and attitudes toward physical activity collected both at the start and end of the three-month training program. He wants the participants to maintain a weekly activity log recording when and how long they exercised each day for the three months after the program ends. There will be a final test of physical condition at the end of the six month study. To help improve adherence to the data recording after the cardiac rehabilitation program ended, the investigator adopted several strategies. First, rather than providing all the logs at one time, they were sent monthly to each participant, and a research assistant contacted the participant to make sure that they had arrived. Between these contacts, the research assistant team contacted each participant in the middle of the month to encourage them to continue completing the exercise log daily. If a previous activity log was overdue, the research assistant also contacted the participant to request that it be returned to the investigator and to provide encouragement to continue recording activities. Finally, to help make returning the logs easy, the investigator provided postage-paid envelopes for the participants to use to return the log.

You should try to get alternative methods for contacting participants in addition to home telephone number, cell phone number, and address. E-mail and text messages might be appropriate but need to be very nonspecific (e.g., reminding a person about an appointment at 2.00 PM the following day, but not specifying with who or about what) unless appropriate security measures are provided. If the participant has a pager or cell phone, then ask if she can be called on those. Ask if it is all right to call her at work, and always ask when the call begins if it is a good time for the participant to talk. Ask the participant for an alternative contact, someone who will know where she is in case she moves or changes her telephone numbers.

You must be flexible in scheduling telephone calls and visits. A participant who is working full time will appreciate being able to come in on weekends or after hours. If the participant is responsible for the care of young children, then the participant may want to come in when someone else is available to watch them. If participants can bring children in with them to appointments, then the study needs to have child care available. Helping with transportation to and from the clinic, such as bus passes and taxi vouchers, can substantially impact the chances of participants returning for follow-up visits.

Adherence problems may arise when participants are asked to follow a certain diet or be fasting before they have a test. In centers that have a specialized research facility for study participants, participants who are required to fast may be asked to stay overnight before the test. This has the added benefit for the participant that he does not have to rise early to get to the center, but the participant may not want to spend a night away from home.

13.5 Use of the Internet

The Internet certainly has the potential to ease participant recruitment, improve participant adherence, and reduce participant dropout.

In certain circumstances it could be used to collect data directly from participants (e.g., daily activity logs), but there are also significant security and confidentiality issues with using the Internet. It is important that you be aware of potential security problems that can be associated with Internet use, mainly the possibility that hackers or others may be able to get into a system, either yours or the one used by the participant, and get information that should not be available to others. This refers not only to medical information but even such information as the participant's social security number, which can be used for financial scams. If you do intend to use the Internet to communicate with participants, and it is allowed by your IRB, you should be able to find out how to secure information appropriately from the information technology group at your institution. You should also make sure that the participant or respondent is using a secure system. Some people do not have computers at home but rely on the ones in a public library, which would not be secure for either sending or receiving information, since others can see the computer screen and also because libraries often use Web-use monitoring software to protect from unauthorized use of their resources.

A more common use of the Internet is for study staff to enter data directly into the study database maintained at a central location (either entered directly or uploaded from a local machine in periodic batches). The same security concerns apply, but as there are a limited number of individuals involved, all of whom are staff, it is much simpler to establish, maintain, and enforce data security procedures.

Finally, using apps on smart phones to collect and transmit data securely from participants over communications network is very common, but there are problems of ensuring security and confidentiality of information.

13.6 Ethical Issues

There are many ethical issues concerning recruitment and retention of participants. Pressuring members of the study pool to participate against their will is unethical and usually counterproductive, since they are more likely not to adhere to the protocol if they feel pressured or coerced. Recruitment by the participant's physician is sometimes considered coercive. Excessive monetary or other rewards for participation are also considered coercive, although it is not unethical to reimburse participants for their time and related costs on a reasonable basis. Your IRB will be able to give you guidance about what is considered reasonable reimbursement at your institution.

Confidentiality must be maintained. When you are contacting participants for recruitment or during the study, do not leave messages that indicate the nature of the call. When you speak to participants, find out if they have concerns about others knowing where you are calling from. You may work out a simple code name that you can use to leave messages if this is acceptable to the participant.

In any interventional study, it is extremely important that participants not be given false hope when trying to recruit them into the study. Participants must be aware that the new treatment is experimental and may not benefit them. We have found this is a common problem, because very often people hear what they want to hear rather than what you say, but you must make every effort to ensure that the participant realizes that most experimental treatments are not successful. In a placebo-controlled trial, it must be clear to participants that they may not be receiving active treatment at all.

Participants have the right to leave the study at any time, and you must honor this right. Sometimes your responsibility for the participant's safety may conflict with this right. For example, if a participant wishes to leave a study while still under the influence of alcohol or another medication that could affect driving ability, you must take steps to ensure that the participant does not drive until the danger is eliminated. If failure to return could be detrimental to the participant's well-being or that of others – as in an interventional study in which participants must be weaned off the intervention gradually – then you must take all possible steps to arrange for the participant to return for a final visit to resolve the potential danger.

KEY POINTS

- A study plan must include plans for identifying, recruiting, and retaining participants.
- Methods of recruitment vary from extremely targeted recruitment in specialty clinics to recruitment from the general population using mass media.
- Recruitment methods should be tailored to the eligible population.
- Participants must not be given false hopes about the efficacy of an intervention.
- Participants must not be coerced in any way to participate.
- If you are treating a patient, you need to be aware that the person might feel coerced into being in your study because of the relationship.
- You may use the Internet for communicating with participants, but you must be aware of the security and confidentiality issues and comply with all institutional requirement to ensure the security of the communication.
- A friendly, helpful staff is essential for both recruitment and retention.

14

Study Data: How Variables Are Used

A study is about information. Information is obtained from data. Investigators collect data, examine this data, describe the values obtained, and make inferences and conclusions based on this data. The conclusions are the information from the study. The individual items collected are the study variables and the values of these variables, which are collected during the study from each participant, are the study data. As the name implies, variables are the items that can vary between study participants. The variables may have different uses in the study. Although you as the investigator usually know why you are collecting specific variables, an understanding of their role helps formulate analysis plans, understand the implications of statistical findings, and present results. In this chapter we define these different uses of variables. The following two chapters discuss these concepts with detailed examples.

14.1 Types of Variables

The study variables are based on measurements taken in the study. These include physical measurements such as height or weight, biological variables measured through chemical assay, genetic information, and emotional and psychological measurements through questionnaires and visual scales. The variables may be these measurements as taken or may be new variables derived from these measurements, such as differences between the baseline and final value of a variable, or composite scores. A variable may be a simple Yes or No response to a question (a binary or dichotomous variable), an evaluation at several levels that may be ordered (from best to worst in steps – an ordered categorical variable), a category (such as race) that is not ordered, a rate or percent, a count, or a continuous measurement that can, theoretically, take on any value in a given range. One variable may be measured or calculated at several time points. Frequently the measurement at the earliest time in a study, usually immediately before the intervention begins, is called the "baseline" value, and values at later time points can be used either as the observed value or as the calculated change from baseline.

Example 14A: A randomized parallel group study of testosterone replacement in hypogonadal men compared a new delivery method, given at two dosages, to a currently approved method of delivery. The participants were treated for six months. Testosterone levels were measured several times during the study, and several summary measures, such as the maximum level and the area under the curve for a given time interval, were calculated. Other hormones, bone markers, body composition, and bone mineral density were measured at the beginning and end of the study and, for some variables, several times during the study. The testosterone measurement was used to create a new dichotomous variable – within or not within the normal range. The primary hypothesis of this study was that the new method would yield testosterone levels equivalent to those calculated for the currently approved method. A secondary hypothesis was that the new method would have fewer side effects than the current method. Mood scores and sexual activity scores were calculated from a weekly diary by averaging each item over the week and then computing a summary score from several items. Expected side effects, such as skin irritation, were measured and recorded at regular intervals if they occurred at or between scheduled examinations.

14.2 Role of Variables in an Interventional Study

A study protocol, along with the Manual of Procedures (MOP: Section 29.3), should specify what variables are to be collected, how they will be measured, what derived variables will be used, why they are considered important, and how these variables will be used in the study. The variables may be grouped into four classes: outcome variables, predictor variables, confounding variables, and safety variables, based on the planned usage in the analysis of the study. The role of these variables depend on the assumptions and objectives of the investigator and are not inherent to any particular variable or method of measurement.

Outcome variables are the basic results of the study. The outcome variables are frequently referred to as endpoints, and the statistical name for them is the dependent variables. Most studies have multiple outcome variables. Frequently one variable is described as the primary outcome variable, and the rest are called secondary outcomes.

Example 14A (continued): The primary outcome variable for this study was the measured testosterone level, dichotomized to normal or not normal. There were also secondary outcome variables spanning many areas expected to be affected by testosterone replacement. The occurrence and severity of certain side effects were compared to test the assumption that the new method would be easier to use than the current method. The other secondary outcome variables, including bone markers, sexual function, mood changes, body strength, body composition, and bone mineral density, were analyzed as changes from the first day of the study.

We discuss outcome variables in more detail in Chapter 15.

Predictor variables are the variables that you think will affect the outcome variables. The statistical name for them is independent variables. In general, the main purpose of a study is to examine the relationship between the predictor variables and the outcome variables. In an interventional study with more than one group, the primary predictor variable is the intervention used, often a treatment for a medical problem. There is frequently a hierarchy of predictor variables similar to the outcome variables, with some being of primary interest. The study design often focuses on the effect of primary predictors on primary outcome variables, particularly when determining sample size. Analysis of the effects of secondary predictors is often seen as exploratory.

Example 14A (continued): The primary predictor variable for both the primary outcome and all the secondary outcomes was the intervention that the participant received. The treatment was assigned randomly when participants entered the study (Chapters 20 and 21).

Example 14B: Investigators are interested in whether a program of diet and exercise, which has previously been shown to reduce cholesterol levels in participants, will reduce the incidence of cardiac events in a group of high-risk individuals. To do this they use a parallel group interventional study, with two groups: one receiving the diet and exercise program, and one following their routine diet and exercise. The incidence of cardiac events would be the primary endpoint, while other outcomes, such as all-cause mortality, would be secondary. The primary predictor is the randomized treatment group assignment.

Confounding variables, also referred to as concomitant variables, are variables that are not manipulated by the investigator and are not a focal point of the study, but may affect the relationship between predictors and outcomes. In other words, they are variables that have to be tested but that usually the investigator has not specified in his hypotheses. These are often demographic variables, such as age, sex, and ethnicity, but other variables may also be confounders in a study. For example, knowing someone is male may predict that he will be heavier that someone who is female.

Example 14A (continued): The primary confounding variable in this study was the underlying cause of the hypogonadism. Since this was a multi-center study, the study site also was a possible confounder. Age was also tested as a confounder. Since this study only involved males, sex was not an issue.

Example 14B (continued): In this study of diet and exercise, age and sex were considered as confounding variables. The inclusion criteria specified a limited age range and the ages were recorded in 10-year intervals. The interaction of age and sex was also tested for an effect on cardiac events.

Predictor and confounding variables are discussed further in Chapter 16.

Finally, safety variables are variables that are not related to the efficacy aims of the study, but are measured to make sure that the intervention is not doing any harm. They are needed only for interventional studies. They commonly include vital signs, lipids, liver enzymes, electrolytes, hematology, glucose and insulin, other measurements commonly included in a chemical panel, and significant adverse events, hospitalization, and death. Other safety variables can be required depending on what effects the treatment could possibly have. The investigators may have to track actual values, or simply categorize a condition as normal or abnormal. A description of adverse events should also be recorded as part of the safety information

Example 14A (continued): Safety variables included the chemical panel described above, as well as a lipid panel. In addition, the investigators monitored prostate size and prostate-specific antigen, which might be adversely affected by testosterone treatment; as both methods involved topical application, skin irritation was also assessed using a standard scale.

Example 14C: In a randomized interventional study, a new therapy was compared to the current standard of care, which was effective but frequently had an adverse effect on lipid levels. The investigators did not necessarily expect the new therapy to be superior to the current method, but they hoped to show that it was at least equivalent and did not adversely affect lipid levels. In this study lipid levels were secondary outcome variables to be compared between groups, as well as safety variables to be monitored.

Example 14D: In studies of steroid supplementation in men with normal levels, mood changes, including increased anger and hostility, may be monitored as a safety measure.

In Example 14A the objective was replacement of abnormally low levels rather than supplementation, and mood changes were included as secondary outcomes with the hypothesis that mood would improve with treatment. In contrast, in Example 14D mood changes reflect a safety concern and need to be monitored for safety reasons.

No matter what the intervention is, one must make every effort to avoid having any safety issues, and must collect appropriate safety measurements. In addition to having procedures in place to avoid pain and injuries during the diet and exercise study (Example 14B), and procedures to handle them should they occur, the investigator also needs methods to record the occurrence of these adverse events.

It is essential that interventional studies include plans for monitoring the necessary safety variables. Many Institutional Review Boards (IRBs) will not approve a protocol without a safety monitoring plan.

In some studies, the safety variables are part of the study objectives, as in Example 14C, which has both that the treatment will have appropriate efficacy but also that lipid levels will not be seriously altered. In these cases, safety variables also have a role as outcome variables, and should be reported as such.

The role that a variable takes depends on your objectives and the role you assign to a particular variable.

Example 14A (continued): Lipid levels were considered a safety variable because the investigator wanted to ensure that they would not be seriously affected by the new treatment. Previous studies showed these levels might be moderately affected by testosterone treatment, but the change was expected to be small and to be acceptable in view of the other benefits.

Example 14B (continued): In this study lipid levels were considered as a secondary outcome for the effect of the diet and exercise program.

In contrast to Example 14A, in Example 14B lipid levels are an outcome variable.

Even within a single study these roles may not be mutually exclusive, and one variable can be used in different ways to explore different questions. For example, outcome variables can be used as predictor variables, to determine if their values are associated with the values of other outcome variables.

Example 14B (continued). The investigators also wanted to determine if any reduction in the incidence of cardiac events is associated with reductions in cholesterol levels. Thus, changes in cholesterol levels will be used as predictor variables in a model for cardiac events and a secondary outcome variable for the effect of the diet and exercise program.

There is a difference in the implications of these associations, however. Although we can never establish cause and effect absolutely, if you modify the value of a predictor variable and then observe an associated change in an outcome variable, then it is reasonable to think that the change in the outcome was caused by the change in the predictor. This is the reason that treatment is randomly assigned, so that there will be strong evidence that the treatment (considered as a predictor) is the reason for the change in outcome. Thus, if there is a reduction in the incidence of cardiac events, then this would be strong evidence that the diet and exercise program caused this reduction. However, we have modified the cholesterol levels only indirectly, as an effect of the treatment. When the predictor is an outcome variable that you have not modified directly, the only thing you can say is that the values are associated. Thus, we can conclude a cause-effect relationship between using the diet and exercise program and changes in the incidence of cardiac events, but can only conclude that the change in incidence is associated with the observed change in cholesterol level. Such findings may lead to another study where the intervention is different values of the suspected predictor to see if a cause-effect conclusion may be reasonable.

There is also some ambiguity as to whether a variable should be considered a predictor or a confounding variable. The distinguishing criteria might be whether the investigator thinks they may be important predictors and has identified them as such in the protocol. The descriptions can overlap, and often the distinction may seem like hairsplitting, but it is important in defining the stated objectives of the study.

Example 14A (continued): Age was considered a confounding variable in this study. However, other studies focus on age-related responses to testosterone treatment, so in those studies age would be an important predictor. The difference is in the objectives of the study.

14.3 Role of Variables in Observational Studies

The previous examples have all been interventional studies, but the same definitions apply to the role of variables in observational studies. In most observational studies the primary outcome is well defined. In a cohort study, secondary outcomes may also be included. In a cohort study, the exposures defining the cohort are the predictor variables; other exposures may be included as confounding variables. Since there is no intervention in these studies, safety variables are not strictly required, but if they can be extracted from the data (in retrospective studies) or added to the protocol in prospective studies, they should be used. Although the safety data may not be as complete as what you would collect in an interventional study, if it is reliable, it should be included.

Example 14E: An investigator would like to see whether young men who played football in high school and had a least one concussion involving unconsciousness had cognitive problems 6 years after graduating high school. This was a retrospective cohort study. The outcome was any one of a series of cognitive problems, such as memory loss. Confounding variables might include such things as age at concussion, number of concussions, other injuries, and other problems in school before the concussion. Since only males were studied, sex was not a predictor or a confounder.

In a case-control study, even though the participants are selected on outcome, the role of the variables would be similar.

Example 14F: An investigator is interested in studying causes of cognitive problems in young adult males in a population. Cases are young adults newly identified with cognitive problems, while controls are selected to match the cases' age. Among the many variables collected as potential causes is medical history of concussion prior to the diagnosis of cognitive problems. In the case-control study, concussion is one of the potential predictors of the outcome variable – presence or absence of cognitive problems.

Examples 14E and 14F illustrate two approaches to investigating a similar problem, but from different directions. In Example 14E, the approach is to start with a cohort some of whom have a particular exposure (concussion with unconsciousness), and determine whether there is an increase in cognitive problems due to this exposure. Once the cohort is formed for this study, it would be possible to expand the research and examine whether other outcomes were related to this exposure. If the cohort is formed with both athletes and non-athletes, it would be possible to assess the effect of other athletic exposures, making this an excellent approach for an investigator intending to focus research on the consequences of high-school athletics. In contrast, Example 14F as a case-control study is focused on the problem of cognitive problems. The study will enable the investigator to examine the role of concussion with unconsciousness as a risk factor, but other potential risk factors can also be examined. As such, this would be an excellent approach for an investigator interested in pursuing research in cognitive problems.

14.4 Measuring Variables

As discussed extensively in Chapter 29, when the study is designed the investigator must specify the sources and measurement methods of all the variables collected in the study. These details include the instruments used for measurement, laboratory methods, even calibration standards and rater training when appropriate. This information, along with operational details, such as exactly how to conduct a test, should be defined in the MOP.

It is the responsibility of the investigator to make sure that the procedures in the MOP are followed by the study team and to monitor the accuracy and timeliness of the data collection. This means that no matter how carefully you specify the variables to be collected, you must make sure that these are measured accurately and consistently and that errors in the measurements are minimized. Chapter 29 discusses ways to ensure that the data you collect is of high quality. In particular,

- The data must be obtained using well-defined, reliable, and consistent methods. In assays of body fluids, a single, validated assay method should be used on all the samples.
- If the data is obtained from several sources, such as the participant's hospital of choice rather than a central laboratory, then care must be taken to ensure that the measurements are comparable.
- If data is obtained via a personal interview, then a single interviewer is the best choice for small studies. If that is not possible, then most studies require that only a limited number of specially trained individuals conduct the interviews, that consistency across interviewers be established before participants are enrolled, and that consistency be monitored during the course of the study.

The data should be as easy to obtain as possible, both for the investigator and for the participant. For example, a measurement obtained from blood or urine would be preferable to a measurement that required spinal fluid. If physical testing is involved, the effort for the participant must be minimized.

Example 14A (continued): Although this was a multi-center study, the hormones and bone markers were all measured using standard assay methods in a single laboratory. Body composition and bone mineral density were measured using validated technology, with the same type of equipment used at each center. An instrument to measure mood changes and sexual function was developed for this study.

14.5 Recoding Data

We present a simple illustration here and discuss recoding outcome variables more fully in Section 15.2. The rationale for recoding data and the methods used apply equally to the other variables in a study when recoding is appropriate.

Example 14E (continued): Cognitive problems must also be defined according to specific medical criteria. But the cognitive problems may also be grouped into classifications, such as memory loss, speech difficulties, behavioral problems, and so on. The number of concussions were presented in the paper, but for purposes of the analysis was grouped into 1, 2, or 3 or more.

14.6 Storing Data

A computer system is the primary method for storage and retrieval of data, although paper copies may be necessary to validate the data in the computer files. In Chapter 30 we discuss some options for selecting a computer database program, although the actual creation and maintenance of a computer database is a technical topic beyond the scope of this book. Having data in a computer, however, does not make it correct, and steps must be taken to ensure that your carefully collected data is correctly recorded in the computer files (Section 30.5).

The most elegant, beautifully designed database or the most expensive, state-of-the-art computer system or sophisticated analysis will not create accurate information unless the data is collected following rigorously defined procedures during the study.

14.7 Ethical Issues

When the data is collected, the investigator must make every effort to ensure that it is complete and accurate. If the data is not reliable, then the study is not good, and you have wasted the participants' time and effort as well as your own. Even in an observational study, the investigator should be confident of the accuracy of the data that will be used and recognize problems with data accuracy and potential bias in any interpretation of the data.

In addition to identifying the key variables related to the hypotheses when planning a study, the investigator must also identify what other variables need to be collected to support and validate the analysis. If confounding variables are not identified and recorded, the conclusions of the study may be affected by the effects of these confounding variables.

For an interventional study the investigator must plan to collect data monitoring the safety of the intervention and adverse events in the study. Although such data is usually not the primary focus of a study, it is critical that the investigator ensures that the intervention is not doing harm to the participants. For this reason, even for very small studies, it is often very useful to have colleagues who are not closely involved in the study do the actual safety monitoring to avoid any potential biases when interpreting the safety data. This is particularly important if you are studying seriously ill individuals, since any safety problem due to your intervention will be hard to separate from the natural course for these individuals. It is often easy to explain away individual adverse events, especially if you are the investigator believing in the benefits of the intervention. For this reasons, many institutions require that even very small high-risk studies be independently monitored for safety by a review panel not otherwise involved in the study.

KEY POINTS

- The purpose of a study is to obtain information to address the hypothesis of the study.
- Information is obtained by analyzing and interpreting data.
- Variables are the different items that are collected during the study.
- Variables may be used in four different ways, which may overlap:
  - Outcome variables are the endpoints in the study.
  - Predictor variables are those that are assumed to influence the value of the outcome variables and are the primary focus of the study.
  - Confounding variables are those that may also influence the value of the outcome variables or relationships between variables, but are not a primary focus of the study.
  - Safety variables are those that must be monitored in an interventional study to ensure participant safety.
- It is critical to ensure that the data are accurate and that methods of obtaining the data are reliable and consistent.
- Data must be collected precisely and recorded accurately.

15

Study Data: Endpoints

In this chapter we discuss the outcome variables, which are the end-points of a study. These are the most critical measurements in the study, as they are the basis for the results that you will present. Although some studies have only a single endpoint, most studies have multiple end-points, of which one is primary. "Outcome" sometimes implies a Yes or No result, and "endpoint" sometimes implies a result after some time interval, but the words are often used interchangeably in practice, and we do so in this chapter as well.

15.1 Defining the Outcome Variables

When you plan a study, you must choose outcome variables that will provide the data needed to answer the questions proposed in the study. Therefore, the selection and definition of these variables is critical. First of all, they must be relevant to the question of interest. They must address the major study questions directly. Moreover, since the human body consists of multiple complex biological systems that interact and overlap, it is likely that there will be other variables that are affected by the intervention or exposures that the participant experiences. For this reason, you may be interested in multiple, related outcomes. You must distinguish between outcomes that will provide information about the efficacy of an intervention and the safety variables that must be monitored to make sure that there are no adverse effects from the intervention.

We emphasize that in any study the outcome variables must be fully specified in advance. It is not acceptable to define an outcome variable after the study is under way. Sometimes investigators will describe an unexpected finding as an unexpected outcome, but this can only be viewed as a chance finding that must be verified in a study designed specifically for that purpose. It is possible that in the course of a study an unexpected result may become so clear and so well explained by the known facts that it may be reported as a valid outcome, but this is rare and needs an extensive justification to be acceptable to the scientific community.

Example 15A: The use of lithium for treatment of bipolar depression was discovered accidentally when investigators were using it for treatment of urinary tract infections and noticed changes in participants with bipolar disorder. Although the results were dramatic and reproducible, a great deal of further study was required to validate the results and to determine a safe and effective dose of lithium for the treatment of bipolar disease.

As you are collecting information anyway, there is a common tendency to collect as much information as you can, even though it is not relevant to the study hypotheses. This puts an unnecessary burden on participants in the study, and can actually reduce the quality of the primary data needed for the study because participants become overwhelmed by the demands of the study, or annoyed at the extensive and apparently irrelevant, and sometimes intrusive, information requested. In addition, if you look at a sufficiently large number of different variables, you are certain to find some results that are statistically significant just by chance.

Example 15B: In the randomized parallel group study of testosterone replacement in hypogonadal men (Example 14A), the primary outcome was the achievement of testosterone levels within the normal range after 30 days. The other outcome variables included hormone measures, bone markers, body composition, bone mineral density, mood, and sexual function. All of these variables were postulated to be affected by hormone replacement, and thus it was valid to include them as secondary outcomes. Variables that were not expected to be affected, such as cortisol or cerebral metabolites, were not measured.

In this example there were many outcome variables, but the primary variable was whether or not the testosterone level at 30 days was within the normal range of men in that age group. Other research goals might use a synthesis of several measurements. The choice of the primary outcome variable depends on the setting of the experiment. It may be related to a particular disease, as well as the investigator's belief as to what is the most critical value.

Example 15C: The term "lipid levels" implies several measurements, including total cholesterol, HDL and LDL cholesterol, the ratio of total to HDL cholesterol, and triglycerides. In most studies, all these variables may be measured; however, for the purpose of defining efficacy in an interventional study, one variable must be selected as the primary outcome. In a study of a lipid-lowering agent that primarily affects LDL cholesterol, the primary endpoint would be changes in LDL cholesterol. In a study of a drug expected to have a lipid-lowering effect on a number of different lipid measures, the endpoint might be the proportion of participants achieving the National Cholesterol Education Program goal.

If the study is an interventional study of a new treatment, then it usually focuses on a single endpoint, and other outcomes are secondary. On occasion, however, such a study will have two equally important endpoints, called co-primary endpoints. If the study is not focused on efficacy, then several outcome variables may be equally important primary endpoints for either an observational or interventional study.

Example 15D: The Collaborative Study of the Psychobiology of depression was an in-hospital multi-center study of the effect of antidepressant drugs on the biological and clinical aspects of depression. Participants who met the study criteria for severe depression, unipolar or bipolar, were admitted to one of six participating hospitals. The study duration was six weeks. After a 10-day washout period, baseline samples of cerebral catecholamines and metabolites were measured in serum, cerebral spinal fluid, and urine for the study. After five more days, participants were randomly assigned to receive one of two different antidepressants, and the biological measures were reassessed after 18 days treatment. Clinical status was evaluated using a battery of behavioral instruments that measured different aspects of depression. Clinical evaluations were done at intake, at baseline, when drug treatment was started, and weekly during the treatment period, including the last day of treatment. The changes in neurochemical and behavioral measures were multiple, equally important endpoints for this study.

An outcome may be measured multiple times, but the frequency of measurements should be no higher than is absolutely necessary to determine the study results. If a variable that changes slowly is measured at short intervals, then this would be a waste of time and resources. Cost, which may affect the size of the study you can do, is also a consideration. For example, MRI and other imaging methods supply information that cannot be obtained through less expensive methods, but their use often limits the number of participants that can be studied.

Example 15E: The effect of treatment in HIV-infected children with abnormal cerebral metabolites was measured by proton magnetic resonance spectroscopy. These children also showed deficits in neuropsychological functioning. The imaging studies are expensive and cause some stress to the children, therefore they were repeated only at long intervals, while the neuropsychological tests caused fewer problems for the children and could be repeated more frequently.

Example 15D (continued). The investigators were interested in the time course of changes due to drug treatment. Because the clinical assessments were minimally invasive and not costly to administer, they were repeated frequently during the study. But the neurochemical assessments, which were very invasive, were only done once during baseline and once during treatment.

15.2 Derived Outcomes

Often, the outcome variable is not one that is measured directly. Sometimes the outcome of interest is one that can take on a large number of values. To give an easily presented response to the study question, the outcome may be recorded into a few categories, most frequently a simple dichotomy Yes versus No or Success versus Failure. Values could be divided into continuous ranges, such as classifying an assay into ranges for low, normal, high, and very high. Discrete variables, such as the number of episodes requiring hospitalization for a sickle cell anemia patient, could also be categorized with a group such as three or more collapsing the data for the few patients with many hospitalizations into a single category.

Example 15B (continued): Although exact testosterone levels were measured periodically during the treatment period, these were used to compute the value for the binary variable addressing normal levels, which was the main outcome variable.

The outcome could be based on a number of different measurements, for example when a response to treatment for depression is based on the change in several measures of depression symptoms. The disadvantages of collapsing data in this way are that it does not use all the information in the original variables, and, from the practical point of view, is likely to require a larger sample size than using the original variables. However it may be the best way of reducing the data to some criteria that can be analyzed.

Example 15D (continued): To determine whether the participants responded to treatment, the investigator used a 50% decrease in a specific instrument, which would be dichotomized into improvement or no improvement. The study protocol also included a more comprehensive dichotomous measure of overall clinical response that would be based on several measurements at the end of the study.

The study design must describe how the data will be recoded. Preferably, recoding would be based on known standards in the literature, as in Example 15B, which used the normal range for different ages. Sometimes theoretical considerations can be used to determine how the outcome should be defined. However, sometimes it is necessary to collect data as part of the study process to know how recoding should be done.

Example 15F: Although there are published standards for many biochemical values in adults, data for children are sparser and are not always age specific. An investigator wanted to study the effects of head trauma on cortisol levels in children. To characterize participants as having normal or abnormal cortisol levels, the first step in the study was the recruitment and testing of a group of control children who did not have head trauma to define the distribution of cortisol in a "normal" population. The investigators used the results from these control children to define the normal range for different age groups, according to a plan specified in the protocol, and were then able to code the cortisol level in the children with head trauma as normal or not normal.

Other types of outcomes may be change from the beginning of the study until the end or a specified intermediate point, or a new variable that combines the results of several variables. The actual change may be used for the outcome, the percent change, or a classification of the amount of change – such as large, moderate, or small – might also be used.

Example 15G: This was a cohort study to determine if participants who exercise before surgery have a better outcome after undergoing joint replacement. After the surgery, the study team collected data from the hospital and the rehabilitation centers pertaining to the participant's recovery of function. The outcome variables were the measures of functioning that were collected as part of the participant's usual treatment. These included assessments by the physician and by the participant himself, as well as standardized physical tests. The results of some of the tests were combined to give a single summary variable measuring overall function, which had been specified in the protocol prior to any data collection.

15.3 Time-Related Outcomes

The outcome variable may be measured several times in the course of the study, and the result of interest may be the time trend in the variables rather than any specific value or the change from beginning to end.

Example 15H: In an open-label extension to the testosterone study of Example 15B, participants who completed the study were invited to continue using just the experimental method in a long-term study. Testosterone, other hormones, mood, and sexual functioning were measured semiannually during the longitudinal study and were analyzed for trends over time.

Example 15I: In another study of depression, participants with major depression were randomized to treatment with one of two antidepressant agents known to be effective or a placebo. Clinical measures were assessed several times in the study. Recovery was defined using the standard method and also a composite variable as in Example 15D. This study focused on comparing the time course of the changes in different measures between the treatments, rather than solely the amount of change that occurred at the end of the study.

Sometimes the primary outcome of the study is not a particular value or response in the participant but the time it takes for this response to occur. If all participants are expected to reach some milestone, then the actual time to occurrence would be the outcome variable. However, there is no guarantee that the outcome will occur in all participants during the period of the study, even though the nature of the disease does not allow the investigator to conclude that the event would never have occurred in a participant. In this case the data from that participant is said to be "censored," meaning the investigator does not know the outcome but does know that the time to event would be bigger than the observation period.

Example 15I (continued): Instead of the pattern of the changes in variables over time, the outcome could have been the time until recovery occurred.

Example 15J: Large-scale HIV treatment studies are done to compare the efficacy, tolerability, and safety of several treatment regimens against each other using a randomized parallel group design. Efficacy and tolerability are assessed as the time to an event, such as the time to treatment failure or the time to discontinuation of the treatment for side effects. Safety, however, is usually analyzed as the number of participants with adverse events rather than the time to the adverse event.

Sometimes the outcome of interest cannot be measured directly. In that case, we use a surrogate variable that is measurable and in some way directly reflects changes or differences in the unmeasurable variable. For example, levels of dopamine in the brain cannot be measured in any acceptable way, so serum and spinal fluid levels of metabolites of dopamine may be specified as the outcome measurement for a study. In some interventional studies the most important outcome is measurable but does not occur frequently enough to provide meaningful results in a study in a feasible time period, so that other variables are used as indicators that the intervention is likely to have the long-term outcome desired.

Example 15J (continued): The ultimate endpoint for treatment of HIV disease is long-term survival. At one time, during the early years of the epidemic when drugs were first being developed, this was acceptable because even the best early drugs only improved survival briefly. Now, however, markers of disease progression, such as time to virologic failure, are used as outcomes. This outcome has been shown to be a reliable predictor of subsequent increased risk of mortality, so that virologic monitoring is done regularly during a study, and participants with virologic failure are switched to a different treatment regimen as soon as it is detected. Time to virologic failure is used as a surrogate for time to death.

15.4 Ethical Issues

We emphasize that in any study the outcome variables must be fully specified in advance. It is not acceptable to specify an outcome variable after the study is under way, and this is especially bad when defined only after the data has been analyzed. This is commonly called "data dredging," with a goal of finding something that is statistically significant to publish. Although the statistical analysis may be correct, the conclusions from any such analysis cannot be trusted. If one does enough statistical tests, one eventually can find something that is statistically significant, but such findings are likely to be due to chance.

Sometimes investigators will describe an unexpected finding as an unexpected outcome, but this can only be viewed as an incidental finding that must be verified in a study designed for that purpose and should be termed an unexpected result. It is possible that in the course of a study an unexpected result may become so clear and so well explained by the known facts that it may be reported as a valid conclusion, but this is rare and needs to be extensively justified to be credible, as illustrated in Example 15A.

Another consideration when selecting the endpoint is how long a study will take to be completed. If the intervention being tested is effective, you want to make it available to all patients with the condition as soon as possible. Using a surrogate endpoint, as in Example 15J is one way to shorten the time needed for a study, but only if the surrogate endpoint is already known to be predictive of the outcome of interest.

Of course, if the endpoint is unobtainable or does not answer the study question, then you have wasted your participants' time and effort, and this is unethical.

KEY POINTS

- The outcome variables must be completely specified in the study design before the study begins.
- An outcome variable can be a single measurement, a measurement coded into classes, or a single variable calculated based on the combined value of several other variables.
- An outcome variable may be measured many times in the course of a study.
- There may be multiple outcome variables in a study:
  - the outcome variables are usually designated as primary or secondary;
  - in an interventional study of a new therapy, there is usually only one primary outcome variable that measures efficacy.
- In observational studies there may be several outcome variables of equal importance.
- When the outcome is time to an event but the study may not be long enough for the event to occur in all participants, then the data is said to be censored.
- Surrogate variables may be used when the outcome of interest cannot be measured with acceptable techniques or within an acceptable time period.
- Incidental findings unrelated to the study hypotheses must be interpreted cautiously.

16

Study Data: Predictor and Confounding Variables

In this chapter we discuss predictor and confounding variables, two categories of variables that are assumed to influence the values of the outcome variables. The difference is sometimes subtle and depends on the stated aims of the study. The effects of the predictor variables on the outcome are the focus of the study, whereas confounding variables are nuisance variables that must be considered but are not of main interest. Like outcome variables, predictor and confounding variables can be direct measurements, recoded values of measured variables, or composites derived from several variables. Like outcome variables, they should be specified in advance in the protocol.

16.1 Predictor Variables

We use the word "predictor" in a very general sense. It does not mean that the value of the predictor(s) will give you an exact value for the outcome. Rather, we assume that the value of the predictor(s) will influence the value of the outcome. From the statistical analysis you can obtain measures to estimate the strength of the predictor on the magnitude or other characteristics of the outcome. In an interventional study, the predictor variables are usually the ones that are manipulated as part of the intervention, and the objective of the study is to see if and how these manipulations affect the outcome. In an observational study, the exposures are the predictor variables. However, predictors may also include variables that describe the participant, such as age, sex, or ethnicity, when these are considered important to the outcome.

Example 16A: Example 15J described a randomized parallel group study to determine the efficacy of several different HIV treatments against each other. The primary predictor variable in this study is the treatment, assigned randomly by a computer program when participants are enrolled.

Example 16B: In Example 15G, a cohort study investigating whether participants who exercise before surgery have a better outcome after undergoing joint replacement than those who do not, the primary predictor was the amount of exercise the participant did prior to the surgery. Because this was not controlled by the investigator, it was necessary to develop standards to classify the type and amount of exercise. The most inclusive categories were endurance, strength training, both, or no exercise. The amount of time was estimated in terms of total hours per week and the number of separate occasions per week. Both the actual times and classifications such as infrequent, moderate, and frequent were used in the analysis.

Example 16C: In Example 15D, a multi-center study of depressed patients, the depressed participants were randomized to one of two drugs and followed for four weeks. Since both drugs were known to be effective overall in the treatment of depression, which drug was used was not considered a predictor of overall outcome. The specific aims were to show that the drugs affected different aspects of depression; therefore, the choice of drug was considered a predictor of change in these outcome variables. The drug was also tested as a predictor of change in biochemistry.

In practice, outcome variables can be used as predictor variables, to determine if their values are associated with the values of other outcome variables, but this must be done with caution. If the investigator modifies the value of a predictor variable and then observes an associated change in an outcome variable, it is reasonable to believe in a cause-effect relationship, with the change in the predictor variable causing the change in the outcome variable. However, when the predictor is an outcome variable that was not modified directly by the investigator, the only thing that can be said is that the values are associated. These findings may lead to another study where the investigator controls the value of the variable of interest to provide more evidence of a cause-effect relationship.

Example 16C (continued): Associations between change in biochemistry and change in the clinical components of depression were also an important part of this study. Although it would not be unreasonable to think of biochemical changes as causing clinical changes, the study was not designed to investigate this.

Example 16D: In Example 15B, a randomized parallel group study of testosterone delivery to hypogonadal men, the primary predictor was method and dose of delivery (the treatment variables). In addition to examining the effect of these different treatments on changes in secondary outcome variables, such as body composition and mood, the investigator tested whether the magnitude of the change in testosterone levels was associated with the magnitude of the changes in the secondary outcome variables. This was not done to generate new hypotheses, but rather to compare the results of this study with the findings and theories of other investigators.

16.2 Confounding Variables

Confounding variables or confounders are variables that are not manipulated by the investigator and are not a focal point of the study, but may affect the relationship between predictors and outcome. In other words, they are variables that have to be looked at, but usually the investigator hopes that these variables are not associated with the primary conclusions about the predictors in the study. In a multi-center study, such as Example 16C, the center where the participant was studied is a confounding variable, and it is important to determine whether it is associated with the outcome.

Example 16B (continued): In this study, since exercise type and amount tend to vary with age and sex, these were considered confounding variables in the study.

Example 16A (continued): In addition to basic demographic variables (age, race, ethnicity, sex), a major potential confounder when comparing

HIV treatments is the severity of the underlying condition, which can be assessed by the CD4+ level, history of AIDS defining illnesses, and viral load at time of study entry.

In Section 21.3.1 we discuss how stratification can be used as part of the randomization in interventional studies to ensure that the treatment groups are similar on confounding variables.

Variables such as age, sex, ethnicity, and site are common confounding variables, since they may affect the results but nothing can be done to affect them. Other variables, such as weight or BMI (in a study of diabetes, for example) or parity (in a study of maternal outcome) are frequently confounding variables in such studies. Disease-specific variables, such as duration of illness, number of episodes, presence of related conditions, family history, and so on may also be confounding variables. It may be possible to match groups on some of these characteristics in observational studies (Chapter 27) to eliminate them as confounders.

Example 16C (continued): Because participants were randomly assigned to drug treatment, age and sex were confounders. Other possible confounders were subtypes of depression, number of previous episodes of depression, and number of previous hospitalizations for depression.

16.3 Predictors versus Confounders

The distinction between predictor variables and confounder variables depends on the stated aims of the investigator. The predictors are the variables whose effects on the outcome are identified by the investigator as the focus of the study. Confounding variables are those that may influence the outcome but are not the focus of the study. They are collected and studied to provide reassurance that they are not affecting the conclusions of the study. To show convincingly that a predictor affects the result, you also must make sure that the differences in outcome are not due to potential confounders.

Example16D (continued): The primary outcome variable is the achievement of testosterone levels in the normal range after 30 days of treatment in hypogonadal men. It is known that testosterone levels tend to decline with increasing age, hence age is a confounding variable. However, the age range of the participants was limited by the inclusion criteria, and the normal range defined in this study was based on men within this age range, so that it encompassed the expected age variation. The investigators thus felt that age would not predict the primary outcome but included it in the analysis as a potential confounding variable.

Example 16E: Investigators were working with the staff of a local school district to encourage the students to have a healthy diet. They developed several alternative menus for the school cafeteria, including changes to the usual foods available from vending machines. The different menus were used for a few months and then they asked the children to rate them using specially designed questionnaires. They believed that menu preferences would be related to age, with older children having more sophisticated tastes. In this study, age was one of the primary predictor variables.

Confounding variables are sometimes referred to as concomitant variables. When an investigator is describing an analysis in which the effect of confounding variables is accounted for, such as age, the investigator will often use a phrase such as "corrected for" or "adjusted for" and then provide a list of variables.

16.4 Ethical Issues

As with outcome variables, the predictor and confounding variables must be specified in advance and rigorously collected. Even though you may be focused on the predictor variables that are the point of your study, it is important to identify the confounding variables, to make sure that they are part of your data collection, and to incorporate them in your analysis. Deliberately not collecting data on known confounding variables, either because they are difficult to collect or because of concerns that they may affect the results of the study, is tantamount to hiding your head under a blanket and hoping everything will be alright. This undermines both the validity of your study and the likelihood that your conclusions will be generally accepted by the scientific community.

However, you should only collect information on potential confounding variables if there is a reason to believe that they may affect the outcome variables. The natural tendency to collect just one more variable because it may be interesting needs to be nipped in the bud. The more variables you collect, the more onerous it will be for participants and study staff. In addition, if the data collection becomes excessive, the quality of the data for the predictor and outcome variables may suffer because the staff may be overwhelmed by the amount of data being collected, or participants may be annoyed about the effort required to provide everything being requested. Finally, if you test enough variables as potential confounders, you will almost certainly find something statistically significant due to chance.

Importantly, incidental findings in investigational studies may be reported if there is some theoretical or existing justification for them, but it would be unethical to present them as if they were predefined hypotheses. You must be clear that these were unplanned analyses and that further research would be necessary to confirm these results. These incidental findings are like incidentalomas when imaging a patient: it is often not clear what, if anything, they mean.

KEY POINTS

- Predictor variables are those that are assumed to influence the outcome variables. They are the focus of the study.
- In an interventional study the predictor variables are usually those whose values are randomly allocated by the investigator.
- Confounding variable are variables that are not the focus of the study but may influence the outcome variables.
- There should be limits on the number of variables that are collected. Variables that have never been shown or proposed to have anything

to do with the outcome variables should be collected only if you are specifically proposing a relationship when planning your study.

- Incidental findings unrelated to the study hypotheses must be interpreted very carefully.

17

Bias

Bias is the single biggest potential problem in clinical research. Bias means that the results observed are consistently influenced away from the true result. Random variation can also affect the results, but bias is different because it consistently influences the results in one direction. If a study is biased, it cannot be valid. Bias is like an infection, which can kill an otherwise healthy study. Even the accusation that bias might exist can cause the validity of the study to be questioned and the results discounted. Therefore, it is critical that a study include measures to avoid not only bias but also the potential appearance of bias. We do not know of any investigators who would consciously bias a study to get specific results, but there are subtle ways in which bias can sneak in to a study. In Chapter 18 we discuss methods to avoid biases.

17.1 Common Sources of Bias

The following sections describe the most common types of bias that can occur during a study. Although these are described separately, there is considerable overlap and interaction between the different categories of bias. A caregiver's perception of how a participant is doing may affect the participant's perception of what is being done to her, and if the caregiver is biased, then the participant's responses may become biased. Some of the biases described apply primarily to interventional studies, while other biases are more often associated with observational studies. Some problems in a study only become biases when they occur differentially between groups. Most importantly, many biases can infect any type of study.

We include publication bias, although it is not a design bias, because it is so often referred to in the literature.

17.1.1 Prognostic Bias

Prognostic bias (also called allocation bias) occurs in an interventional study when participants are selected or assigned to treatment based on certain characteristics. The characteristics in this discussion are different from those specified in the inclusion and exclusion criteria (Chapter 12); instead, they are characteristics that would influence the results of the study. Assignment of healthier appearing participants to the new treatment would create a bias in favor of the new treatment. Although this specific bias should not occur in a properly implemented randomized interventional study, it can arise when the study is not randomized. Importantly, randomization implies that the treatment assignment of a participant is independent of the participant's characteristics and can be known only after the participant is enrolled in the study (Section 20.1).

Example 17A: In a comparative study of high-dose oral fluconazole versus standard of care therapy for cryptococcal meningitis in AIDS patients, the investigators might use the oral fluconazole in all participants able to take oral medications, while participants unable to take oral medications received the standard of care (an IV therapy). Thus, healthier participants would be assigned to the oral fluconazole group rather than to the standard of care group. Such a study would be very biased.

Prognostic bias is much more common in observational studies. A case-control study can be biased when the control population is different from the cases in ways that affect the outcome. In Chapter 26 we state that controls should be as similar to the cases as possible, with the only differences being those of outcome. If the controls have healthier lifestyles or a healthier environment than the cases, then the study is biased in favor of a larger difference between the groups, which could be attributed falsely to exposures. If the controls are worse on these factors, then the study is biased in the other direction: a difference due to the exposures of interest may be obscured by the adverse effect of the controls' general environment.

Example 17B: In a case-control study of adult males with a congenital hormone imbalance, data was collected from a multi-item questionnaire and the focus was on social and cognitive problems. The cases were to be compared to a group of "healthy" men – those without the imbalance or related problems – with the same age distribution. The investigators recruited employees from their institution for controls. When the data was examined, it was seen that almost all the controls in the study had a bachelor's degree or at least some kind of training certificate and therefore probably did not have cognitive problems. Therefore, the study was biased in favor of finding a difference in cognitive function between cases and controls.

A cohort study may be biased by the selection of the cohort or by differences between groups in a comparative cohort study. A bias can occur in comparing ethnic groups when one group has a higher socio-economic index than the other, which may result in a healthier lifestyle, improved access to health care, or other factors that would influence their outcome. This is similar to the type of bias noted earlier in this section for case-control studies. Even within a single cohort, if the sub-group of unexposed participants differs from the subgroup of exposed participants in ways other than the exposures of interest, then the result may be biased either for or against a particular result.

Example 17C: The Million Women Study was a cohort study to determine if there was a link between hormone replacement therapy (HRT) and breast cancer. The cohort was comprised of women who were invited to enroll when they had routine mammography. They were followed up for breast cancer incidence and death. The study showed an increased risk of cancer in women who used HRT. However, other investigators observed that women who have routine mammography are not representative of the general population; they are more likely to be using HRT and also more likely to be at risk for breast cancer. Thus the study was biased toward finding an association that may not exist in the general population.

Example 17D: In this famous example an investigator tried to show that high doses of vitamin C were an effective treatment for cancer. The investigators treated 100 advanced cancer patients with vitamin C, beginning the treatment at the time when they were diagnosed as "untreatable," and recorded their survival history. The control group of 1,000 patients was selected from records of patients from the same hospital who were not treated with vitamin C, and the researchers computed their survival time from when they were diagnosed as untreatable. However, further investigation showed that the two groups were not comparable. In addition to not being matched by important prognostic factors, the average time from the initial diagnosis to "untreatable" status was shorter in the patients treated with vitamin C. Therefore, they would have begun vitamin C treatment earlier after the diagnosis of their disease, and thus the study was biased toward their living longer. Subsequent properly designed analyses showed no benefit of vitamin C in cancer treatment.

Historical controls can be a source of prognostic bias due to the fact that circumstances change over time. Changes in the diagnostic criteria, environmental factors, and population demographics may introduce systematic differences even though the major criteria appear to be the same. The methods for measuring key parameters and the standards for defining normal laboratory measurements may change over time.

Example 17E: As part of a study of the effects of changes in the American diet, investigators wanted to determine if the prevalence of glucose abnormalities had changed. However, the standards for diagnosing Type II diabetes or impaired glucose tolerance from a fasting glucose or Oral Glucose Tolerance Test have changed over the years, with the threshold for diabetes or impaired glucose tolerance being reduced. Thus, the same glucose levels could cause an individual to be identified as "normal" in a historical control population but to be diagnosed as "abnormal" in the current population, biasing the study toward showing that the rate of abnormalities had increased in the current population.

17.1.2 Selection Bias

Selection bias can refer either to self-selection of individuals to be a participant in a research study or selection by the investigators of study participants to support a particular hypothesis, which would be a nonrandom sample. Selection bias is obviously related to prognostic bias: the major difference is that selection bias refers to bias in the overall study population, whereas prognostic bias generally refers to bias in selecting or assigning groups for comparison.

Example 17F: In 1998, a British researcher published a paper claiming that there was a link between the administration of the measles, mumps, and rubella vaccine and the appearance of autism and bowel disease. The paper reported on 12 children who were observed by this pediatrician before and after having the vaccination. This link could not be reproduced in other studies, and further investigation showed that the original paper had many flaws. These included the fact that 5 of the 12 children showed symptoms of neurological problems before they were given the vaccination. Since the researcher was also paid by lawyers who were acting for parents suing the providers of the vaccines, the integrity of the researcher was questioned and his choice of participants was seen as a case of selection bias.

Example 17G: Academic researchers in psychology often use students as study participants to investigate behavioral reactions or help develop psychometric scales or norms for behaviors. But these students are a special population: they are literate, educated, English speaking, usually young (under 30), and often knowledgeable of the implications of some of the questions they are asked or situations they are asked to respond to. Thus, there is selection bias in these studies.

If you are requesting volunteers for a study using an outreach method, selection bias from the participants may occur. Individuals may volunteer for a study because they are hoping for a free physical examination even if they do not meet the criteria asked for. Individuals who have good health care will be less likely to volunteer for a study unless they meet the requirement. This can be particularly true if you are recruiting volunteers through public media, such as newspapers or radio announcements.

Example 17H: Investigators want to estimate the prevalence of a certain disease in an area. They put notices in the local paper asking persons with certain characteristics to volunteer for the study. However, in this area there are several neighborhoods where most of the residents are non-English-speaking immigrants. If there are no newspapers in the immigrants' languages available, these people will be underrepresented in the study, which may bias the prevalence estimate to be either low or high.

17.1.3 Participant Bias

In an interventional study, if the participant is aware of what treatment he is receiving, this may influence his reporting of symptoms and response. To a certain extent, we all see what we expect to see, and a participant who knows he is receiving an active drug may take a more optimistic view of his progress, and may also be more sensitive to possible side effects. A participant who knows he is not receiving active treatment may tend to exaggerate his lack of progress.

Two additional types of participant bias are well known and potentially pervasive, and so we discuss them specifically: recall bias and bias due to the learning effect.

17.1.4 Recall Bias

Recall bias occurs when participants are asked to recall information and the accuracy and completeness of their recall may differ due to their circumstances related to the study questions. Although all interventional studies are basically prospective, the participant is still asked to recall adverse events that occur between visits.

Example 17I: In a study comparing the effects of exercise versus no exercise, the participant must be aware of his treatment. Participants are interviewed every month and asked about any problems since the last time they were interviewed. A participant who is exercising may be more likely to remember any aches and pains, whereas a participant who is not exercising may see them as part of normal living, and may forget about them.

This type of bias can be an especially serious problem in observational studies. In case-control studies, cases may have more reason to focus on the past than do controls.

Example 17J: In a case-control study to examine the association of prenatal events with a class of birth defects, cases were mothers who had given birth to infants with the defect; controls were mothers who had given birth to healthy infants. The mothers were interviewed within 1–2 months of delivery and were asked about nutrition, activity, and any health problems or injuries during the pregnancy. In this situation, it is likely that the mothers with affected infants would have been thinking more about what happened during their pregnancy and have possibly discussed it with friends and relatives who might remind them of small, possibly harmful incidents. The mothers of normal infants would probably just be thinking about managing with a new baby. Thus the study would be biased to show more prenatal events in the group of mothers with affected infants.

Similarly, in comparative cohort studies, differences between groups, such as ethnic differences, may affect the impact of experiences and cause differences in recall.

The accuracy and completeness of recalled information is an issue in any retrospective study, but it is only a bias when it consistently influences the results in one direction, as in the above examples. Inaccurately recalled information is not a bias, however. In many studies where part of the evaluation consists of food consumption over some time period, most investigators agree that people tend to underestimate the amount of food consumed, so the accuracy of the information is questionable. If the study is comparing groups where one group might be more likely to underestimate or underreport the food consumed, however, this may introduce bias.

17.1.5 Bias Due to the Learning Effect

When participants are repeatedly given the same or similar tests or questionnaires, their performance at one period may be affected by their recall or learning from the previous periods. This is an expected effect, called the learning effect. High school students who take college entrance examinations are encouraged to take the test more than once on the theory that their test-taking skills will improve, and only the highest score will be reported to colleges. This is problematic in an interventional study when the evaluation is related to cognitive improvement, however, because an apparent improvement may not be due to the intervention, but simply to the participant's needing less time to understand the instructions, remembering the questions from the last test and having asked or thought about what the answers should be.

Example 17K: In a study of treatment of children with HIV, the children were given a series of cognitive tests at the beginning of the study which were then repeated every 6 months. The results showed some improvement, but it was not clear if this was due to the treatment or to better understanding of the test process by the children.

Example 17L: In many therapeutic studies, improvement in motor control may be an important outcome. It can be evaluated by physical tests such as dot-tracking, trail-making, and mechanical tests. If the tests are repeated, the participant's performance may improve simply by being more comfortable with the test. Thus there may be a bias toward apparent improvement which is not due to the therapy.

Another effect of repeated testing or evaluation most frequently occurs in a subjective evaluation, such as evaluations of mood or perception. In this case a participant may try to remember responses from the previous test and attempt to repeat them in order not to appear inconsistent.

Like recall problems, a learning effect may not always be a bias. If it occurs in both cases and control participants in a case-control study, or if it is expected and controlled for in an interventional study, it would not be a bias.

17.1.6 Care Provider Bias

The care provider's knowledge of which treatment a participant is receiving may affect the way the physician deals with the participant. For example, if a physician knows the participant is receiving the experimental treatment, then she may ask more questions about side effects and, perhaps subconsciously, show more concern for adverse events. Conversely, if it is known that the participant is not receiving the active drug, or is receiving a well-studied standard of care, the caregiver may pay less attention to adverse events. Knowledge of the participant's treatment may also effect how the physician treats the participant, particularly whether she treats mild symptoms, such as occasional headache, aggressively or adopts a watching mode.

These differences in behavior may in turn affect the participant's perceptions. More concern on the part of the caregiver may evoke more concern in the participant, which may tend to focus the participant to exaggerate even mild symptoms, or develop real problems due more to stress than to the treatment.

17.1.7 Assessor (Rater) Bias

By assessors, or raters, we refer to those who administer tests or questionnaires or interview participants to evaluate the participant's progress or final results. Frequently, the assessor may also be the caregiver, and the comments of the last section also apply here. If the raters know, or think they know, which treatment the participant is receiving, this may affect their perception of the results, particularly if the assessment has a subjective component. They may look more closely for changes and be more likely to identify changes as positive results in those they believe are receiving the experimental intervention. Alternatively, they may be more rigorous in evaluating participants who they believe or know are on the experimental intervention to avoid seeming biased, and thus miss real changes. If the assessment is done at interim periods in the protocol while the participant is still being treated, this may also lead the participant to think he knows which treatment he is receiving, and thus introduces more participant bias, as described earlier. Even if the participant's treatment is not an issue, different raters may have differences in their standards for a subjective measurement.

Assessor bias may induce recall bias in the participant, by prodding the participant to continue to think about the past and giving clues to help recall events.

Some observational studies can require that investigators or their staff review hospital charts or other documents to derive some of the study measurements. This is another situation where rater bias can be a problem. If the assessor knows that the participant is a case or a control in a case-control study, or knows the exposure or subgroup membership of a participant in a cohort study, this may influence the rater's interpretation of the records in the same way that knowledge of treatment would influence them.

17.1.8 Laboratory Bias

Laboratory personnel are also assessors in a study. Knowledge of the treatment a participant receives may influence the rigor with which tests are run and the interpretation of the results. Not all laboratory tests are precisely graded either by programs in a computer or precise, numeric standards. Some tests are less objectively graded, for example color intensity, leading to the same potential bias as other subjective assessments.

Example 17M: Frequently laboratory personnel or other raters review the results of assays and decide that some may be in error and should be rerun. These judgments can be subjective and might be influenced by knowledge of the participant's treatment. In many studies, multiple samples from each participant are saved to be run together in a single batch at a future time. If the laboratory personnel know that a group of samples come from the same participant, this may also influence decisions to rerun a specific sample as an outlier.

17.1.9 Analysis Bias

When data is analyzed, it is necessary to identify the different participant groups and indicate to which group each participant belongs. Analysis bias occurs when the personnel performing or directing the analysis know which is the treatment group or the affected cases and tailor the analysis to try to come up with findings that fit a particular hypothesis. This can include performing multiple different analyses until a statistically significant result is found, which can lead to reporting spurious results. Sometimes investigators, including statisticians, are too eager to accept results that fit the hypothesis, without a careful evaluation of whether other factors could explain the results. Alternatively, there can be extensive data dredging done to explain why a negative finding is actually due to confounding of some sort. It is frequently possible not to reveal the nature of each group, which can be simply identified as group A or group B for analysis purposes, although often this requires that other types of data such as side effects be similarly disguised.

17.1.10 Interpretation Bias

Many clinical trials have a procedure for interim monitoring of results and have designated individuals, serving on a Data Safety and Monitoring Board (DSMB), outside the study to review these results (Section 2.4). The DSMB is regularly presented with data from the study, which usually is in terms of groups, but the groups need not be identified. If the individuals are aware of the treatment groups, then there is a possibility for bias when the results fit the expectations of the DSMB. If they expect a new therapy to be much better that the standard of care, and the interim results appear to support this, they may be more willing to halt the study and declare that the new treatment is superior. Similarly, if they have reservations about the new treatment, they may halt the study because of a difference between the groups in adverse events.

17.1.11 Publication Bias

Publication bias refers to the fact that studies with negative results may not be published. Although publication bias is not a bias for your individual study, if you are doing a review or a meta-analysis of existing studies, then the lack of availability of negative results will lead to a more positive evaluation than would be produced if the results of all studies were known. It is true that journals are often unwilling to accept negative articles, but this bias also often occurs because an investigator does not try to explore or publish negative results on the theory they know the manuscript will not get accepted. This is a recognized problem and is being addressed by various organizations at this time. As an investigator, your role is to try to assure that all results are disseminated, whether positive or negative, statistically significant or not. Thus, negative findings should be presented in some venue, perhaps as a poster or talk at a meeting if it cannot be published in a journal, even though it may not seem worth the effort.

17.2 Non-Differential Bias

In the previous section we described biases that influence the study results in a single direction away from the truth. Non-differential bias occurs when opportunities for variation or measurement errors are equivalent in all study groups or at all time points and are not in a single direction. This results in an increase in the overall variability or "noise" in the data. When hypotheses are tested (Appendix A), the difference in question should be large relative to the variability to be considered statistically significant. Therefore, non-differential bias can hide real differences between study groups or changes over time. Because the null hypothesis is usually one of no difference, non-differential bias is often referred to as bias toward the null hypothesis.

Example 17N: Blood pressure is very variable within an individual over time, and thus the variability in the measurement can swamp any effect of a treatment. There are several ways of reducing this variability. One simple method is to take blood pressure several times (usually three, a few minutes apart) and use the average of the multiple measurements rather than using an individual measurement. Since the average has less variability than a single measurement does, this helps reduce the impact of the measurement error on the conclusions from a study.

Example 17O: In a study with several assessors, it is essential that the raters be cross-trained to assure that there is no variability in measurement due to the rater. Even if each assessor sees participants from all groups so there is no bias in favor of any group, a difference in standards will contribute to variability in the data that will act to obscure the statistical significance of differences between groups.

17.3 Ethical Issues

A deliberately biased study is unethical. To trust to luck and not take all steps possible to reduce bias is sloppy research, at best, and in extreme cases indefensible. Techniques to reduce bias, as described in the next chapter, should be part of the protocol, and it is incumbent on you, the principal investigator, and all other study personnel, to make sure that these methods are followed at all times.

Publication bias is a serious ethical problem for the scientific community because it may lead to patients being given useless therapies, or investigators spending time investigating hypotheses that have already been tested and found false. When results are not published because the investigator or the sponsor does not want them known, then this is deliberate deception. Action has been taken to require that results for all later-phase studies of drugs and devices conducted under U. S. Food and Drug Administration oversight as new drugs or investigational devices be made publicly available.

KEY POINTS

- Bias is the single biggest potential problem in clinical investigations.
- Bias is different from random variation, because bias consistently influences the results in one direction.
- Even the possibility of bias can cause the validity of a study to be questioned.
- Although deliberate bias is unethical, inadvertent and subconscious biases can occur.
- There are several categories of bias that can affect an individual clinical study:
  - prognostic bias;
  - selection bias;
  - participant bias;
  - recall bias;
  - learning effect bias;
  - care provider bias;
  - assessor (rater) bias;
  - laboratory bias;
  - analysis bias; and
  - interpretation bias.

- Non-differential bias is expected to increase the variability of the differences found in the study, and may cause a real difference to be obscured.
- Study design and implementation must include methods to reduce bias.
- Publication bias is a more general bias in the scientific literature, and affects reviews and meta-analyses but not individual studies.

Avoiding Bias

This book is about creating a valid study, and a study must be unbiased to be valid, so in some sense this whole book is about ways to avoid bias. We highlight some of the important measures in this chapter, including population selection, randomization, and blinding, also referred to as masking.

18.1 Selection of Study Population

The choice of an appropriate population for a study is critical, yet it is sometimes difficult to locate and recruit participants for a study. Selection bias (Section 17.1.2) can be avoided by a realistic assessment of the populations that form the study pool and careful review of the criteria for inclusion and exclusion to ensure that it does not result in a biased population (Chapter 12).

It is up to you, the investigator, to use your best judgment: be honest with yourself as to what you can achieve. If you can only work with a limited population, then this must be acknowledged as a limitation in the presentation of the results of the study (Section 12.4). In Chapter 13 we gave some ways to reach potential participants outside your immediate environment.

Example 18A: Example 17C described a cohort study of the link between hormone therapy (HRT) and breast cancer. This study was considered biased because the women in the study were more likely to be at a higher risk for breast cancer and were more likely to be taking HRT than the general population. The Woman's Health Initiative subsequently studied many of the same questions. There were 40 centers in different areas of the United States, including 20% minority enroll-ment. The investigators at each center had to devise plans for recruit-ing women in their entire geographical area, not just from their patient base, and for recruiting women with a diversity of health risk and health problems. The results of this study, which supported a link between HRT and breast cancer, were consistent across centers and were gener-ally considered to be unbiased and representative of the U.S. population.

Often in a case-control study it is tempting to use the most readily available population as controls, but they may have demographic and economic characteristics that are not representative of the population at large. Although it might be easy to recruit graduate students and col-leagues, they are a very select group in terms of age and education, and sometimes economically. This may result in a control population that differs from your cases in ways that are associated with the outcome of interest, and thus confound the comparisons of exposures.

Example 18B: Example 17B was a case-control study of adult males with a congenital hormone imbalance where controls were employees from the investigators' institution and almost always had at least some kind of training certificate and often a bachelor's degree or higher. The investigators thus also recruited a second control population from out-side the institution in environments where they would expect to find a population that was more like the general population in cognitive function.

Recall bias is a common risk in a case-control study, because affected participants may have more reason to remember past events than do controls. One way to mitigate this effect is to select a control population that has characteristics that are different from the outcome of interest but that would still induce equal levels of recall.

Example 18C: Example 17J was a case-control study of prenatal events to determine their association with certain birth defects. It was believed that mothers with healthy infants would be less likely to recall events during the pregnancy than would the mothers of the cases. Therefore, the investigators added a second control group that consisted of moth-ers of infants who had birth defects different from those being studied.

Another way to minimize the effect of recall bias is to use a structured interview or questionnaire to ask about specific events, rather than just use open-ended questions. The interview may include specific methods to assist in recalling events.

Example 18C (continued): The investigators were particularly interested in nutritional intake during pregnancy. The participants were asked what vitamin supplements they took and, if they had any left, to read the contents to the interviewer. They were also asked about the amount and frequency of eating other foods such as breakfast cereals and fortified bread.

Use of historical controls can introduce bias due to changes in methods of evaluation, such as assay methods or assessment instruments. Diagnostic criteria and the timing of diagnoses may be different. For example, many conditions may be identified earlier in the development of the disorder now than in the historical controls and more cases may be identified due to increased vigilance. Frequently there is limited information about the controls so that you may get summary statistics about age and sex but not the actual distribution or the age by sex distribution. We are generally not in favor of using historical controls for any study, and definitely not for an interventional study unless there is a uniform outcome from the disease. However, they might be used in observational studies if the investigator is careful to ensure that the populations are comparable in prognostic factors and exposures and that the outcomes of interest were evaluated using equivalent methods, but the use of historical control often raises concerns about potential bias.

18.2 Randomization

As we have stated in many places in this book, we believe that randomization is needed in interventional studies in all but the most extraordinary circumstances. Furthermore, we have never heard an investigator present an "extraordinary circumstance" that was not, ultimately, a way of saying it was too much work. This work is essential for a valid study. Randomization after enrollment is the single most effective way to rule out the possibility of prognostic bias. However, more than just random treatment allocation is needed: the treatment allocation cannot be assigned until after the participant is enrolled and completed screening for the study, and even then the actual treatment should be known by as few individuals as possible (see Section 18.3).

Example 18D: Consider the dilemma an investigator would have if the treatment assignment were known prior to enrolling and screening patients, for instance if the envelope containing the treatment allocation of the next participant had inadvertently been opened by an assistant. Suppose an investigator knew that the next participant would be given the experimental intervention. As is typical, this investigator believes that the experimental intervention will be more effective than the standard treatment being used in an interventional study, and his personal belief is that this is especially true for more severely affected individuals. The investigator has several patients scheduled as potential participants that day: the first is a patient with a relatively mild case, the second is a patient with a more severe case. The investigator knows that he needs to do everything possible to act the same to both patients when attempting to recruit them into the study. It will be extremely difficult for this investigator to do so, however, as he will feel it best if the first patient does not enroll and the second patient does, so that the second patient receives the benefit of the experimental therapy.

Because the investigator knows what treatment the next participant receives, even if it has been determined randomly, the situation has enormous potential for prognostic bias. For this reason, when we talk about randomization, we specifically mean that the treatment allocation becomes known only after a participant is enrolled and fully screened for the study.

Example 18D (continued): The investigator decides, after considering the problem and discussing it with a colleague, that he will not be able to treat the two potential participants the same way. Therefore, he skips the next treatment assignment, marking it as unused. When the potential participants do arrive later in the morning, he then can act the same to both of them, as he does not know which intervention they will receive until they consent for the study, complete screening and are enrolled.

Investigators must have compelling reasons to justify a non-randomized interventional design, such as an extremely small population with the condition, no current effective treatment, and a known, disastrous outcome for untreated patients, as illustrated in Example 5B. Chapters 20 and 21 treat randomization in more detail.

18.3 Blinding

Blinding is an attempt to obscure some information from study participants and study staff. This is the classic term used to describe studies (a single-blind study, a double-blind study, and so on; see Section 22.2 for details), although many people now prefer the term masking. This is especially true for studies involving the eyes. Sometimes blinding is used to refer to individuals, such as participants or raters, and masking is used to refer to data, but this distinction is not fixed, and we will use the terms interchangeably. In interventional studies, a double-blind study, in which the participants, the caregivers, and the assessors are all masked, in combination with randomization after enrollment is an effective and important way to minimize many of the participant and rater biases at several levels. Blinding reduces the problem of biased reporting and evaluation at every level where it is used.

In Chapters 22 and 23, we focus on blinding of interventional studies at the participant and rater level, as these are critical. Masking of laboratory personnel and, to some extent, of the data managers and statisticians as well, is important to reduce the possibility of bias. Generally the statistician must know what group the participant belongs to but does not have to know which group is which (e.g., that group A is active drug and group B is control). Even when a study cannot be completely masked, it is recommended that it be blinded as much as possible.

Example 18E: In a study to determine whether exercise plus testosterone improves muscle mass more than exercise or testosterone alone, the participants are randomly assigned to four groups: exercise, testosterone, both, or neither. The drug treatment was blinded to both participants and raters: all participants received a matching gel, with testosterone included for participants assigned either to the testosterone or both group. It was, of course, not possible to blind participants to exercise, but it would be possible to mask the exercise intervention from the raters. The investigators felt, however, that because there would be a considerable amount of interaction between raters and participants concerning their well-being, it would be difficult to maintain this blind. Therefore, they did not attempt to blind the assessors to exercise, although laboratory staff and statisticians were blinded to both testosterone use and exercise.

Although blinding is most common in interventional studies, it can and should be used to reduce assessor bias in observational studies as discussed in Chapter 28. Although information about the participant (whether a case or a control in a case-control study; whether exposed or not exposed in a cohort study) cannot be hidden from the participant, the interviewer should be masked to this information. This will reduce any tendency of an interviewer to ask questions differently of cases and controls (or of those exposed or not exposed in a cohort study), which may lead to biased results. If the study involves a review of historical material, then the outcome the participant has experienced in a cohort study should be masked from the rater, or to the status of the participant as a case or control in a case-control study. This is also true if any laboratory assessment is part of the protocol for both intervention and observational studies.

Example 18F: In a case-control study to determine if an early childhood experience leads to subtle learning difficulties in later life, the protocol includes review and evaluation of academic records by a cognitive specialist. The specialist is not told whether the records being reviewed are from a case or a control. The database includes a code for group (A or B), but the statisticians are not told which group is the cases and which is the controls.

18.4 Assessment Methods and Training

Other ways of reducing bias include the methods of assessment used in a study and the procedures, training, and management of the study personnel. A detailed Manual of Procedures (MOP; Section 29.3) reduces the opportunity for rater bias to occur. Assessor (rater) bias may be reduced by the creation and use of data collection instruments that are as objective as possible. This is relatively easy for many physical measurements that use standard instruments; it is less easy and thus more critical for measurements that require some interpretation on the part of the assessor. Instruments that require an assessor's evaluation of a participant's condition usually contain a subjective component. A structured interview is an excellent tool for reducing both rater and participant bias. A structured interview will define the focus of each question and limit the range of responses. Also, it will include additional prompts or instructions that the rater can use if the participant requests clarification. This not only improves consistency between assessors but also may assure that the participant's responses do not depend too much on the interaction of the participant with the rater, and that the participant will be answering the same question when the assessment is repeated over time. Chapter 29 provides more details on designing interviews and questionnaires. Validated structured interviews for specific conditions may be available from the literature.

Example 18G: Diagnosis has often been described as an art, and there is usually a subjective component to it. This is particularly true of psychiatric diagnosis, which cannot yet be determined by physical evidence. Thus the American Psychiatric Association has developed a manual defining psychiatric diagnoses and very detailed criteria for assigning them to a patient (Diagnostic and Statistical Manual of Mental Diseases [DSM], currently in its fifth edition). Since the criteria can be subjective, the Structural Clinical Interview for DSM has been designed to elicit information in a way to minimize rater bias.

Implementation procedures are critical to avoid participant and rater biases. Extensive cross-training of assessors will help reduce bias due to individual differences between the raters.

Example 18H: In a study of major depression, the investigators used videotapes of structured interviews to train raters and to evaluate the reliability of the data collection instruments when used by different raters. The raters all viewed the same tapes and completed the instruments for each taped participant. The results were compared between assessors to identify weak spots such as missed ratings, or raters who were consistently different from the others, and further training was initiated as necessary.

Another source of participant bias is what is known as the learning effect. This occurs when tests or questionnaires are repeated over time. A participant may appear to improve in cognitive function, but this may be a result of remembering the answers or just being more familiar with the instruments and therefore able to work more quickly. Similarly, a lack of change may be artificial: the participant remembers what was said last time and just repeats it, rather than thinks about how he feels now. Sometimes the participant does this deliberately because he does not want the raters to think she is inconsistent. This is a difficult bias to eliminate, but there are steps that can be taken to reduce it. The number and timing of assessments should be minimized and spaced as widely as possible consistent with the study goals. Some instruments are designed to mitigate this effect by mixing questions on different topics; this makes it harder for the participant to remember what was said last time. This also has the benefit of encouraging responses that are independent of the response to previous questions, and therefore more likely to be true. Instructions to the participant to not think about their responses at the last evaluation are helpful but not always effective.

18.5 Data Monitoring during the Study

An important mechanism for catching potential bias is to validate data throughout the study rather than review it only at the end. This is discussed in Section 30.5, but as this is important to avoid potential bias, we present an example here.

Example 18I: In a study of geriatric patients, several potential tests could be used to assess physical performance. The participant and the assessor jointly decide which of the three tests (from hardest [standing on one foot] to easiest [standing on both feet spread wide apart]) the participant would be rated on. There were detailed instructions for the test, and the three assessors were trained on how to do the test. During data review, however, it was found that participants with one assessor were generally doing easier tests, with the response of "unsafe/unwilling to try" for the harder tests. Many of these participants were seen by other assessors at other visits and tried the more difficult stances. This assessor was being more conservative than the other assessors in interpreting the instruction that for the first question began with: "If safe, ask the participant ..." Unlike the other assessors, who asked all the participants they tested whether they were willing to try standing on one foot, this assessor only asked participants when she thought they could do it without difficulty.

Example 18I illustrates why it is important to review the data while the study is ongoing, so that such problems can be identified and mitigated quickly. This is commonly done for multi-center studies, where variability between sites is a major concern, but also should be done even in a single-site study if more than one assessor is being used. In this case, the bias was non-differential, but it could still obscure a real effect because of the increased variability in the measurement.

18.6 Ethical Issues

A deliberately biased study is unethical. Avoiding bias requires extra effort on the part of the investigators and assessors, such as a more extensive recruiting effort or extra training of the staff. Some methods, such as blinding, may involve some deception of the participants and must always be done with their knowledge of and consent to the masking after Institutional Review Board (IRB) approval of the study and the study procedures, including the blinding. Some participants may feel nervous about being inconsistent in responding to repeated assessments, or even consider the techniques used to eliminate recall bias as "trying to trick them" into giving different answers. The participants should be made aware of the importance of these methods and assured that they will not be judged on their consistency. Ultimately, if a study is biased, then the conclusions are not valid and all the effort going into the study, both yours as the investigator and all the participants, is wasted. A study in which reasonable and standard steps are not taken to prevent potential bias is at best sloppy research. You are using participants in a study despite knowingly and deliberately risking that the study results will not be valid.

KEY POINTS

- Bias is the single biggest potential problem in clinical studies.
- There are specific methods an investigator can use to avoid bias in a study:
  - Recruiting a control or comparison population that is similar to the affected population in all ways except for the outcome in a case-control study;
  - If some assessments require the participant's recall of events, the potential for accurate recall should be the same in all groups and techniques to assist participants should be standardized for all participants;
  - Randomization of participants in interventional studies;
  - Blinding at as many levels as possible, including laboratory and data analysis personnel;
  - Use of measuring instruments that are as objective as possible;
  - Design of measuring instruments to minimize the learning effect; and
  - Training and evaluation of raters to identify individual biases in assessor ratings.
- If historical controls must be used, attempt to ensure that they are similar to the current population and were assessed in comparable ways, recognizing that the use of historical controls often raises issues of potential bias when attempting to publish a study.

Part IV

ADDITIONAL CONCEPTS FOR INTERVENTIONAL STUDIES

19

Describing the Intervention

It might seem easy to define the intervention you want to study, but it rarely is. Although you know what the intervention will be, such as a specific drug, device, or therapy, you must also specify how it will be used. Often you need to consider how the intervention is actually used in practice so that you can specify how it is to be administered within your protocol.

19.1 Problems in Describing an Intervention

There are often complexities in taking a medication. A medication may require that it be taken in the morning after getting out of bed, or at night just before going to bed. Some medications must be given with meals, and others must be taken at least two hours after (or before) meals. Some must be taken with other medications, and others cannot be taken with specific other medications or with specific foods. Some medications are titrated to individual responses, so they are increased if a participant does not respond. Other medications are reduced (but not eliminated) if there are side effects. We are unaware of any medications that must be taken on a specific calendar day or date, but are aware that some medications are prescribed that way (always take on Sunday, or take once a month on the first day of the month) to help patients remember to take their medicine.

When providing the details of the intervention for your study, you need at least to think about the following items, and to specify all relevant ones in your clinical protocol:

- when the medication is taken;
- how the medication is taken;

- how the medicine is dosed;
- what the medication is taken with;
- what must be avoided with the medication;
- how the dose or dose schedule is adjusted for toxicity;
- how the dose or dose schedule is changed for inadequate efficacy; and
- what should be done when a dose is missed.

This needs to be done for every treatment involved in the intervention. If your intervention is being added to a standard of care, then you need to give all the information necessary to describe the use of the standard of care as well.

Example 19A: A new drug is found to be excreted renally. Thus, dosage of the agent is defined based on a participant's creatinine clearance assessed using a procedure specified in the study protocol or the more detailed Manual of Procedures (MOP; Section 29.3).

Example 19B: A new drug is being tested, which is titrated to the individual participant's response, like insulin is adjusted in diabetics. The protocol or MOP needs to specify when dose adjustment is considered, how the decision to adjust doses is made, how the new dose is determined, and how frequently it may be changed. This includes what measurements are made to decide whether the dose needs to be adjusted and how these measurements are interpreted to determine what the next dose should be.

Example 19C: A new drug is taken once a week. If a participant misses a dose and remembers later, the participant is instructed to take it within three days of the day it was due. Otherwise, the participant is instructed not to take a dose until the next scheduled treatment day, to avoid taking two doses too close together.

Example 19D: A drug is known to have certain side effects in some participants. For some of the side effects (such as rash), if the side effect is mild or moderate, participants should continue taking the drug as scheduled, at the regular dose. Although the participant may continue taking the drug if a rash is mild or moderate, the drug must be held back if the rash is severe. Thus, there need to be rules defining what a severe rash is. If the drug could be restarted later, there would need to be rules about when the drug could be restarted, and how the dose would be adjusted for the participant. For another potential side effect (change in liver enzymes), even if the side effect is mild, the participant needs to discontinue the drug because the side effect may rapidly become more serious.

Example 19E: In many oncology studies, multiple medications are taken. The protocol must specify for each medication the dose used, any pretreatment needed for a medicine (e.g., to minimize allergic reactions, fluid loading, etc.), and what needs to be done for adverse reactions. In addition, when more than one medication is being given, the order of the medications needs to be specified if they are taken on the same day. There must also be rules about side effects, including rules for deciding which drug should be considered the cause for different specific toxicities and thus needs its dose adjusted. As in Example 19D, rules for dose holding, adjustment, and restarting are also needed.

Example 19F: Some interventional studies assess the additional benefit of the new intervention when added to the standard intervention. One example would be assessing the effect of a new chemotherapy agent being added to a standard regimen for a specific cancer. As in Example 19E, dosing information is needed for each of the drugs in the regimen, not just the experimental intervention.

19.2 Determining the Control Intervention

There are two basic types of control groups that can be used in an interventional study: an active control group, which would receive a currently used standard treatment for the condition (standard of care); or a placebo control group, that is, a control group in which the participants only receive placebo medication. Sometimes the experimental intervention is being added to the standard of care, as in Example 19F. In this case, the control group is the active therapy with a placebo for the new intervention if the study is blinded, while the intervention group is the active therapy plus the intervention. Since all participants are receiving the standard of care, such a study does not raise ethical issues unless there is potential toxicity from the interaction of the new treatment with the standard of care or risks from the administration of the placebo treatment (e.g., if it required a lumbar puncture to administer).

Using a placebo control group potentially raises significant ethical issues. There is a general consensus that placebo controls cannot be used if there is an established therapy for the disease and the disease being studied can lead to death or irreversible damage, even if the possibility of these adverse events or death is extremely low. For slowly progressive diseases, a placebo control group may sometimes be allowed if the study period is brief relative to the rate of disease progression, so that disease progression would be minimal.

There is also a general consensus that a placebo control group would not be appropriate for very painful conditions or severe symptoms if a treatment exists that will control or alleviate those symptoms, again with the possible exception of very brief studies. Generally, the more severe the disease or the symptoms, the more scrutiny a placebo control group should and would receive. An exception, however, might arise when the benefits of the standard therapy are not clear-cut, such as if the benefit is very marginal or there are many complications and side effects from the standard therapy.

Another problem using a placebo control group is that you are comparing the new treatment to doing nothing, as if there were no other choices. But if a standard of care exists, then the results for the new treatment should be compared to the standard of care to see if there is any benefit to the new therapy.

Example 19G: The Antihypertensive and Lipid Lowering Treatment to Prevent Heart Attack Trial (ALLHAT) was a long-term, multi-center trial conducted on a large group of participants ages 55 and older with hypertension and at least one other cardiovascular disease risk factor. It was supported by the U. S. National Heart, Lung, and Blood Institute. The treatment for hypertension had originally used low-cost diuretics; more recently, newer and more costly medicines had been shown to be effective, but they had not been compared to the earlier drugs. The ALLHAT hypertension study compared these newer drugs to older treatments.

Even though the clinical efficacy of the treatment might be slightly less than the clinical effect of the standard of care, the new treatment may still provide other benefits such as being easier to use, having fewer side effects, and being less costly or less visible. The acceptable size of the decrease in clinical effect, known as the "non-inferiority boundary," must be defined in the protocol.

Example 19H: In this study of testosterone supplementation, a new delivery method using a gel applied directly to the skin was compared to the existing method, which used a different formulation applied with a skin patch. The gel application did not result in skin irritation, which the patch caused, and the gel also was not as obvious as the patch that sometimes embarrassed patients. Because of these benefits, the FDA was willing to accept the gel if the percent of men with normalized testosterone was not more than 10% lower than the current standard of care.

If there is an established standard therapy for the disease, the control group will often be the standard therapy rather than placebo. One complication arises, however, when there are different therapies that can be used, all of which are considered standard of care. In such a situation, picking which of the standard therapies should be used as the active control group can be quite difficult, and we would encourage you to talk with your colleagues to help make this decision. In general, you would try to pick a control therapy that is considered the standard for the conditions addressed by the intervention therapy. Similarly, if the intervention targets a certain demographic group, then the control therapy should be the one that is most commonly used in this target group.

The acceptance of studies using a placebo control group has decreased over the years, as their disadvantages and the better information obtained when using an active control group have become apparent.

Example 19I: At one time placebo-controlled studies in osteoporosis were the norm. When a large multiyear study was being started, no issues had been raised by any of the Institutional Review Boards (IRBs) about the use of a placebo control group. Over time, however, therapies to treat the condition became widespread. Thus, a reviewer raised concerns about the ethics of using a placebo control group when results of the multiyear study were submitted for publication.

19.3 Describing the Control Intervention

In addition to specifying information for your new intervention, you need to specify the same factors for the control intervention. Nothing additional needs to be specified if you are doing a placebo-controlled study: the regimen for the placebo should be as similar as possible to that for the active drug, even when things are not necessary, such as avoiding other medications. However, if you are doing an active controlled trial (e.g., comparing one medication to another), you need to provide details for the active control as well, considering all the same factors as for the interventional medication.

Example 19J: Some oncology studies compare several different regimens to one another. In these cases, information needs to be provided for each of the regimens, even if one is considered standard of care, to ensure that the control arm is administered in a precise manner. This would include all the details needed for the experimental arm: how and when each of the drugs in the regimen is taken, what, if any, pretreatment is needed, the order of the different drugs if more than one is administered on the same day, how the different drugs are adjusted for various toxicities (including which drug would be considered associated with each toxicity), and what toxicities would lead to discontinuing the drug.

Depending on the details of how the standard of care is administered, or of the side effect profile, it may be impossible to maintain the blind for many or all participants.

Example 19K: In a study of two regimens for treatment of cancer, the two regimens differed significantly in their known side effect profile. In one arm of the study, mild or more significant rash was expected in about 80% of participants, while in the other arm, hypertension (or elevation of currently controlled hypertension) was expected in the majority of participants. To minimize the impact of this on maintaining the blind, the informed consent document listed the common side effects of both arms in a single list. The primary outcome of the disease was its radiographic progression, which was determined by a radiologist who had no access to the side effect information.

We discuss this problem further and offer more details on some potential solutions in Section 23.3.1.

19.4 Ethical Issues

A clear definition of what intervention is being studied is critical for several reasons. First, there is no justification for exposing any participant to a treatment that cannot be well defined, since at the end of such a study it would not be possible to describe what was studied. Thus, such a study could not contribute knowledge, nor, if some participants apparently benefited from the intervention, would it be possible for them to actually continue an ill-defined intervention. Second, as illustrated in the examples, sometimes the precise treatment varies depending on participant characteristics, participant behavior, and results of the intervention (both efficacy and safety) in the specific participant. Finally, if you cannot clearly describe what you are proposing to study, how could an IRB ever approve the study?

The use of a placebo control group raises ethical concerns when there are established therapies for the disease. These concerns increase as the disease becomes more severe, the potential adverse outcomes without treatment become more serious, and the duration of the study increases, lengthening the time that participants are without standard treatment.

Whether the control group is placebo or is the standard of care, the participant must be aware that he will be randomly assigned to a treatment group. If a placebo control group is used, the participant must be willing to take the risk of being assigned to a placebo. If the participant is blinded in the study (Chapter 22), the participant also must accept that he will not know what treatment he is receiving during the study. This should be made clear as part of the informed consent process (Chapter 3).

KEY POINTS

- A clear definition of the intervention, what is being studied, is needed before beginning a study.

- Often the definition of the intervention requires specifications for numerous contingencies, such as dose adjustment for toxicity and instructions for missed doses of a medicine.
- Defining the rules for the intervention becomes even more complicated when a treatment regimen, rather than a single medication, is being studied.
- Using a placebo control group potentially raises many ethical issues and may not be acceptable when there is at least one established therapy for the condition.
- The participant must be aware that intervention will be randomly assigned among the possible treatments.
- If the study involves a placebo arm, the participant must be aware that there is a possibility that she will receive only a placebo for the condition.

20

Randomization: What and Why

Einstein is often thought to have said that "God does not play dice with the universe." Without entering either in the scientific or theological issues of this statement, there is at least one place where you should "play dice": when making treatment allocations in an interventional study. This process, called "randomization," is used to minimize the chance that the groups in the study differ on any important prognostic factors, and thus to avoid prognostic bias. Randomization implies that a chance process under the direction of the investigator is used to determine which of the two or more specific interventions a participant receives. This does not mean, however, that the investigator controls which treatment is assigned to a specific participant. In a randomized interventional study, participants are enrolled into a clinical study and randomized after giving informed consent and completing the screening process, which ensures that the participant meets the enrollment criteria for the study. In this chapter we discuss what randomization is and why it is essential, while the next chapter discusses how randomization should be done.

20.1 What Is Randomization?

Randomization involves the random allocation of something to the participants. We are deliberately using the awkward word "something" here, because the something might be whether the participant receives an active intervention or is studied without an intervention, or which of several interventions the participant receives, or it might be the order in which different interventions are given. For convenience throughout this book, when we talk about an intervention, we may mean any of these somethings.

Randomization implies that

(a) there is a random process allocating the intervention;
(b) the process is under the direction of the investigator; and
(c) no one knows what the intervention will be until the participant has completed all the screening and is enrolled into the study.

All three are essential. The process being random means that there is no pattern – that is, that no one can predict in advance what intervention the process will assign – so knowing the history of the process (that is, all the assignments until now) does not help you predict what the treatment assignment will be for the next participant. A computer algorithm that simulates rolling a die or tossing a coin (but not a person doing that!) is used to determine the intervention allocation. The result is generally called a "randomization table" or "randomization schedule." The second item on the list means that you cause a randomization schedule to be created and applied when participants are enrolled in the study. But importantly, the third item means that neither you nor anyone else involved with participant screening or care knows what intervention a participant will receive before they have completed the screening process and are enrolled into the study and randomized. Although you direct the process, you do not control the assignment to a specific participant. This is important, since generally inclusion and exclusion criteria for a study allow participants to be excluded if they are "unsuitable." If you know which treatment the next participant will receive, you may decide, consciously or unconsciously, that a participant is unsuitable for the study because of the treatment the participant would receive if enrolled. See Chapter 21 for how randomization can be implemented. Most randomized studies also include blinding (Chapter 22), if possible, so that the investigator does not know what treatment a participant receives until after the study is completed.

Example 20A: An investigator wants to assess whether a new drug is better than the standard of care. The investigator decides that certain participants will receive the new drug and certain participants will not, so that the investigator will have a comparison group. Perhaps the investigator believes that the new drug will be better for some patients while the standard of care is better for others. This is not a randomized study, since the investigator assigns the treatment. Even though the investigator may try to make the groups as similar as possible, this procedure is subject to potential prognostic bias, either conscious or unconscious, leading to systematic differences between the two groups, which could confound any effect of the intervention.

Example 20B: Instead of assigning certain participants in the study to receive the drug and others not to receive the drug, the investigator decides to use the participant's birthday to decide which treatment the participant will get. Although this is not predictable and may or may not be known before the participant is accepted into the study, this process is not under the investigator's direction, so this is not randomization.

Example 20C: Instead of using birthdays to determine which participants receive the drug and which do not, the investigator decides to actually toss a coin. Tossing a coin seems random, and since the investigator is doing it, it is under the investigator's direction. However, appealing as this is, a coin can be biased, and there are people who can toss a coin to come up heads (or tails) in a nonrandom sequence.

Example 20D: Instead of tossing a coin, the investigator uses a computer program to prepare a randomization table (that is, a list of the treatment assignment for each participant) to determine which participants receive the drug and which do not. As the investigator has prepared the list of assignments, however, the results are known to the investigator before a participant is enrolled, so this is not a randomized study.

Example 20E: The investigator has someone who has nothing at all to do with seeing potential participants (in our experience this might be a statistician, pharmacist, spouse, secretary, lab assistant, someone down the hall) use a computer program or a table of random numbers to develop a numbered list that specifies active treatment or control in a random order. The investigator will assign participants a Study ID number (Section 29.1) when they are screened for the study. Once they have completed screening and been accepted into the study, they will be assigned the next treatment on the list, based on the order in which they completed screening. The investigator has thus directed the process but has not been involved in the treatment allocation. This is a randomized study!

Randomization is often considered only in the context of the classic therapeutic clinical trial. Participants are randomized to one of two (or more) intervention groups, with the treatment intended to benefit the patients who are participating in the trial. Randomization, however, is not limited to an intervention that is intended to treat an underlying condition. It can and should be used in any study in which the investigator wants to assess the differences between two or more interventions on any type of outcome.

20.2 Why Randomize?

Randomization protects against allocation or prognostic bias (Section 17.1.1) between the interventional groups, in which one group has a better prognosis in general then the other group. It also protects against selection bias (Section 17.1.2.), when participants are recruited based on their expected response to the intervention. Theoretically it also provides balance on all unmeasured prognostic variables.

Example 20F: An investigator has decided not to randomize participants in a study, but instead to assign them alternately, as they are recruited, to the experimental treatment or the standard therapy, since randomization is "too much work." Assume that the assignment is known and that the next participant will be given the experimental intervention. Both a relatively sick person and a relatively healthy person come to the clinic for the study. Some investigators, attempting to ensure that they are being as objective as possible in assessing efficacy, might try to enroll the relatively sick individual more aggressively into the study. This could lead to prognostic bias, as participants with a worse prognosis would be in the experimental arm, potentially negatively biasing the efficacy assessment in the experimental group. Other investigators might decide on the basis of the potential toxicity that the relatively sick individual should not be recruited into the study.

This is an example of selection bias, selecting participants based on their expected response (in this case, to avoid toxicity), but this could also bias the efficacy assessment.

Even if an investigator is scrupulously objective, and does try to recruit both individuals equally hard, how compelling would such an assurance be to others when appraising the validity of the project?

Example 20G: An investigator in a study has decided not to randomize participants, but rather to assign them systematically, as they are recruited, alternately to the experimental treatment or the standard therapy. Assume now that the intervention assignment is not known, but that the next participant will be given treatment A, and that there are a number of participants in the study already. Both a relatively sick person and a relatively healthy person come to the clinic for the study. Again, the issue is whether the investigator would make an equal effort to recruit these individuals. Although the investigator will not know for a fact which treatment is which, she will have seen a number of participants with one treatment (the first, third, fifth, seventh, ninth … participants enrolled) and a number with the other treatment (the second, fourth, sixth, eighth, tenth … participants enrolled). One group seems to have more toxicity than the other group, and also somewhat better efficacy, which might be what is expected from the experimental treatment. So the investigator may not know which group is which, but will certainly have a hunch, even if it is based on an impression of the data, and even if the hunch is wrong.

This example indicates the danger of prognostic bias. Depending on the direction of the bias, this could mean that the experimental intervention looks better than it should compared to the control group (since participants with a better prognosis went into the experimental arm) or worse than it should compared to the control group (since participants with a better prognosis were recruited more aggressively into the control group, to "bend over backwards" to be fair.) However "bending over backwards" – a term an investigator used to one of us in another context – is not in any sense fair. It is a deliberate bias against the experimental intervention. So if the experimental intervention fails, it might be because it was not effective, but it might also be because of the attempt to "bend over backwards," which biased the conclusion.

Even if there is no bias, which is always questionable without randomization, it is impossible to provide compelling evidence that there is no bias without randomization. In fact, even with randomization, a common question is whether the treatment groups are comparable, but at least with randomization the question is whether the results were consistent, not whether the entire study is fundamentally flawed.

20.3 Why Randomize Individuals?

Suppose that an investigator is convinced that he needs to randomize participants but feels that it is logistically too hard to randomize each person individually. Instead, the investigator does a convenience allocation, where you allocate people by some known pattern. One example could be date of birth (some birthdays [day of month] assigned one intervention, some birthdays assigned another intervention, as in Example 20B. Another common example is allocation by day, so that all participants enrolled in the study on the same day would receive the same intervention. Finally, some studies have allocation done by study site, where participants in one site get one type of intervention and another site get a different intervention. Why do these methods potentially create problems?

First, there might be conscious or unconscious bias, knowing the allocation rules, to recruit aggressively or not recruit certain people depending on their birthdays or the day they come to the clinic. Although the day that someone comes to the clinic might be random, as the investigator knows the treatment that the person would receive if recruited, this is not randomization. Again, people reading about your study have to believe that it is not biased. Convincing people is very hard.

Second, even if many people are studied, the results need to be analyzed based on the number of randomization units. So in the extreme case, where everyone at one clinic receives the experimental arm and everyone at the other clinic receives the control arm, you are really comparing just two numbers: the summary results at each clinic, and not the individual results of each individual participant.

Finally, if the assignment of one individual becomes known, then very often the assignment of others can be determined as well, leading to the potential for all kinds of participant and rater biases to occur, even if the study is intended to be blinded. Example 20G illustrates this general problem with assignment using an external pattern, such as order of entry, date of birth or day or week, rather than true individual participant randomization. This again raises questions for others about the validity of the study.

20.4 Ethical Issues

Arguments have been made that randomization is fundamentally unethical in trials testing therapies for a disease (a therapeutic trial), because the investigator as physician usually has a belief as to which of the two interventions being assessed will be better for a specific individual, as illustrated in Example 20A. We certainly agree that if a physician actually knows which treatment is better for a patient then randomization is unethical. However, having a belief is not the same as having knowledge. If there is a general consensus of how best to treat a specific type of patient, then the study's inclusion and exclusion criteria should be written so that such patients would not qualify for the study. The fact that there is not a general consensus implies that there is inadequate data to justify the physician's belief, so the physician does not know which treatment would be better for the specific participant. As illustrated by Example 10C, even when some groups "know" that one treatment is better, other groups may "know" the opposite. Randomization is ethical.

Randomization is essential in an interventional study because it eliminates the possibility that an investigator, or other member of the study team, can consciously or unconsciously assign participants to a specific treatment, which would potentially bias the study results. Thus, randomization helps ensure that the results of a study provide the information physicians need to know which treatment is likely to be better for a specific patient in the future.

Moreover, any interventional study poses risks and costs to participants. If nothing else, it costs time, and time is valuable. Even coming to an appointment imposes costs from missing work or paying for child care, and general risks involving commuting. But interventional studies involve possible risks from a potentially harmful treatment, as well as risks from the procedures involved in the study. Even drawing a small amount of blood poses a risk.

Given that participants will be exposed to some risk, it is necessary to believe that the study will have some benefit overall – that it will provide useful information about the intervention being studied. Moreover, this needs to be information for the wider scientific community, not just for your personal use. Failing to randomize intervention assignment poses a virtually insurmountable credibility hurdle for an interventional study, making it inherently flawed. As such, failing to randomize participants among the available treatments makes your interventional study unethical, since it cannot provide convincing information to the scientific community.

KEY POINTS

- Randomization requires that the intervention group is assigned by a process under the investigator's direction.
- Randomization requires that there is no pattern to the allocation of participants to a specific group.
- Randomization requires that neither the investigator nor anyone else knows in which group the participant will be until after the participant has completed all the screening processes and is enrolled in the study.
- Randomization is not limited to studies in which a therapy is being given for a disease, but should be used in any study in which two or more interventions are allocated to different participants.
- Randomization should be done on each individual participant.
- Randomization eliminates two major sources of bias: prognostic bias, where one treatment group has a better prognosis than the other group; and selection bias, where participants are selected for treatment based on their expected response.
- Randomizing participants is an essential procedure for gaining credibility for your results from the general scientific community.

21

Techniques for Randomization

In this chapter we describe methods for creating a randomization schedule for interventional studies. The definition, rationale, and importance of randomization are discussed in Chapter 20. Randomization is closely linked to the use of blinding, which is described in Chapters 22 and 23.

21.1 Requirements for a Valid Randomized Study

There are three basic requirements for a valid randomized study, as we discussed in Chapter 20. An additional requirement applies when the study is blinded (Chapter 22). Blinding, in which knowledge of the specific treatment is kept secret after enrollment, ideally from the participant and everyone working with the participant, is an important method for avoiding bias in a study, and should be used whenever possible. In this chapter we assume it will be a component of most randomized studies.

Requirement 1: There is a random process allocating the intervention. This implies that there must not be any pattern or structure in the randomization schedule (also called the "randomization table," the "randomization list," or the "treatment assignment list"). This means that assignment cannot be based on such things as day of birth, day of the week that individual entered the study, and the like. As mentioned in Chapter 20, although a given participant may chose to enter the study on a random day, this is not randomization.

Requirement 2: The process is under the direction of the investigator. This means that the investigator is responsible for how the allocation of one intervention or another to a participant is made – that is, how the randomization schedule is created. This does not mean that the investigator has access to the randomization schedule before or during the study.

Requirement 3: No one knows what the intervention for the next participant will be until the participant has completed all the screening and is enrolled in the study. When an individual is screened for eligibility for a study, the individuals making the decision on the participant's eligibility must not know what intervention the person would receive if enrolled. This is true even if the study itself will not involve any blinding. This is why there cannot be any pattern in the treatment assignment schedule, as it could lead to manipulation in various ways. Knowledge of a pattern could result in the subconscious introduction of selection bias (Section 17.1.2).

Requirement 4: As an additional requirement in a blinded study, the randomization schedule must be kept secret from all the individuals involved in the study who are to be blinded. This gives another reason for not having a systematic component to treatment assignment. Sometimes it is necessary to break the blind for a specific participant, and if the assignment was systematic, breaking the blind for this participant could reveal the treatment for other, possibly all, participants in the study.

21.2 Creating a Randomization Schedule

In a study with randomization, participants actually have two distinct ID numbers. The first, which all participants have in all studies, is the Study ID number (Section 29.1). This is a number that is used on all the participant's case report forms. This number is assigned when a participant is enrolled into the study (generally when the consent form is signed). Even participants that fail the screening criteria will usually have a Study ID number, as it is important to be able to account for screening failures when preparing the study for publication.

The second number is the randomization number, which is linked to an intervention. There are actually two separate lists that are needed. We use the term "list" since in theory it could be done on a piece of paper, but normally there would be two different computer files. One file contains the case report form that links the Study ID number with the randomization number. The second file would be the computer file linking the randomization number with the treatment group. Without this second computer file, the randomization number by itself cannot tell you the intervention a participant has received.

The following sections are written as if you, the investigator, are creating the randomization schedule. In practice, very often a statistician, a computer specialist, a pharmacist, or someone else in your institution who will not be working with the participants will create the schedule according to your needs.

Generally, you would make a sequential list of numbers for the randomization numbers. You generally create a list with many more numbers than you are actually likely to need for the study, in case a large number of participants drop out of the study and you need to recruit more participants than expected. Often sample size is determined for the number of participants completing a study, and then enrollment is adjusted for the expected dropout rate. If more participants drop out than you initially planned when designing the study, more participants will need to be recruited to have enough participants completing the study.

Example 21A: In a study of treatment of patients with COPD with one of two alternative therapies or a placebo, there are three treatment groups. The study design specifies 40 participants completing in each group. The investigators estimate that no more than 20% of the participants will drop out of the study, so if a total of 150 participants are enrolled, and 20% (30 participants) drop out before completing the study, then there would be 120 participants left, approximately 40 in each group, the number determined to be needed when the study was designed. In case the actual dropout rate is higher than 20%, however, the statistician creates a randomization list using blocking (see Section 21.3.2) for 200 people, to ensure that the randomization list is long enough to ensure that enough participants can be enrolled to get the target of 120 completing the study.

If you use strata (see Section 21.3.1), there would be a separate list, one for each stratum, and often the first number on the list would show the stratum. As an example, for a study of 200 participants in total, the list for stratum 1 would be numbers 1001–1200, the list for stratum 2 would be numbers 2001–2200, and so forth. If there are only 200 participants in total, obviously some of the randomization numbers will not be used. Most of the participants might come from a single stratum as in the second continuation of Example 21C at the end of Section 21.3.1.

You then need to create a list of treatment assignments. The simplest way to do this is to use a computer program to generate a list of random numbers that determine the intervention group. The first randomization number is assigned the intervention determined by the first random number, the second randomization number is assigned the intervention determined by the second random number, and so on. If stratification is used (see Section 21.3.1), then this process is done once for each of the stratum, so the treatment order will vary between different strata.

Example 21A (continued): Since there were three equal-sized treatment groups, the statistician used a computer program to generate random numbers, with a uniform distribution from 0 to 3. A uniform distribution means that any number in the range is equally likely, so the chance of the next number being 2.000000 or 0.343629 is equal. If the number was between 0 and less than 1, the treatment was the control group; if the number was between 1 and less than 2, the treatment was the first experimental treatment; and if the number was between 2 and less than 3, the treatment was the second experimental treatment. These treatment assignments were assigned to the sequential list of randomization numbers.

As participants are enrolled in the study, they are assigned the next randomization number on the sequential list; if strata are used, the number is assigned from the list for the participant's stratum. Once a randomization number has been assigned, it should not be used for any other participant. In some studies, a set of treatment materials for the entire study are prepared in advance for each participant so that if a participant begins treatment but then drops out, there will not be a complete set of treatments for that randomization number if it is used again. This is another reason that the sequential list contains many more randomization numbers than are specified in the study design as the total number needed for the study.

Example 21B: In a placebo-controlled study comparing drug treatment of depression, the participant is given a series of escalated doses over time until the maximum dosage is reached. Individual sets of the active drug or placebo are prepared by the manufacturer labeled according to the dosage schedule, and given to the investigator, identified by randomization number but not contents, so the study is blinded (see Section 23.1.1). If a participant drops out of the study after one week, he will have used part of the set for his randomization number.

In most cases, computer programs can be used to generate the complete randomization schedule. The user enters some parameters specifying the total number of participants to be randomized and the number of intervention groups, and the program generates a series of random numbers based on a statistical distribution that may be built into the program or may be selected from a list of choices by the user. Technically, these numbers are pseudo-random numbers, since they are systematic, but in most programs the pattern will not begin repeating until more than 4 billion distinct random numbers have been generated. Even statisticians are comfortable with considering this as acceptable.

Most computer programs assume equal-sized groups, but some have the ability to generate schedules for unequal allocation of treatments. The randomization is usually done by someone who has no interaction with the study participants, to avoid the problems of prior knowledge or compromising the blinding. Most often a statistician, familiar with available computer resources, is asked to create the schedule, as done in Example 21A.

21.3 Adding Special Features to the Randomization Schedule

As we stated in Chapter 20, the major purpose of randomization is to have prognostic factors balanced between groups. We recognize that, due to chance, not all factors will be balanced; indeed, 5% of all the variables measured at baseline would be expected to be statistically significantly different (at $P < 0.05$) between groups by chance alone. But there may be prognostic factors that are so important that they could confound the effects of an intervention if they are unequally distributed between the groups, and the investigator may not be willing to rely on chance to balance these factors. Supplemental methods are needed to create groups of participants with the required balance while maintaining the randomization within groups. These methods are known as stratification and blocking. Stratification is used to help balance these prognostic factors between intervention groups. Blocking is used to avoid potential confounding from temporal changes, which might occur if less sick patients start to enroll in the study over time.

21.3.1 Stratification

In a stratified randomized design, the values of important prognostic factors are used to classify participants into two or more groups, called strata when they are enrolled into the study. The strata may be for a single characteristic, such as sex, or for a combination of factors, such as sex and age group, and are determined before participant recruitment begins. Ideally, stratification criteria should be specified as part of the study design, but sometimes they are recommended by a statistician who was not involved in the study design but is asked to produce the randomization schedule. The most common strata are sex, age, ethnicity, or disease state, but other factors related to the course of the disease may be used for stratification.

Example 21C: In a comparative study of two treatments for blood pressure, participants are stratified by age (less than 60 years, 60 or older), sex, and BMI (25 or less, greater than 25). This results in 8 strata: for example, younger, slimmer females and older, heavier males

As Example 21C shows, the strata for dichotomous factors, such as sex, or for variables that can only take on a few values are usually based on the actual value of the variable. For factors that have several values, such as BMI and age, they are usually grouped into a small number of categories to keep the number of strata reasonable. It is very easy to have too many strata in a study, so the tendency to include variables just in case they might be important must be avoided. As you select factors and levels to stratify on, remember that the number of levels are not added but are multiplied.

Example 21C (continued): This study has been stratified on age (2 levels), sex (2 levels) and BMI (2 levels). The number of groups is 8 because you have 2x2x2 combinations of the levels. The investigator initially considered adding another factor, ethnicity at 3 levels, which would have resulted in 24 strata (2x2x2x3), and stratifying age into 3 groups instead of just 2, creating 36 strata (3x2x2x3), but decided this would be too many strata for the size of the study.

This shows how quickly the number of strata increases as you increase the factors of interest. At some point the ratio of participants required by the protocol to total number of strata may get very small. If this happens, you must reduce the number of strata, either by not using a specific variable for stratification or reducing the number of levels for a variable, or preferably both. Some variables can be accounted for in the analysis without seriously compromising the study results; a statistician can help you decide which these are.

Once the strata are defined, a separate randomization schedule is prepared for each stratum. In most cases, different ranges of the sequential randomization numbers are used for each stratum, and the ranges should be large enough to ensure there will be no overlap. Even if the expected number of participants in each stratum is small, you might start the randomization numbers for one stratum from 1001, the next from 2001, then 3001, and so forth. As participants are accepted into the study, they are assigned the next sequential randomization number in their stratum. The individual responsible for implementing the randomization is responsible for making sure that the correct randomization schedule is used for each participant. Assignment is still based on the participant's randomization number, but the randomization numbers are only sequential within strata.

Stratification does not require that the number of participants in each stratum be equal, nor does it specify the number of participants that each should contain. The number of participants in each stratum may be, and frequently is, very different. The purpose of stratification is to ensure that these factors are balanced equally between treatments. It is common to allow for a large number of randomization numbers in each schedule, even though most of them will not be used.

Example 21C (continued): In this study, it is expected that the younger, slimmer groups will probably have fewer participants than the older, heavier groups, but the males and females will be enrolled in roughly equal numbers. Rather than attempting to make randomization schedules with different sizes for the various strata, a table allowing for half the total population is prepared for each of the 8 strata to ensure that the tables are large enough for the most likely strata, the older, heavier individuals.

In most studies you can assume that there will be fewer participants in some strata than in others, and this may make achieving a balanced randomization problematic.

21.3.2 Blocking

Blocking is a method for maintaining the balance between treatment groups in the randomization on other factors. Essentially the randomization schedule is set up so that after a given (small) number of participants are randomized, there will be the appropriate ratio of participants in each group. There are several reasons for doing this. First, this controls for temporal or seasonal changes during the study, with the same proportion being recruited into each intervention group in each time period. Although this is especially important when these factors are known to affect the disease, this is always a possibility that needs to be considered. For studies in which recruitment is expected to take a long time, there can easily be a change over time in the type of participants recruited.

Example 21A (continued): The COPD study was conducted in a city where seasonal pollen counts and allergies are a major concern. Therefore, to avoid a seasonal effect confounding the treatment effects, the randomization schedule was blocked in groups of 6. That means that after 6 individuals have been enrolled, there were 2 participants assigned to each treatment; after the next 6 there would be 2 more in each group, after 18 individuals had been enrolled there were 6 participants assigned to each treatment, and so on. This means that the final groups will be balanced with respect to season when they entered the study. This does not mean there will be equal numbers of individuals enrolled in each season, but that the distribution of seasons will be approximately the same in each group.

Example 21D: When an investigator started a study, he used stringent inclusion criteria, limiting the study only to patients with severe disease. Because of recruitment problems, however, the investigator modified the inclusion criteria to allow for less severely affected patients to be included. As the study did use blocking, roughly equal numbers of the severe patients (recruited early) were in each treatment group, and roughly equal numbers of the less severe patients (recruited later) were in each treatment group as well, so overall the treatment groups were similar in terms of the severity of disease. Without blocking, it would have been possible that an intervention group might have contained a substantially higher proportion of participants with severe disease.

When a randomization schedule using blocking is created, the randomization numbers are sequentially grouped into blocks of some length. If equal-size groups are used, this would be a multiple of the number of intervention groups, but if unequal randomization is used (see Section 21.4), then the block size would be a multiple of the effective number of interventions. The length of each block, defined as a multiple of the number of effective interventions, may vary within each of the strata. This helps mask the treatment allocation rules if the study is not blinded. For example, if the study has three intervention groups, the block sizes may be 3, 6, or 9, depending on the total size of the study. If stratified randomization is used, then each randomization schedule must be blocked separately and the block size may vary between different strata. As with stratification, the block sizes should be determined when developing the study plan.

Blocking becomes especially important when interim analyses are planned or when the possibility exists that the study may be terminated before recruitment is completed. If a study is terminated before recruitment is completed, using blocking ensures that the different intervention groups, although smaller than planned, would be roughly the same size, which provides the best chance to find differences between the interventions.

If stratified randomization results in small numbers of participants in some strata, then varying the block size in different strata will help create a balance of treatments within each strata. If you expect only a very few participants in one stratum then you might use the number of treatments as the block size, although you would use a larger block size for a stratum expected to have many participants. This way you can expect to have approximately equal numbers of individuals from each stratum in each treatment group.

Example 21C (continued): Because the expected number of participants in the young, slim strata was much smaller than the expected number of participants in the older, heavier strata, the randomization schedule for participants in the young, slim stratum was blocked using a block size of two and four (one or two in each treatment group when the block was completed), whereas the other groups were blocked using a block size of four and six (two or three in each treatment group when the block was completed) because they were expected to be more common. The block size was determined randomly as part of the program creating the random allocation for the blocks.

21.3.3 Benefits and Pitfalls of Stratification and Blocking

Stratification and blocking, together or separately, can help improve the validity of your study by adding balance across study groups with respect to key prognostic factors and temporal changes. The results will not be perfect, however. Participants may drop out, upsetting the balance between treatment groups. A single stratum may not have exactly the right number of participants to complete a block. When all the participants needed have been recruited and randomization is completed, there will probably be incomplete blocks in some strata. This can be taken into account when planning the study, by using different block sizes for different strata. For example, in a stratum expected to be large, you could use a large block size, while a smaller block size would be appropriate for a stratum expected to be small. If, when recruitment is completed, you have 63 participants in a large stratum with two treatment groups and you use a block size of 6, then the worst you could have would be a ratio of 33/30 participants in the two treatment groups, or

10% difference. If you had only 9 participants total, you could have an imbalance of 100% (6/3), but with a smaller block size the imbalance would be reduced – to a 25% difference (5/4) with a block size of 2 or 4.

Use of these methods requires some additional effort in planning and implementing the study. However, the value of using these methods greatly exceeds this effort. Most statisticians have had experience with stratification and blocking and can help you make good decisions. They also have computer programs that can generate blocked schedules. Many programs are designed to implement stratification; if not, then the programs can be rerun (but not repeating the last schedule) to obtain separate randomization schedules for each stratum.

We recommend that blocking be used in all studies, because studies do get stopped in the middle (often for recruitment problems), and having roughly equal numbers in each treatment group provides the most information for the total number of participants in the study. We also believe that stratification, if used judiciously, can be helpful. However, you must be careful not to use too many stratification levels. As you chose different variables on which to stratify, the number of different strata multiply rather than add. If you think it would be good to stratify on 3 age groups and 2 genders and 2 centers, then the total number of strata is 12. If there are 2 treatment groups and the protocol specifies 50 individuals, if things worked out perfectly, on average you would have just 4 participants in each stratum. In most cases you will not have exactly 4 participants in every stratum so will not achieve the balance you had hoped for. We have both been involved in studies in which too many stratification factors have been used, so our advice is to use stratification very cautiously, only for factors that are critically important to have balance, and even then the impact of all the different stratification factors must be considered on the size of the smallest stratum before proceeding with stratification. If there is any doubt whether a stratification factor is really needed, our advice is not to use it.

21.4 Unbalanced Randomization

Randomization is often assumed to require imply an equal number of participants in each of the intervention groups. Randomization, however, does not require nor imply that the intervention groups are the same size. A randomized study can be done with unequal randomization. For example, if a 2:1 randomization is done, with 2 participants allocated to one group and 1 participant randomized to the other group, the effective number of interventions would be 3. This is often done for logistical or practical considerations in clinical trials because it is thought that it is easier to recruit participants for a study if they have a better chance of receiving the new intervention (participants feeling that a new intervention is likely to be better than the existing one).

Example 21E: A professor uses an assessment of the effect of time of day on a speed of performance test as a practical example in his research design course. All students in the two sections of the course are expected to participate as part of their course work. The professor has found that the results are much more variable in the early morning, so that he wants 2/3 of the students to be tested in the morning and 1/3 in the afternoon. The professor makes a list of all the student ID numbers in order separately for each of the two sections. A computer program allocates the time of assessment to each of the two lists randomly. In this randomization, the effective number of interventions is 3, and the approach described in Example 21A can be used. If the random number is between 0 and less than 1, the randomization number is assigned to the afternoon test, while if the random number is at least 1 and less than 3, the randomization number is assigned a morning testing period. In addition to providing the 2:1 randomization that the professor wanted, this example illustrates stratified randomization. About 2/3 of each section is doing the morning testing so the students feel that the two sections are being treated equitably.

21.5 Ethical Issues

We extensively discussed the ethical issues associated with randomization (or more precisely, with the lack of it) in Chapter 20. Here we only point out the ethical issues involved in using the randomization schedule. No one involved in determining the eligibility of a potential participant should be involved in creating or reviewing the contents of the final randomization schedule used in the study. It is critical that procedures be in place so that the staff can only access this information after the participant has completed all screening procedures and is enrolled, ready to be randomized to an intervention. After that, some members of the staff may need information about the intervention for a participant. In this case the staff should only have access to the information about the intervention for this single participant. It is far better if the intervention can be kept blinded to all the staff if possible (see Chapters 22 and 23 on blinding). The randomization schedule should be guarded and protected throughout the study; often the person who created the schedule will also keep a copy. Losing the randomization schedule in a blinded study means that you will never be able to interpret the results of the study, as you will not know which intervention the different participants received. Even if the study is not blinded, attempting to recreate the treatments received at the end of the study may be exceedingly difficult.

KEY POINTS

- Intervention assignments in a randomization schedule cannot have any pattern.
- Personnel screening individuals for participation should never know the intervention assignment before the participant has completed all the screening procedures and is enrolled in the study and the participant randomized.
- If blinding is used in the study, no one who is supposed to be blinded should ever see the randomization schedule.
- Stratification can be used to balance the intervention groups with respect to important prognostic factors, but caution is strongly advised to avoid too many stratification factors.
- Blocking may be used to balance the intervention groups with respect to temporal or seasonal factors, and to ensure roughly equal numbers in each intervention group should the study be stopped early.
- If the randomization is complicated, the advice and assistance of a biostatistician or other specialist in planning and developing the randomization schedules is recommended.

22

Blinding in Interventional Studies

Many measurements in clinical studies have a subjective component that may be influenced by knowledge of the participant's treatment. Blinding, also called masking, is a process that is specified in the study protocol to keep such information secret from the participants themselves, the physicians and other clinical assessors, the laboratory personnel, and even the statisticians. Blinding may occur on several levels, from none (an open-label or unblinded study), to single-blind (only the participant or the assessors are blinded), to double-blind (both the participants and the assessors are blinded), to studies in which everyone working with the participants or with the data is blinded (completely blind). The double-blind study is the standard for interventional studies. In this chapter we discuss different levels of blinding in interventional studies and how they may be part of a study design. In the next chapter we give specific methods for implementing and maintaining the blind. Although blinding is most commonly associated with randomized studies, it should also be used in observational studies, as assessor's knowledge of a participant's clinical status or prior exposures can bias results. Blinding in observational studies is discussed in Chapter 28.

22.1 Why Blinding Is Used

In the ideal world of scientific research, all outcomes would be measured by precise and reproducible criteria and judgments would be completely objective. However, we do not live in an ideal world. Many measurements in clinical studies have a subjective component, such as an assessor's assessment of a participant's mood, the participant's assessment of her well-being, or a relative's assessment of the participant's level of functioning. For brevity, we will use the term "assessors" to refer to all those who evaluate or interact with the participant. This may include examining physicians, nurses, psychologists, nutritionists, exercise therapists, and laboratory personnel.

Even objective tests, such as muscle strength, depend on how hard the participant tries to do the test. It is difficult for anyone, either the assessors or the participants, to be completely objective when they have strong ideas or hopes about what the effects of a treatment will be. Similarly, a participant may not be able to assess his physical or psychological responses objectively if he is aware of what treatment he is getting. Thus, the results of a study can be biased if either the participant or the assessors know what treatment the participant is getting. To prevent this, we use masking so that the information is not available to bias the participant or the assessor. Blinding is one of the most important ways to avoid bias in any comparative study. Even if you are convinced that you and your associates can be completely objective in a study, if you choose not to use masking whenever possible, you will have difficulty convincing reviewers, referees, and readers of the validity of your study.

22.2 The Hierarchy of Blinding

Often it is not possible to mask everyone in a study. There is a natural hierarchy of blinding, from the open-label study with no blinding to the completely blinded study in which, in addition to the participants and all assessors, the data management staff and biostatisticians are also blinded, even though they do not do any participant assessments.

In interventional studies the intervention is masked. In the following sections we begin with the double-blind study, which is the standard for interventional studies and should be used whenever possible. The completely blinded study is an extension of the double-blind study. We follow with examples of single-blind studies and finally open-label studies that have no masking at all. These are presented with the understanding that you must deal with the limitations of these approaches, but we emphasize that efforts to increase masking in a study will greatly benefit the reliability and credibility of the results. Methods for implementing blinding are discussed in the next chapter.

22.2.1 Double-Blind Studies

In a double-blind study neither the participants nor the assessors know the treatment the participant is receiving. This is the standard for an interventional study, since it minimizes both potential participant biases and potential assessor biases. It should be used whenever possible, which is whenever it is ethically permissible to mask the participants.

Example 22A: In a classic double-blind study comparing a new oral treatment for Type II diabetes to an existing treatment, the treatments are both administered as identical white tablets. Participants are in the study for 1 year. The primary outcomes are monthly average morning glucose levels and periodic HbA1c measurements. Participants measure and record their own morning glucose levels. Blood samples are drawn for insulin, glucose levels, and HbA1c as well as safety measures at monthly visits. The participants are also assessed for ophthalmologic problems at the beginning, at six months and at the end of the study, and have complete physical examinations at the beginning and last visit. All the laboratory tests use standard methods, and the samples are identified only by a study code. The persons assessing the ophthalmologic status of the individual and the physical examination are also masked to the participant's treatment.

Sometimes one or more of the assessors cannot be masked if the treatment would be obvious from some of the laboratory tests or if treatment knowledge is needed to ensure appropriate handling of side effects. The study may still be considered double-blind if these unmasked individuals are not involved in assessing the endpoints of the study.

Example 22B: In a placebo-controlled study comparing two treatments for depression, both participants and assessors were blinded to treatment. It was necessary to monitor drug levels to make sure the participant was achieving therapeutic levels and to adjust drug dosage accordingly, and it was clear from the magnitude of the levels what the medication was. The samples of treatment drugs were given a separate drug sample number that was linked to the participant's study number. The drug levels were assayed by an outside commercial laboratory and the results were sent to one individual to review. The person who reviewed the drug levels was only aware of the participant's drug sample number and did not interact with participants at all or perform any assessments. The pharmacist was given all changes only by the drug sample number that could be linked to the study number. Thus the study was double-blind.

In Example 22B, as in many studies, the pharmacist had no contact with the participants or their data, knew only the drug sample number, and was not an assessor. Therefore, it was not necessary that the pharmacist be masked to the medication.

Example 22C: Assay results must be checked for values beyond known limits or unreasonable differences between replicates. The discrepancies may be flagged by a computer system, but the report must be reviewed by a human. Discrepant values can be accepted, deleted, or recommended to be assayed again. All laboratories have standard quality control procedures to handle such decisions for routine tests. For specialized assays done by members of the study team, the review (like the assays themselves) needs to be done by someone blind to the treatment given to each participant. Assays should be identified by a laboratory number that is different from the participant's study number. If the information in the assay values does not reflect the treatment, then a member of the study team could do the review, otherwise an individual not associated with the study should be the one to make decisions about the laboratory data to maintain the blind.

22.2.2 Complete Blinding

A study is completely blinded when all personnel who evaluate the participants or analyze the data are masked to the participant's treatment. This is an expansion of the double-blind study described in the previous section. The additional masking would refer to personnel who do not see the participant or create data, such as the data management and statistical staff. Although data management is probably the most objective activity in a study, blinding these staff members prevents their inadvertently disclosing the participant's status to another staff member. In addition, it ensures that data from all participants receive equal scrutiny. The study plan sometimes requires that statisticians make decisions about the direction of the analysis after the data is collected, and thus the statisticians should be masked to ensure that the analysis is not directed toward a preferred conclusion.

Statisticians usually have to be able to identify participants as members of different groups (e.g., group A, B, C, etc.), but they do not need to know which treatment is associated with each letter. In practice, at some point, if the treatment is effective, it may become clear which group is which, but this should not be used to modify the data analysis.

Example 22B (continued): The drug levels were assayed for therapeutic reasons in an outside commercial laboratory, but all other serum samples were assayed in a laboratory associated with the principal investigator's institution. Although the existence of drug in the serum would indicate the participant's treatment, this information was not known to the laboratory staff. Therefore, the laboratory staff was blinded to the treatment for the samples they assayed. The drug serum levels were not entered in the database used for the primary analysis, so the data analysis staff did not have access to this information, and so they remained blinded as well. After the primary analysis was completed, analyses using the drug level information were made to determine if the drug level affected the outcome.

22.2.3 Single-Blind Studies

In a single-blind study, either the participants or the assessors are masked, but not both. Ideally, the assessors would be masked to the treatment and the participants would not be masked because it would be impossible for the participants not to know the intervention they are receiving.

Example 22D: An investigator is studying the effect of different types of exercise on disease progression. Participants are randomized to one of two exercise routines: endurance training or strength training.

Obviously the participants will know which type of exercise they are doing, and some other investigators will know, such as those responsible for doing the training. The physician who gives participants the physical examination or the psychologist that evaluates the participant's current mood can be blinded, however.

A study in which the participant is not blinded but the assessors are blinded puts some extra burden on the participant to keep the secret from the assessors. The participant must be made aware of the limits on what he can say to or ask of the assessors. The reason for blinding should be carefully explained to the participant, and he should be reassured that this requirement is only to improve objectivity and rigor of the study and does not imply any concerns about the treatment. If the participants are young children, or adults with mental problems that would limit their understanding, then this will probably not be effective and another approach to masking may be necessary.

Example 22E: Participants are randomized to receive either drug treatment or psychotherapy for minor depression. Participants receiving medication receive it from a treating physician, who is not involved in assessing participant outcome. The participant can freely discuss the medication and any possible side effects from the drug with the treating physician. The treating physician would be responsible for reporting side effects from the drug for the study. Similarly, participants receiving psychotherapy would meet with a therapist, and could freely discuss any issues with the therapist, who would be responsible for reporting adverse events. There would be another individual, who had no knowledge of the participant's treatment, who would be responsible for assessing outcome in both groups of participants. The participants would be told that they should not discuss the treatment that they are receiving, including side effects from the medication, with the blinded assessor, and reminded of this at the start of each visit with the assessor.

In most studies, some amount of friendly interaction between the participants and the assessors is part of the protocol. This is important to enhance the participant's adherence (see Chapter 24), encourage honest answers to questions, and retain the participant in the study. But this same interaction may lead the participant to break the blind for the assessor accidentally.

Example 22F: In this single-blind study of a chronic condition, participants are randomized to exercise or no exercise. The participants meet with the investigators biweekly to review their progress. Meetings start with a friendly "How are you today" and a discussion of general problems. In this situation it is possible that the participant may say something like "I feel a lot better since I started exercising" or "My legs hurt from yesterday's workout." Although participants will be instructed to avoid saying things like this, not all participants will remember to adhere to this request.

In rare cases, the participant may be masked to treatment but some assessors may not be because of the need to adjust medication, the medication affecting laboratory values, potential side effects, and so on. In most studies these factors can and should be monitored by an unblinded person who is not involved in assessing outcome, as described in Examples 22B and 22E. If the same person both adjusts the medication and assesses outcome, then there is the risk of both caregiver and assessor bias (Sections 17.1.6 and 17.1.7) from this individual. Methods of adjusting medication without breaking the blind are discussed in Section 23.1.2.

Single-blind studies involve a trade-off between the advantages of having the assessors blinded versus the problems that would ensue if the blind were broken for some but not all participants. Although the blind may be broken in double-blind or completely blinded studies, it is more likely to occur in single-blind studies such as Example 22F, where the participant is aware of the treatment received. Even if some investigators need to be unblinded for participant safety, the outcome assessments should be made by a blinded assessor.

22.2.4 Open-Label Studies

In an open-label study, no one is masked. Single-blind studies are preferable to open-label studies, since at least some sources of bias are eliminated, but on occasion this may be impossible or unnecessary. All single arm studies are open-label. Most open-label studies are pilot studies or Phase I clinical trials, when only one treatment at one dose is given at a time. Dose-ranging studies may also be open label. Sometimes a study cannot be completely masked either to the participant or to the assessors, such as a comparison of different invasive procedures. Sometimes an open-label phase may follow the blinded phase of a comparative study.

Example 22G: Investigators are evaluating a new treatment for a rare disease, which is very debilitating, progressive, has no known treatment, and is always eventually fatal. As there are no known severe adverse effects of the treatment, the investigators feel that it would be unethical to deny treatment to any participant, because the study potentially has significant benefits and no known severe risks. Therefore, the treatment was studied in a single group in an open-label study.

Example 22H: In a double-blind study of testosterone replacement, hypogonadal participants were randomized to either the standard or a new method of testosterone delivery for six months (Example 14A). At the end of the study, a new phase was initiated. All participants were given the opportunity to use the new method for another 2 years in an open-label extension. The purpose of this second phase was twofold. First, the long-term effects of the new method could be evaluated during the extension period. Second, participants who might refuse if they felt they would only receive the standard treatment were assured that they would eventually have access to the new delivery method, improving recruitment and retention.

Example 22I: Investigators wish to determine if pharmacological treatment of a specific condition may be sufficient some of the time. The standard of care is surgical treatment. Participants begin on pharmacological treatment and continue to surgery if the condition is not resolved by a certain time or worsens. The outcome is the percent of participants who do not need surgery. This is an open-label study in a single group of participants.

Obviously, there is an opportunity for bias in these studies. To illustrate this problem, in the pilot study or Phase I clinical trial, participants know that they are on an experimental therapy. They may over- or underreport side effects, may overestimate the efficacy of the treatment simply because they are happy to be getting some treatment, or may underestimate the effect because they are expecting more of a benefit. Assessors are also susceptible to bias because of their knowledge of the treatment. In Example 22G participants and assessors might overestimate the magnitude of the effect simply because something is being done. In Example 22H, the potential bias would be limited to the second phase during the open-label extension, so the primary comparison at the end of the double-blind phase is protected. In Example 22I if the standards for needing surgery are not very specific, then an assessor's preference for treatment may affect the results.

22.2.5 Multiple Levels of Blinding

Not all studies fall neatly into the previously defined categories. Some studies examine the interaction of several interventions on an individual and different levels of masking may be used for each intervention.

Example 22J: In a study of the effects of hormone supplementation and exercise training on muscle mass and strength in healthy participants, participants were randomized to four groups: supplementation only, exercise only, both, or neither. The participants and assessors who evaluated them were unblinded with respect to exercise, but a placebo control was used for the hormone supplementation, so that the study was double-blind to hormone use. Since hormone levels were monitored and entered in the database, laboratory, data management, and statistical personnel could be blinded to exercise use but potentially could identify participants who were taking supplements by increased hormone levels.

22.3 Monitoring Safety and Breaking the Blind

The expression "breaking the blind" is used to describe revealing the intervention information about one or many participants. In most circumstances this does not occur until the study is completed and the data are analyzed. However, in an interventional study, there must be a mechanism to disclose the treatment a specific individual is receiving in case of an emergency. Therefore, there must be at least one person associated with a study who can provide treatment information when needed. In most cases, this person should not be involved in any of the study assessments. Sometimes, this may be the person who prepared the treatment allocation schedule used to randomize participants after they are enrolled (Section 21.2).

Ongoing monitoring of safety may require breaking the blind in a non-emergency situation. In any clinical study involving an intervention at least one person is the designated safety monitor and is required to review safety data and adverse event reports. Frequently there are several people reviewing different aspects of the data as part of the Data Safety and Monitoring Board (DSMB; Section 2.4). If the safety data includes levels of the study drugs, the person reviewing it will be unblinded. The safety monitor also reviews adverse events to determine if the action taken was appropriate or if further action is needed. In many cases this will not require breaking the blind, since the drug may be discontinued without participants or assessors knowing which drug it is. If there is a possibility of interaction between the study treatment and the recommended action, the blind may have to be broken.

The need to occasionally break the blind for an individual is another good reason not to use convenience methods for assigning participants to treatment, such as "all odd numbered participants get treatment A" (Section 20.3). If this method were used, then once the blind is broken for one participant, the entire scheme is known.

22.4 When the Blind Is Broken

If a blind is broken for some participants, either deliberately as described above or inadvertently, as may happen in a single-blind study, then this may have some impact on the analysis and potentially on the number of participants available for analysis and therefore the power of the study (Appendix B). If unblinding is a rare event, so that blinding is maintained for virtually all participants, it needs to be mentioned in the study report but is unlikely to have a substantial impact on the results. If a substantial fraction of participants are unblinded, however, this may impact the scientific credibility of the study.

Example 22F (continued): It is likely that assessors will find out that some participants are definitely exercising, but is less likely they will find out that some participants are definitely not exercising. Therefore, the blind is likely to be broken only in one group. When potential bias is limited to one group, group comparisons become more complicated and less reliable, and the integrity of the study might be questioned if the assessors are unblinded for a large number of participants, although this is still better than having potential (and differing) biases in both groups.

22.5 Ethical Issues

Blinding contributes to the validity of a study by enhancing the objectivity of assessments. Therefore, it should be used whenever possible, even when this requires more effort, more paperwork, and perhaps additional staff to implement. If blinding a participant would require that mock interventions be used on the participant, then the risk of these interventions would need to be incorporated into the risk-benefit calculation to determine if they are warranted. If masking assessors requires an additional unblinded individual be involved in the study to ensure individual participant safety, this should be done, if at all possible. In some circumstances, immediate knowledge of the participant's treatment may be needed, and plans to provide this data should be established when the study is being developed. This can usually be handled by the use of an unblinded person, as well as established procedures so that the blind can be broken quickly in case of an emergency.

If masking is used in a study, then this must be disclosed to the participant when obtaining informed consent. Often participants are uncomfortable with the notion that they will not know which intervention they are receiving. The informed consent should mention that procedures exist for disclosing the intervention to their physician if this information would affect the medical care the participant needs during the study.

KEY POINTS

- Blinding is an important way to maintain the objectivity of study assessments.
- Blinding may occur at several levels.
  - A double-blind study is one in which both the participants and the assessors are blinded. This is the standard expected in interventional studies.
  - A completely blinded study is one in which in addition to the participants and assessors, data management staff and statisticians are also blinded.
  - A single-blind study means that either the participants or the assessors are blinded as to treatment, but not both. In these studies, it is almost always the assessors who should be blinded.
  - An open-label study is one in which there is no blinding.
- A study generally requires that there be an individual or committee to monitor the safety of the study. These individuals may be unblinded in special circumstances.
- There must be a procedure to determine the participant's treatment in case of emergency.

23

Techniques to Blind Interventional Studies

In the previous chapter we described the purpose of blinding and the different levels used. In this chapter we describe some techniques to implement and maintain the blind. These techniques may be used in single-blind, double-blind, and completely blinded studies as needed. Although blinding is usually associated with interventional studies, it should also be done for observational studies whenever possible. We describe methods for blinding observational studies in Chapter 28.

23.1 Masking the Intervention

We assume that a randomization schedule has been generated according to the methods in Chapter 21 by an individual not involved in the assessment of participants, and that participants accepted into the study are sequentially assigned a randomization number that is linked to the randomization schedule and that determines the allocation of the specific intervention. To protect privacy, each individual is given a study number when first identified as a potential participant (Section 29.1), but the randomization number is only assigned when the participant has passed all the screening criteria for the study, and it is different from and unrelated to the study number.

Blinding methods in randomized studies include not only physically masking the material that is used in the intervention but also ways of masking other information, such as laboratory results, that might reveal the intervention.

23.1.1 Masking a Pharmaceutical Intervention

There are many techniques that can be used for creating the material to blind an internal or topical pharmaceutical intervention. The simplest case is when there is a single intervention, which we will refer to as the active treatment, and a placebo, and the placebo can be created in the same form as the active treatment – as a tablet, capsule, cream, or liquid. The placebo should be identical to the active treatment in physical appearance and have similar taste, smell, and consistency. Often the manufacturer of the active drug will prepare matching placebos for use in randomized studies. In a similar way, a study involving different doses of the same medication can be blinded by giving each participant the appropriate mix of active drug and placebo tablets or liquids.

Example 23A: Participants will be randomized to one of three groups in a study to determine optimal dosage levels for a new use for an existing drug. The drug levels, 5 mg, 10 mg, or 15 mg twice daily have been shown to be safe. The drug is manufactured in 5 mg tablets. The manufacturer will provide the identical placebo tablets. All participants will take three tablets each time, but they will be given a combination of active drug and placebo tablets to achieve the correct dose.

If the protocol is a comparison of two drugs, such as a new treatment versus standard of care (SOC), and the two treatments are administered using equivalent vehicles, it may be possible to administer medications that contain either the test or the SOC treatment but are identical in appearance. If the two treatments have different forms or may be distinguishable for other reasons, such as taste or texture, then there should be matching placebos for each treatment, and a participant would be given the correct combination of placebo and active drug according to the randomization. This method can be used even if the method of delivery of the two treatments is different. For example, a participant could receive both a liquid medication and a tablet, one of which would be a placebo.

Example 23B: A study is designed to examine the additive effect of two different treatments; one is administered as a tablet and the other as a gel. The design calls for four groups; placebo only, the first treatment only, the second treatment only, or both treatments together. Each participant is given the appropriate combination of active or placebo tablet and active or placebo gel, depending on the assigned group.

If a treatment or treatments can be prepared in capsule form, then this may be very useful in maintaining the blind. A capsule can conceal some easily identifiable characteristics, such a strong taste, that might be hard to duplicate in a placebo. A capsule can also often be created to contain different doses of a drug without any visible change.

Example 23C: In Example 22B two treatments for depression were compared. The treatments were administered in capsules. The capsules were identical in appearance and could contain different dosages. This method also meant that if dosage changes were required, the pharmacist could simply change the content of the capsules without any visible changes to the capsules.

23.1.2 Maintaining the Mask When Dosage Levels Change

Sometimes the study protocol defines a periodic evaluation of the drug efficacy and dose changes, either up or down, for some participants. In this case, the blind can still be maintained. The evaluation and decisions about doses are made by an outside unblinded investigator and the treatment changes will also be determined by the same or another unblinded individual. If the testing and adjustment is on a fixed schedule, then each participant will have a change in the physical amount of medication, although the actual active drug may not change.

Example 23D: In a placebo controlled interventional study, the drug levels may be adjusted after three months. The manufacturer has supplied identical tablets with either 0 mg, 2.5 mg, or 5 mg of drug. Each participant begins by taking one tablet with either 0 mg (the placebo) or 5 mg of drug. The dosage may be adjusted either up or down based on clinical or laboratory results. After three months in the study the number of tablets each participant receives is increased by one. Participants in the placebo group will receive two placebo tablets. Participants in the active drug group may have their dosage increased by either 2.5 mg or 5 mg, but may also have their dosage decreased by replacing the 5 mg tablet with a 2.5 mg tablet and a placebo. Participants on active drug not needing a dosage change will simply be given an additional tablet containing placebo.

In Example 23D the testing could be repeated and the dosages further adjusted after a suitable period.

Some studies require that dosage modifications be done only as required, not on a regular schedule, and only for participants who require change. If only those participants receiving the active drug have dosage changes, then it will be clear that they are being treated with active drug. One way to maintain the blind in these circumstances is to create a schedule in which participants are randomly selected for an apparent dose change, usually the addition of a placebo. Depending on the study design, the investigators might also appear to reduce the amount of "medication" the participant is taking.

Example 23E: For a study similar to Example 23D, drug levels were monitored every four weeks and changes were made when necessary. The biostatistician generated a randomized schedule of changes. This identified which participants would get a dosage "change" in the form of an additional placebo tablet and the time when they would get the change. Real changes would be implemented as discussed in Example 23D. If the participant had had a real change in the prior interval, there would be no dummy change to avoid unnecessary anxiety, but real changes would be made as needed. Participants could receive up to two additional tablets. If more dosage changes were needed, these would be implemented by changes in the dose of the tablets given.

23.1.3 Masking for Non-Pharmaceutical Intervention

Blinding for studies that use other than oral or topical treatments is more difficult and tends to raise ethical issues. Nutritional studies may be blinded if all food is to be supplied by the investigators and the difference is not detectable, such as a tasteless supplement that is mixed with food. If the procedure is invasive, then it is usually not ethical to perform a non-active equivalent. Studies in which a placebo IV infusion, using the same carrier as an active infusion, have been allowed, but this might be problematic. The risks of a sham infusion are generally higher than those of an oral placebo therapy, particularly if the participant is unusually fragile. Studies with sham surgeries have also been done, but they are rare because of the risks to the participant. Most studies involving invasive procedures are single-blinded, but particularly for very aggressive therapy such studies are at significant risk of participant bias (Section 17.1.3).

Example 23F: Investigators wished to evaluate the efficacy of transcutaneous electric nerve stimulation (TENS) for treatment of chronic back pain. They wished to compare TENS alone to TENS with and without stretching exercise and no treatment. They were able to develop a sham unit with lights, dials, and wires that was identical in appearance to the TENS equipment, so that participants and most assessors were blinded to whether or not the participant actually underwent TENS. The assessors were also blinded to stretching exercises, although the participants could not be.

23.1.4 Masking Laboratory Staff

Blinding of laboratory staff brings up some additional complications. If the substance to be measured includes drug levels, then the staff cannot be blinded to the participant's treatment. Ideally, it would be preferable that the laboratory staff not know if two samples come from the same participant; however, sometimes it is necessary that all samples from a participant be assayed in a single run, to minimize inter-assay variability. Problems may be reduced if samples from several individuals are assayed in a single run and both the participant and time order is masked within the run. In many studies, the samples that go to the laboratory are assigned a different set of identification numbers, not tied to the participant's study identification number or to other samples from the participant.

Example 23G: In a study comparing two different delivery methods for a drug, serial sampling was performed at the beginning and end of the study to determine the pharmacokinetic properties of each delivery method. The protocol required that all assays for one individual be done in the same run. The assay procedure required review of the samples for quality and possible decisions to reject or rerun some values. In addition to using sample numbers so that the laboratory personnel and reviewer were blinded to the participant and treatment, the temporal order of the samples was masked so that the reviewer would not be influenced by the relationship between samples that were taken sequentially.

Example 23H: In a multi-center study of the psychobiology of depression, each center was supplied with sheets of nine-digit random numbers. Each random number was printed on two labels. When blood and urine samples were collected from participants and allocated into tubes for assay by the central laboratory, one label was attached to the tube as its only identification. The other label was attached to a form that contained the participants study ID, date of the sample, substance being assayed, and other related information. The sample numbers and the study information were reconciled when the database was created. This procedure blinded laboratory staff but not data management staff and statisticians.

23.1.5 Masking Data Management Staff

Blinding of data management staff has similar problems to that of blinding laboratory staff if data that will identify the treatment must be entered or reviewed. Many studies have a single person who is authorized to enter these data. This person may also be the one who enters the group assignment into the database. File protection, such as password protection, can restrict access to this or other sensitive data. Many laboratories can send assay results directly to a computer database without anyone manually entering the data, so that the data management staff does not have to see the values. The analysis staff must have some code that identifies participants as belonging to the same group, but data that would break the blind may be limited to one individual, at least during the initial analysis. If the actual treatment received rather than solely a group identifier such as "A" and "B" must be included in the analysis, then it must be released to the statisticians. Even if the groups are identified only by a letter code, however, it is possible that the results overall will be sufficient to unblind the study statisticians while the analysis is on-going.

23.2 Providing the Intervention in Blinded Studies

Once you have a randomization schedule and methods for masking the intervention from the participant and assessor, the next question is how the interventions can be physically provided to the participants so that the blinding is maintained. There are three general approaches: allocation by the treatment manufacturer, allocation by the pharmacy at the site, or allocation by study personnel.

23.2.1 Treatment Allocation by the Manufacturer

Allocation by the manufacture is most commonly used when the treatment manufacturer is providing both active treatment and placebo in identical form (Section 23.1.1). The manufacturer may create the randomization schedule and provide the study site(s) with a method for assigning study identification to each participant, or they may be using a schedule derived from an outside source. In either case, they will create packets for each randomization number with the contents as specified by the randomization schedule, and forward these packets to the study center to be given to the participant without modification.

Example 23I: Investigators wished to determine if an existing oral preparation currently approved for one condition will mediate the symptoms of another chronic condition that is unrelated to the condition for which the medication is approved. The design was a double-blind, parallel group, placebo-controlled intervention study with participants from three different centers treated for six months. A randomization schedule for each center was prepared by a biostatistician and sent to the manufacturer. The manufacturer prepared packages containing all the medications for the six months in weekly dispensers. The packages were identified only by the randomization number and were sent to the centers in batches, beginning with the first 20. Centers were instructed to collect unused medications and, if an individual was randomized but not treated, to return the package and not use it for other participants.

23.2.2 The Institutional Pharmacy

Many institutions have pharmacies that have some staff members who are available to work with researchers and are trained in supporting blinded studies. The pharmacist is given the randomization schedule. If a manufacturer is supplying both the active drug and the placebo, then the medications may be sent to the pharmacy using job lot numbers or some other key to distinguish them. Frequently the hospital pharmacists will create the different vehicles. When a participant is accepted for the study and given a randomization number, the pharmacist is sent an order for medication for the study for a specific participant, which is then filled with the medications according to the randomization schedule.

Example 23J: In a randomized, double-blind, parallel group study a new medication in tablet form was compared to the current standard, which was a liquid. The manufacturer of the new medication supplied both active drug and placebo tablets in identical form to the pharmacist. The pharmacy purchased the current standard and created a matching placebo. The randomization schedule was given to the pharmacist who used the standard procedures at the institution to keep it masked from other individuals. The treatment orders, identified by randomization number, were sent to the pharmacist who selected the correct combination of active drug and placebo. The pharmacist kept records of the medication dispensed in a secure file.

23.2.3 Allocation by a Member of the Study Team

In some studies the treatment may be allocated by an unblinded person on the study team, who has the randomization schedule and also the means of identifying the products. This may occur if the study is very small, a pharmacist is not available, or there is not adequate funding to support the pharmacist. In this case, the person allocating the treatment should not be evaluating or interacting with the participants after treatment allocation.

Example 23K: In Example 22D participants were randomized to either endurance exercise or strength training. The study was single-blind and there were no pharmaceuticals involved. Therefore, the investigators decided that one member of the study team, who was involved in recruiting and screening, could also inform the participants about their exercise mode according to the randomization schedule. This staff member would not be aware of the randomization assignment before the individual was accepted into the study, and would not do any evaluation of the participants once they were in the study. The record of randomization was kept in a locked cabinet in this person's office, and the computer record of randomization was created by this person and password protected.

23.2.4 Keeping the Randomization Confidential

To avoid the possibility of others learning what intervention participants are assigned to in a blinded study, the study protocol should specify procedures for protecting this information. Any paper copy that contains this information should be kept in a locked drawer or cabinet with limited access. In a pharmacy, this access should be limited to the pharmacist who dispenses the medications. If the allocation is done within the group, then no other member of the study team should have access. Similarly, computer records of participants' assignments should be created by a single person and be secured by whatever method is operational in your facility. An individual's potential assignment should not be known until the individual is enrolled into the study and given a randomization number. This can be done if the person who creates the randomization schedule gives the person who allocates the treatment a set of opaque sealed envelopes, with the randomization number on the outside and the treatment on the inside, and the envelope is not opened until the individual is accepted into the study. Periodic envelope checks can help ensure that they are not opened prematurely.

Example 23K (continued): To avoid potential prognostic bias (Section 17.1.1), all of these procedures were used. Individual treatment assignments were stored in sealed envelopes, prepared by the biostatistician who prepared the randomization schedule. The staff member who was doing the assignment was instructed not to open an envelope until the person had been accepted and the randomization number assigned in the computer record of randomization, maintained by the staff member. Periodically, the biostatistician checked that envelopes had not been opened until a participant was randomized. This way the recruiter would not know the results of the randomization in advance and could not be suspected of being biased in the recruitment process.

With adequate resources, randomization can be done using a web-based or interactive voice randomization system. After a participant has completed all the screening procedures, a study staff member enters the participant into the randomization system. In addition to the Study ID, this would normally include additional data to ensure that the participant was correctly identified and would include all of the stratification variables used in the study. After this data has been validated (usually a real-time process in these systems), the randomization information would be provided to the study staff member. In a double-blind study, this would be only a randomization number for the pharmacist who would provide the treatment. In a single-blind or open-label study, the appropriate additional information would be given to the staff member, or provided to caregivers needing to know the intervention the participant was to receive.

There are several advantages to such an approach. Most importantly, it provides additional assurance that the treatment was not known prior to the participant's enrollment. In addition, it avoids some of the security concerns about paper and local computer files storing information about randomization. It can provide a more systematic and secure mechanism for randomization across a group or institution using such a system. It also eliminates all the work involved with using sealed envelopes for randomization.

23.3 Common Problems Maintaining Masking

23.3.1 Side Effects

Side effects are one of the major ways in which the blind is broken, particularly when an active treatment is compared to a placebo. When side effects are observable by the participant, it is much harder to blind him to the fact that he is getting an active treatment. There are significant ethical problems in inducing side effects in participants to mask the fact that they are receiving placebos. Side effects may be an instant tip-off to the physician as to what treatment is being used, as well as participants given their widespread use of the Internet, even when the protocol specifies comparing two treatments, or different doses of one treatment.

The impact of side effects on maintaining the blind may be reduced by stating the types of side effects expected very broadly in the informed consent or combining the side effects of all the potential therapies into a single list, but this may lead to ethical problems if the amount of information does not meet the standards of informed consent. At least partial blinding may be maintained in the presence of side effects by excluding all side effect information in the records used by any assessors who do not need to be aware of them. The protocol of some studies may specify maintaining multiple medical records, one without side effect information, the other without outcome data, and study staff will use the appropriate records for their activities.

Example 23L: In an interventional double blind parallel group study the two treatments being compared had very different side-effect profiles: one drug caused hypertension in many individuals receiving the drug, while the other drug caused a rash in most individuals. Thus, all outcome assessments were done by assessors who had no knowledge of the participant's side effects.

23.3.2 Efficacy

Some new treatments represent major advances. A truly effective treatment can be recognized by its efficacy in participants. When this happens, it is usually very clear which treatment a participant is receiving, at least for the health care providers involved in the trial. Although this is a problem that most of us would not mind having, it can affect the trial integrity in a longitudinal study in which the participant may be reevaluated several times after the initial response. In most studies, new treatments are not that potent, and placebo effects do occur. If a new treatment is so obviously superior, then it is likely that the study will be stopped early for ethical reasons and the new treatment offered to all participants.

Example 23M: In Phase III studies of surfactant for the treatment of respiratory distress in premature infants, the differences were so dramatic that the treating physicians could tell the treatment from the infant's response. These studies were stopped early by the Data Safety and Monitoring Board because of the overwhelming evidence of efficacy.

23.3.3 Leaks and Guesses

There are occasional investigators who consider it a game or a challenge to try to guess what treatment a participant is on in a blinded study. Most investigators do not do this, recognizing the importance of maintaining the objectivity that comes from being blinded and also being too busy to play games. It has been our experience that, in a parallel group study with 1:1 randomization, the guesses are right about 50% of the time, which is about what they would get by tossing a coin. Whether or not a guess is correct, it may result in a biased rating, not only from the specific investigator but from anyone else influenced by the investigator's attitude or with whom the investigator has shared the supposed knowledge.

Another problem occurs when treatment information is inadvertently leaked to assessors or participants. This is fairly easy to avoid by good control of the randomization information and proper staff training. You must make sure the staff understands the importance of blinding, the need to protect it, and the damage that can be done by not maintaining it properly, emphasizing the danger that compromising the blind may destroy the integrity of the whole study.

Another source of leaks originates in a single-blinded study, when an unblinded participant inadvertently or deliberately gives a blinded assessor information about the treatment. This is illustrated in Example 22F. The best way to avoid this is to make sure that the participant understands why blinding the assessors is important and is aware of what must be done to avoid leaking the information. The assessors should also be trained to avoid any questions that might lead to breaking the blind.

23.4 Ethical Issues

Blinding is an important part of study validity, and should be implemented whenever possible, even when this involves extra study costs or time. There must be adequate methods to assure that the blind is maintained throughout the study to preserve study integrity.

The use of placebos raises several ethical issues, which are discussed in Section 19.2. If a current standard of care exists, it should generally be used for control groups. This should be the best treatment available, even if this creates difficulties in maintaining a blinded study. In all cases, the participants must be informed in clear, direct language that they are not guaranteed to receive the new treatment, and if placebo is an alternative, they may not be getting any active treatment at all.

It is unethical for the study staff to try to guess or otherwise find out what treatment the participants are receiving in a blinded study, or to encourage the participants to guess at their treatment or respond to pointed questions unless such guesses are anticipated in the study design and systematically collected at the end of the study as part of the study procedures.

KEY POINTS

- Blinding of treatment may be done in several ways:
  - using placebos that are identical in appearance to the active drug;
  - if different drugs are being compared, using a placebo for each;
  - giving each participant a combination of active drug and placebo in studies comparing different doses of the same medications; and
  - giving dummy changes to everyone when changes in medication are necessary, or giving dummy changes according to a randomized schedule of changes.
- Provision of treatment in a blinded study may be done in several ways:
  - the drug manufacturer may create packets with the appropriate medications identified by the randomization number;
  - the institutional pharmacist may keep the randomization schedule and prepare the appropriate medications; and
  - the allocation may be done within the study group by a person who is not involved in evaluation of the participants.
- The protocol must include methods to protect information linking the participant to the intervention.
- Documents that contain information about the blinding must be kept in a locked cabinet.

- Computerized data must be password protected and meet all other security requirements set by your institution.
- Problems with maintaining the blind that may occur in a blinded study include:
  - side effects of the medication;
  - obvious efficacy; and
  - leaks and guesses.

24

Adherence and Compliance

You, the investigator, want the participants to comply with your study procedures, which involves coming back for study visits as scheduled and participating fully in every assessment, and may involve taking medications at home in an appropriate manner for an extended period of time. The participant, however, decides whether to follow your requests or not. Following these requests is called "adherence to the protocol." You have no real control over whether or not the participant adheres to the study protocol, or even ever returns for another study visit. Thus, you need to define what participant adherence actually means for the study, how you will measure it, and what is "good enough." Then you need to implement procedures to maximize participant adherence. If you cannot obtain reasonable adherence to the protocol, you may be unable to interpret the results of the study. We focused on a critical component of adherence, retaining participants, in Section 13.4, and here we focus on other aspects of adherence. As retention is such a critical component of adherence, however, we also briefly discuss methods to improve retention of participants in this chapter as well.

24.1 Efficacy versus Effectiveness

In the simplest possible case, you give a single dose of an intervention under direct observation and wait to observe the change in some measure within a participant. With a single dose of an IV infusion, what happens if a participant wants the infusion stopped in the middle, or has a reaction to it? First, you have to stop the infusion immediately. Second, you have to include the adverse reaction in the results of the study, since all safety problems need to be identified and reported. But what do you do about any outcome measures? If you exclude this participant's results on the outcome measures from the results of the study, you would be assessing efficacy: the effect of the intervention in those who followed the study protocol. If you include the participant's results, despite getting only a partial dose of the infusion, you would be assessing effectiveness: the effect of the intervention in the entire population in the study, whether they received the full infusion or not.

Efficacy assesses the actual biological effect of the intervention on the outcome. Thus, participants who do not get the full intervention are excluded from the analysis. Before an intervention can be thought to be potentially useful, efficacy has to be demonstrated. If there is not a biological effect, then the intervention cannot have a real benefit. However, efficacy alone is not enough. Even when an intervention is efficacious when used properly, if participants and later patients will not use the intervention because of tolerability or convenience issues, then the intervention will not be effective. Effectiveness measures how useful an intervention will be in actual practice.

Example 24A: You are studying an existing therapy for the treatment of a new indication. You recruit 10 participants with the condition for your study. One problem, already known about the therapy, is that it tastes awful. Among your 10 participants, 3 take the medicine with every meal, as they are supposed to, and all 3 of them show substantial clinical improvement of the condition. This suggests that the therapy is efficacious for the condition. The other 7 participants, however, take the medicine irregularly, or stop after one or two doses, because of the horrible taste. These 7 participants show little or no clinical improvement. Overall, then, the effectiveness of this medicine is rather poor.

This has implications on how you consider describing your intervention. For efficacy, you would be focusing on those who are adherent with the intervention. These participants use or take the intervention reliably, follow the instructions for use reliably, and in general would be considered good participants. You would use what is sometimes termed a "per protocol" analysis, summarizing the outcome only in those participants who followed a set of prespecified criteria. These criteria do not mean that the participants have to be perfect, however. For many oral medications, missing no more than 1 in 5 doses, so adherence is at least 80%, is considered good adherence. However, this level of adherence might be considered very low for some illnesses.

Example 24B: You are studying a new medication regimen for patients who are HIV positive who have failed multiple previous therapeutic regimens and are currently not virally suppressed. The new medication regimen needs to be taken twice a day, based on pharmacokinetic data, and is very intolerant to missed doses. In an early study seeking to show that the medicine can work, you would focus on the efficacy of the regimen in participants who adhere to the protocol. Thus, you might require at least 95% adherence for a participant to be considered adherent, so you would only include participants who took the medicine every day, twice a day, missing less than 1 dose every 10 days, when you analyze the results.

The initial studies were very promising, with remarkable efficacy in this population. Thus, an effectiveness study was begun.

Example 24C: Another study with the same medication regime as in Example 24B evaluated the effectiveness of the medication. Therefore, outcomes were analyzed for all participants, whether or not they took the medication regimen regularly or reliably. Furthermore, as is common in many studies of effectiveness in HIV medications, if participants did not complete the study, they were assumed to be failures, so that effectiveness would be conservatively measured.

24.2 Adherence: How Is It Assessed?

Adherence is a relatively new term, replacing the older term of "compliance" to describe participants' behavior with respect to the protocol requirements. Compliance seemed to indicate a passive role for the participant in letting the study personnel do things to them. Adherence includes the actions and responsibilities of the participant as part of the study team. Adherence is assessed for all aspects of the study protocol, to assure that the participant is using the intervention as it is supposed to be used and participating in other protocol activities. As the investigator, you would like participants to be perfectly adherent. This includes

- following timing and dosage regimens faithfully;
- recording information as required, such as recording reactions to the treatment, food intake diaries, exercise activities, etc.;
- participating in specific activities, e.g., exercise classes, during the treatment period;
- attending all clinic visits; and
- participating fully in all evaluations designed to assess the effectiveness of the treatment.

As you realize that no one is perfect, you need to set minimum standards for what would be considered acceptable adherence. The first aspect of adherence would seem simple to assess: Are participants adhering to the study treatment or not? But even in the simplest case, when you are directly observing whether the participant follows the treatment, defining acceptable adherence is often quite difficult.

Example 24D: In a study to assess the effects of an exercise program, participants are supposed to exercise three times a week, under supervision, for twelve weeks. Thus, a participant should attend a total of 36 exercise sessions. As the investigator you need to consider what you would consider adequate participation to demonstrate the benefits of the intervention. Is it a minimum number of sessions, such as 24 sessions over 12 weeks, which could be 3 sessions a week for 8 of the 12 weeks and nothing for the last 4 weeks, or is it a minimum number of weeks with at least 2 sessions?

In Example 24D, it is simply the presence at an exercise session that is being considered to define adherence. But exercise programs require more than mere presence to have an impact on the participant. It might appear that having the research assistants involved in the training program determine how actively the participant is involved would be useful. However, doing so means that the research assistants would have to make a judgment about the participant's effort (the participant is trying or not), which would be subjective at best. More importantly, it is not clear how such assessments could then be used in the exercise program, without risk of coercing the participant to try harder.

Assessing treatment adherence is even more difficult when participants are not being directly observed, which typically is the case.

Example 24A (continued): The medication with the terrible taste must be taken regularly and, in accordance with the treatment instruction, with meals. Traditionally, the amount of medication taken is assessed by counting how much remains at a study visit. You must define how often medication needs to be taken for the participant to be considered adherent to the therapy. In addition, you must implement procedures to assess whether the participant is taking the medication with meals. A simple way to do this is with a medication diary, recording when and under what circumstances the medication is taken. There are also special medication bottles that record when a pill is taken out of them. Finally, a periodic text message asking when the participant last took the medication and if it was with a meal would be useful if this is acceptable to the participant.

Pill counts are often used to assess whether a participant is taking the medication. Unfortunately, a correct pill count is not necessarily an indication of adherence to a dosage schedule. The participant could forget to take a pill one day and, in order not to upset anyone, just throw that pill away. Similarly, a participant can record that the medication is taken with meals, even if it was not. For some interventions it is possible to use periodic tests of drug levels in the blood to determine if the right amounts have been taken, but this is yet another test for the participant. This requires that the expected levels of drug in the blood be well established and that individual variation be taken into account.

If the participant is required to supply information about activities or events that are not directed by the protocol, such as a food diary or exercise plan, then it is difficult to assess the accuracy and timeliness of the information.

Example 24E: In a study of the use of a new statin for cardiac health, participants are asked to fill out a weekly food diary. There are two problems: one is that the participants may not remember what they ate on any particular day; and another that the participants may report what they think they should have eaten rather than be embarrassed about or scolded for what they really did eat.

Adherence to the clinic schedule is relatively simple to assess: either a participant returns or does not return as scheduled. But there are complications even in this simple dichotomy.

Example 24F: In a study of a treatment for HIV infection, viral load is measured every 12 weeks during the study, with target windows of plus or minus 4 weeks; that is, the week 24 visit should occur between weeks 20 and 28 after enrollment, and the week 36 visit should occur between weeks 32 and 40. When a participant comes at week 30, rules need to specify how to determine if this data is used for the week 24 visit or the week 36 visit or neither, and whether the visit is considered adherent for either visit.

Many procedures for assessing results of the intervention require that the participant do something. How do you assess whether the participant is actually engaged, trying as hard as possible, or just going through the motions?

Example 24G: In a study of a new treatment to reverse muscle wasting, the study will assess the effect of the treatment using 10-meter walk time and time rising from a chair, two standard measures of physical performance. It is quite hard to assess whether a participant is trying as hard as possible to perform the tasks, particularly as such a study is being done in participants who have trouble doing these tasks. Thus, this aspect of adherence cannot be reliably assessed.

This situation is similar to that in Example 24D in that it might be desirable for the rater to judge the participant's efforts. Usually, however, no attempt is made to do so, and the results, whatever they are, are taken as the participant's best effort.

24.3 Overall Measures to Improve Adherence

Although it may seem trite, the most important factor in participant adherence is the relationship between the participants and the study personnel who interact with the participants. When study personnel are supportive and encouraging of participants, the participants are more likely to fully commit to participating in the study. Partially, this reflects individual personalities, but some factors seem to be common to the best study personnel. Most importantly, effective study personnel are actively interested in the participants themselves, not just as participants in a study but as whole people, with lives outside the study. We have observed some of the best study personnel making notes after participant visits about non-study material – the participant's plans for vacation, family events, and so forth – and reviewing these notes prior to the next visit to reinforce the personal relationship with each participant.

Effective study personnel are not feigning interest in the participant – they are interested in the people as people, recognizing that they happen to be participating in the study. The study personnel are not focusing their interest on retaining the participant. Rather, the participant's adherence is a by-product of the study staffs' interest in them as people. We have seen coordinators visibly distressed after visits when participants are having problems in their personal life. The staff you have working with participants – and your own attitude toward participants if you are working with them directly – seems to matter far more than almost anything else you might do to enhance participant adherence.

There are, however, some basic things that might help with participant adherence by making it either easier for the participant to adhere or less likely for the participant to fail to adhere by chance. These can be considered standard features which should be incorporated into any study when possible.

First, both the duration of the study and the demands of the study on participants need to be minimized as far as possible. These are related: the longer you want a participant to remain in a study, the easier it has to be for the participant to adhere to the study requirements. Many exercise studies are relatively intense (three or more exercise sessions a week under the supervision of an investigator) but also relatively short (4 to 12 weeks). Longer exercise studies often allow participants to exercise when convenient at a facility of their own choosing, making the exercise component less standard, but improving retention compared to a

more standardized exercise program that required participants to visit
the study site three times a week.

Second, are all the measurements being made actually needed? We
are not talking about how many assays are done on a blood specimen,
but about how many tubes of blood need to be drawn at visits. More
tubes increases the time a participant must spend at a visit. This especially applies to questionnaires and interviews, where "just one more
question" seems like a small and reasonable idea to an investigator –
even when the questionnaires can take more than three hours to complete. It is unlikely that all the information is essential. The reality is that
almost certainly some of this data will never be analyzed.

Third, each procedure in the study should be as simple as possible
for the participant. For a study where weight is an outcome measure
(such as a weight loss study), is the requirement to change to a hospital
gown multiple times worthwhile? It will reduce the variability in the
measurement which allows the sample size to be smaller. The increase in
retention by measuring weight in normal street clothes without shoes,
however, might more than compensate for the increase in sample size.

Example 24H. Participants in a diet and exercise study are asked to
complete a three day food and exercise diary once a month, each month
between study visits, which can be as much as six months apart. Rather
than giving a participant all the diaries at a visit, the investigator sends
the food and exercise diary to the participant each month with a postage-paid envelope as a way of reminding the participant about this and
making it convenient for the participant to return it. An alternative, if
allowed by the Institutional Review Board (IRB), would be to have a
web-based or app-based data collection system, so that reminders about
the diaries and the data collection would be even easier for participants.
Study staff contact participants two weeks after the material was sent out
if it had not been completed to encourage the participant to complete
the material if they were willing to, but also to encourage the participant
to continue in the study even if they did not have time to complete the
form this month.

Example 24H illustrates how considering everything that you hope
the participants will do for you, and thinking creatively about how

to make it as easy as possible for the participant to adhere, can make adherence less difficult for the participants, likely increasing adherence to the demands of the study.

24.4 Measures to Improve Retention in the Study

In addition to the attitude of study personnel to participants, there are a host of adaptations of study procedures that can improve participant adherence, especially with return visits. Reminding participants of upcoming visits should always be done if the participant allows for this contact. Participants, just like everyone reading this book, are busy, and sometimes people do just forget. After missing an appointment, some participants might dropout rather than be embarrassed about forgetting an appointment. Having evening or weekend appointments whenever a participant needs that accommodation and making arrangements for child care when requested will also improve retention. Without these accommodations, if may be quite hard for some participants to remain in the study.

Helping with transportation to and from the clinic, such as bus passes and taxi vouchers when needed, can increase retention. It might seem that reimbursing participants after the fact for their transportation expenses is perfectly reasonable and ensures that these expenses are justified. We recognize that if bus passes are provided in advanced a few might be misused, but we also know that for some participants these costs are just another small hurdle which makes returning for a study visit just a little bit too hard.

Study visits should be scheduled in such a way that participants should not have to wait a long time to see study staff. If participants arrive on schedule, then the wait should be minimal. Ideally a staff member would greet the participant by name as the participant is arriving at the registration desk, waits while they register, and then takes them to a room to start the visit.

Regular contact with participants, particularly checking in with them between visits when the visits are months apart, can help keep participants from being lost to follow-up. Some suggestions for maintaining regular contact are described in Section 13.4, as are some other methods for encouraging retention in the study.

24.5 Ethical Issues

To be ethical, a study should provide results that are credible and useful to the target population. If not, then the study is a waste of the participant's time and effort. When considering adherence with the treatment regimen, the difference between efficacy and effectiveness must be kept at the forefront of all analyses and interpretations. If you are requiring a certain level of adherence of participants for remaining in the study and including them in the analysis, then you really must recognize, and any reports you make of the study must specify, that you are considering efficacy in a potentially very select and special group of individuals. Providing extensive support to your participants to adhere to the treatment regimen may lead to very good efficacy, but such support is rarely provided to patients in general clinical practice, so claims about how effective the therapy would be in general practice are unwarranted. On the other hand, if you do not make any effort to enhance adherence to the treatment regimen and the results of the study show a lack of efficacy, then this may be because the demands of the protocol are too onerous for general use, but may also be because the participants were not given a reasonable level of encouragement.

There is a slippery slope between encouraging participants to return and almost coercing them to return for a visit by playing on their guilt for not doing their part. We have seen investigators and study staff sliding down this slope on several occasions without being aware of what was happening until it was pointed out to them. Similarly, there is a difference between encouraging a participant on an assessment by saying, "You did great and I'm sure you can do it again for the repeat measurement" and saying, "Good work, but I'm sure you could do better next time," which is judgmental.

You cannot force a participant to adhere to the protocol. If refusal to comply may endanger the participant's health, then you must do what you can to find a way for the participant to ease out of the protocol, such as tapering the medication until it can be safely discontinued.

KEY POINTS

- You cannot force a participant to adhere to the protocol.
- Although you want participants to adhere to your study requirements, it is up to the participants whether they will adhere or not.
- The distinction between efficacy and effectiveness is critical when planning and interpreting a study.
- If you provide support to help participants adhere to the treatment regimen, and limit analyses to those who are adherent, you must recognize that you are assessing efficacy in what may be a very select and special group of participants.
- There are multiple methods to help improve adherence and to encourage participants to try hard when doing assessments, but it is important to be aware of how you can cross from being encouraging to becoming coercive.
- If a participant wants to discontinue the study, you must ensure that this is done safely.

Part V

ADDITIONAL CONCEPTS FOR OBSERVATIONAL STUDIES

25

Defining Populations for Cohort Studies

Chapter 6 presented an overview of cohort studies, which are observational studies of the relationship between exposures and outcomes in a specific population. Part of the study design is determining what population should be studied, the availability and quality of information about the cohort, and, for prospective studies, the potential for long-term follow-up. These are more general concepts than the specific inclusion and exclusion criteria that are described in Chapter 12, which addresses individual characteristics. We start by discussing a study with a single cohort. The principles apply to a study with multiple cohorts as well, which is discussed in the last section.

25.1 Data Availability

In addition to defining detailed criteria for inclusion or exclusion of individuals in the protocol, it is important to think in general terms about the population in which you are interested. In most studies you will be collecting data over some interval of time. It may be historical data for a retrospective study or follow-up data for a prospective study. Perhaps you are interested in following a population with a specific disease who attend your clinic. You propose a prospective study where you will follow individuals and collect data over time. The key issue is whether these participants can be followed for the required interval of time. What follow-up mechanisms need to be in place to achieve this? Will participants be expected to be seen on a regular schedule by medical personnel as part of their regular care? How much of the information that is required for the study will be available from regular care, and what evaluations must be done specifically as part of the study protocol?

Example 25A: Investigators wished to do a 5-year follow-up study of women who have gestational diabetes to determine if they will develop metabolic abnormalities after the delivery. The women are in a special high-risk pregnancy program and, as part of the program, are expected to visit a clinic 6 months after delivery for a follow-up examination, including an oral glucose tolerance test, and then annually after that. This center is treating an immigrant population, which is very mobile, and the expected loss to follow-up, even for the first follow-up evaluation, is high. To improve the follow-up, as part of the protocol, the investigators proposed to employ a bilingual research assistant to call patients and remind them of their appointments and ask if they can help with any problems. The women were also asked to supply the name of another individual who should be able to reach them in case they moved or changed phone numbers.

In a retrospective study, the key issue is whether the information required for the study can be retrieved from existing data. This means that not only the exposures and outcomes but also potential confounding variables must be available. In most studies the availability of information varies with the individual, but in some populations and for some data items there may be special problems obtaining information that must be considered in the design.

Example 25B: Investigators studying risk factors for cardiac disease know that family history is an important contributor to risk. However, there is often a problem obtaining accurate family history for some populations. For immigrant populations from less developed countries, family members may not have been tested or diagnosed. Moreover, if the family members are not in this country, little may be known about their past. In addition, in all populations, some illnesses are considered shameful and not discussed.

Before any data can be extracted, it is important to ensure that both Institutional Review Board (IRB) approval is obtained (Section 2.3) and the requirements for patient privacy are met (Section 2.1.2).

25.1.1 Data Sources

Data may be obtained from existing sources or collected during the course of the study. Existing resources include, but are not limited to, information from the participant, hospital or clinic records, public health records (such as death certificates), private physician records, teachers, or school counselors. Often a family member or someone close to the participant can provide relevant information. This person is often referred to as the "best informant." Institutional records are a good resource for many studies. Many retrospective studies have used data from large community-based medical centers with stable populations, such as the Mayo Clinic in Rochester, Minnesota, which is known for excellent tracking of and record keeping about its patients. Health Maintenance Organizations, such as Kaiser Permanente, also provide a valuable resource for longitudinal observation studies, such as cohort studies, for investigators with access to their database. Other sources include the Veterans Administration, larger secondary and tertiary health centers, and public records of births and deaths.

Example 25C: Investigators want to study the effect of repeated fever in young children on growth in later life. They work at a large regional health center that serves most of the residents in an area and maintains a database on all patients. The population is relatively stable. Therefore, the investigators believe they can get adequate and complete information from the institution's electronic medical records.

Prospective studies often begin with current or historical information, and then continue collecting information from interviews, tests, and from new medical records when the participant allows access.

25.1.2 Stratified Sampling

Stratified sampling, also known as targeted sampling, is a method used to acquire a cohort with specific characteristics, usually demographic. The purpose is generally to create a cohort that is more similar to the general population than would be expected through random, untargeted samples, and thus improve the generalizability of your study (Section 11.1).

The investigator must first define what important subgroups exist in the target population and what percent of the total population they represent. Then a plan must be developed to enroll participants from the different groups in the same proportions into the study.

Example 25C (continued): The investigators will not use the total population, which is very large, but will take a sample of 3,000 participants. They would like this cohort to have the same ethnic and sex composition as the total population; therefore, they will ask the data management personnel to identify the group membership of each participant, then select a specified number of children at random within each ethnic group.

In Example 25C the method of achieving the targeted sample was straightforward; however, if you are recruiting participants from the public, some populations are more likely to volunteer to participate than others are. Therefore, you may have to make an extra effort to recruit from some of the targeted groups. Methods for reaching specific populations are described in Section 13.3.

25.2 Quality of Information

Information for either retrospective or prospective studies can come from several sources. In a retrospective study investigators are dependent on historical data. In a prospective study you may also do some of the assessments yourself as part of the study, but you could make use of other sources to reduce costs, reduce the burden on the staff and participants of the study, and possibly save some time. Of course, when the assessments are part of the protocol, they will be done with precision and care as described in Chapters 14 and 29. However, many or all of the assessment methods may not be under your control, and so as part of the planning, you should evaluate the quality of information you can get.

There are several questions that can be asked about information obtained from others. What method was used to obtain the data? For example, were glucose measurements obtained from a laboratory blood sample or a monitoring device? What methods were used to assay hormone samples? If the result was reported as a coded category rather than as original data, what were the criteria for coding? How exactly was a diagnosis made, since standards may change over time? What standards were applied to define overweight and obese when the data was collected?

Things become much more complicated when considering physical exposure measurements. It is often not clear how the exposure was measured and how the findings were reported. Sometimes exposure can be recorded as a simple yes or no response, but at other times there may be different levels of exposure, which may not be clear in the records. Exposure may be identified as the appearance of symptoms, but what symptoms are recorded? What about the time period for continuing exposures? These could be reported as a cross-sectional measurement of exposure at a specific time point, cumulative exposure over a given time interval, or peak exposure during a specific time period.

Example 25D: In a cohort study of mortality and cancer morbidity in workers manufacturing specific chemicals for the rubber industry, to be in the cohort the workers had to have a minimum employment period of 6 months and have had some employment during a specified period. The exposure level for one of the chemicals was calculated for each job and department title by calculating the average exposure for several periods. The cumulative exposure was calculated by computing the product of duration of time on a specific job and the average exposure and then summing these over the time the worker was employed.

You must consider how reliable the information is. There are often problems with recall bias, in which the recall may be affected by subsequent events (Section 17.1.4), or just poor recall, particularly of repetitive events.

Example 25A (continued): The women were asked if they had gestational diabetes in prior pregnancies. However, sometimes they were not tested, either because that was not the practice where they had the earlier delivery or they did not have any predelivery care. Although investigators believe the size of the infant provides a clue about gestational diabetes, often this information is not very accurate. A woman may not have a feel for the relative size of the baby, particularly if it is her first. Also, not all countries have birth certificates with length and weight recorded, so the mother's knowledge of these measurements might not be accurate.

Example 25E: In a study of a chronic episodic disease, the participant is often asked how many prior episodes they have had. If there were many, then the exact number may not be known. Often investigators prefer to recode the results cutting off at the limit of expected reliable recall, such as none, 1, 2, 3, 4, and more than 4.

Because the information in existing records is not under your control, you need to determine whether the data will be of good enough quality to use for a study (Section 9.1.2). If a data item is missing for a large number of participants, it may be better to exclude it from the analysis or try the analysis with and without this variable. There are statistical methods for handling these problems, but the amount of missing data may still diminish the credibility of the study, and the consequences must be considered. You may choose to analyze participants with complete data as a separate subgroup, but often these participants are different from the rest of the cohort in other ways, so that you cannot generalize conclusions from this subgroup to the entire cohort. If missing data is a problem, you should, if possible, consult with a statistician about how to approach the problem.

Example 25A (continued): An investigator may think that potential participants who lack important information about their medical history or who might be difficult to retain in the study should be excluded. However, these women may have differences in their diet and amount of exercise compared to women with more access to medical care in general and to prenatal care in particular. As diet and exercise are believed to be important in glucose metabolism, limiting the analysis only to mothers with reliable information would potentially bias the results of the study.

25.3 Study Time Line

In an interventional study, participants are entered into the study after they are screened; that is the entry date, and the assessments for the study and the intervention are conducted on or after that date. In a cohort study, there is also an entry date, often preceded by a screening process, but even in a prospective study some of the exposures of interest may have occurred before the entry date. In a retrospective study, all of the exposures will have occurred and been assessed before the date the study begins, so that the entry date refers to a time in the past.

The exit date for the study should also be defined. It may be an exact date or based on a time following the exposure or entry date. Some very large prospective studies, such as the Framingham Heart Study, are open-ended; that is participants are followed at some level throughout their lifetime and subsequent generations may also be followed. In many cohort studies, the exit date is defined to be either the occurrence of a specific event or a given number of years in the study. Often in retrospective studies the exit date will be before the study starts. Many of these studies require that special analytic techniques, known generally as survival analysis, be used.

Example 25F: In a prospective study of patients who presented at a hospital center with acute myocardial infarction (MI), the investigators wished to study the effect of different treatments as well as demographic and other medical diagnoses on the patient's health in the five years after the acute MI. Participants were enrolled at some time after they entered the hospital, but the study was considered to have begun on the day they presented with the MI. Participants were followed until they had another cardiac event (defined in the protocol), death by any cause, or for 5 years after presenting with the MI.

The frequency and timing of measurements during the study period should be defined. Sometimes it is not only the timing of measurements individually but the timing of an exposure relative to an outcome that is critical. If so, you must determine whether the exposure was measured at the right time for the outcome of interest.

Example 25G: The effect of exposures during pregnancy may differ depending on when they occur during the pregnancy. A lack of folic acid affects development in the first trimester, but not usually in subsequent trimesters. Note that here the "exposure" refers to a deficiency: the lack of enough folic acid. Later in the pregnancy, other exposures, such as maternal smoking, may affect development.

25.4 Multiple Cohort Studies

The simplest cohort study includes only a single group of participants, and the relationships between exposures and outcomes are examined for the total group. But a study may have multiple cohorts, in which comparisons may be done both within and between cohorts or just between cohorts. These types of studies are often called "comparative cohort studies." The cohorts have the same entry criteria except for the variable of interest. If the cohorts are to be matched, then one group must be identified as the index group, and the other groups matched to the index group. The cohorts may be matched either individually or on frequency. Matching in observational studies is discussed in Chapter 27.

A comparative cohort study may be used to assess the effect of an exposure when an interventional study is not possible. In this design, one group would consist of participants who have had the exposure of interest; the other group would consist of participants who were similar to the first group in all important factors except the exposure. Thus, the non-exposed group would serve as a control group for the study of the exposure. Usually the cohorts are matched, with the index cohort being the group of exposed participants. In a sense, this design is similar to the case-control design, but in the case-control design groups are defined by outcome rather than by exposure as done in the comparative cohort study. Like the case-control design, there can be more than one control group (non-exposed group in the comparative cohort study; without the outcome in the case-control study).

Example 25H: Investigators used a comparative cohort design to investigate whether exposure to benzene, even at concentrations below the current limit on exposure, would have harmful effects on blood cells. They identified a cohort of workers in a shoe factory where they were exposed to low levels of benzene. The comparison cohort was comprised of workers with similar demographic characteristics who worked in a clothing factory and had never had any known exposure to benzene.

Other comparative cohort studies do not select on exposure, but on some other characteristics, such as ethnicity, to see if the relationships between exposures and outcomes are the same in all groups. In these studies the groups are often analyzed separately and then the exposure-outcome relationships found in individual cohorts compared between cohorts.

Example 25I: Investigators have prior evidence that specific alleles of certain genes may be associated with a tendency to develop alcoholism. There is also some data suggesting that both the rate of occurrence of the allele and the effect of the allele on alcoholism may be different in Mexican Americans than in non-Hispanic Caucasian groups. Therefore, the investigators planned a study of two cohorts of males in the age range of 20–55 years of age. One cohort would be identified as Mexican American and the other as non-Hispanic Caucasian, based on the origin of both sets of grandparents. The rate of alcoholism and the response to certain chemical challenges related to alcohol metabolism were measured in participants with and without each specific allele and compared both within each cohort and between cohorts, while the prevalence of the alleles was compared only between cohorts.

More complex designs may be seen in some of the very large prospective cohort studies, such as the extensions to the Framingham Heart Study which has become a multigenerational cohort study. There may be several cohorts and subcohorts selected within the total sample population, as well as nested case-control studies (Section 26.3.2) within the total study.

25.5 Ethical Issues

The ethical issues associated with cohort studies are covered in detail in Section 6.5. Although you are not doing an interventional study, you must first have your study approved by your IRB, determine if an informed consent is needed from the participants or it is waived, and whether there are privacy rule concerns before you begin your research. If so, they must be resolved before any data can be released to you. As in any study, you need to preserve the participant's confidentiality.

If you do have contact with an individual, it costs time and effort for the participant to provide the information, and this should be kept to a minimum. There is also a potential for distress due to being asked to recall difficult memories. On occasion, you may need to contact someone other than the participant, such as a relative or close friend, to provide information on a deceased participant. Again there is a concern that the study will cause distress to these individuals as well as possible violations of the deceased's privacy.

KEY POINTS

- IRB approval or waiver is required before beginning the research.
- In a prospective study the population must be accessible for follow-up for the required period of time.
- Exposure and outcome data for the population must be available from existing records or must be collected during the study.
- The data must be reliable and must be adequate for the intended purposes.
- The timing of study entry, exit, and measurements during the study must be specified.
- Comparative cohort studies are used in two ways:
  - to compare results between exposed and unexposed participants; and
  - to compare results in different groups with selection on characteristics other than exposure.
- An informed consent and release of protected health information may be required from individual participants.

26

Participants in Case-Control Studies

Case-control studies are designed to assess whether there is a link between one or more exposures and a particular outcome. The purpose of the control group is to determine whether this exposure is equally common in individuals without the outcome compared to individuals with the outcome. The study must do this without introducing bias or potential confounding that could either mask or accentuate the relationship. Ideally, individuals would be controls only if they would have been included as cases if they had the outcome of interest. Often it is desirable to have more than one control group, selected in different ways, to provide more convincing evidence for the relationship.

26.1 Identifying Cases and Controls

26.1.1 General Considerations

Both cases and controls must be selected according to inclusion and exclusion criteria. The criteria will be the same between the groups, with the exception of the outcome. There should be a great deal of confidence that the cases have the outcome of interest. This can usually be ascertained through records and physicians' referrals. Equally important, there should be no evidence that the controls have the outcome of interest. This may be determined by an interview with the potential control, but sometimes controls must be tested to confirm that they do not have the outcome of interest. Moreover, it is critical that there be no other differences between the groups that would bias the results. The potential for deliberate or subconscious bias is particularly strong in case-control studies because the outcome is known. Even if bias is not intended, it may be present when cases and controls are obtained from different populations.

When there are multiple control groups, the criteria that define the different control groups will include a specific criterion for each of the control groups in addition to the general control criteria.

26.1.2 Identifying Cases

Cases are defined by specific inclusion and exclusion criteria (Chapter 12). For some studies, cases may be identified by appealing to the general public for volunteers with the outcome of interest. Methods include mass mailings, advertisements in the media, or posters in selected sites, such as senior centers, day care centers, clinics, religious organizations, and the like. This may be the best way to identify potential participants if the outcome of interest is not one that would be recorded in a clinical or public record. The disadvantage of this method of identifying cases is that you may have to screen many individuals to get even one individual who fits the criteria for being a case in the study.

Example 26A: To study the effect of certain foods on the development of osteoarthritis (OA), investigators placed advertisements for individuals with OA in several local newspapers. It was not clearly specified that the condition had to have been medically diagnosed, so they were flooded by responses from people with some kind of pain in their joints, hoping for a free consultation. Even after the specification of medical diagnosis of OA was added to the advertisement, there were many calls from individuals who did not meet this basic criterion for cases.

When the outcome being studied is a condition that is likely to be underreported, such as drug or alcohol dependency or childhood sexual abuse, then a general call may be the best way to recruit participants. Recruitment through support groups and rehabilitation programs is possible, but this would only identify a subset of the population. Although confidentiality is required in all studies (Section 2.1.2), it is a particularly sensitive issue for these participants, and the text of the advertisement should emphasize that privacy will be respected. Sometimes it is possible to get special authorization to guarantee confidentiality to participants even from mandatory legal disclosure; your local Institutional Review Board (IRB) will be able to give you more information about this, which is termed a "certificate of confidentiality" in the United States.

You may introduce some bias with a general appeal because the people who respond may be different from the general population with the condition, particularly if the media used reaches only a specific population. There may also be a problem obtaining adequate, reliable records for ascertaining some of the study exposures.

Example 26A (continued): The investigators worked in an area with a large immigrant population. Therefore, they placed the advertisements in several different foreign-language newspapers as well as English-language newspapers. Because they required medical records to confirm the diagnosis, the investigators had to exclude many individuals who had recently arrived in the country and did not have any records of their medical history.

Most investigators prefer to identify cases through health care providers. This can include individual physicians who treat patients with the condition, as well as clinics or hospitals. Potential cases identified in this way are more likely to have the condition of interest. Moreover, these individuals are more likely to have records of medical problems and treatment available. If the participant is recruited through a hospital or clinic, normally there will have to be institutional approval of the record screening (either for this specific study or as a general policy that patients have already allowed their records to be used for medical research). The investigators will normally provide material for the health care provider to give to patients, which specifies that the patients are under no obligation to participate and should contact the investigators directly if they wish to participate. IRB approval of the precise material the health care provider will forward to potential cases is required, and for advertisements in general, in addition to IRB approval of the study itself. The investigators will have to obtain informed consent as necessary and must protect the privacy of the individual in accordance with government regulations (Section 2.1.2) for protecting patient privacy. More detail on recruiting participants is given in Chapter 13.

Public records, such as birth or death certificates, registries, and health surveillance files, can provide a large pool of potential participants, but the information may be limited and it may be necessary to find other sources to complete the exposure information. Most of these public records are computerized, and investigators can obtain access under specific conditions, but usually the identification of the participant is not included, which may be a problem if you need more data.

Example 26B: In a case-control study of non-Hodgkin's lymphoma, cases were identified from the area's rapid case ascertainment system and from monthly surveillance, epidemiology, and end results program abstracts. This should represent virtually all cases in the area. These systems allowed cases to be contacted through their primary health care provider. After consenting to participation, a subset of cases had their diagnosis verified by an independent review of the pathology.

Another source of cases is laboratory specimens, including autopsies. This would of course not require consent from the participant, but you may have to contact family members if additional information is needed, which may present disclosure issues as well. Another disadvantage is that the specimens needed may only be available for a limited time or cannot be found.

Example 26C: To study the activation of microglia cells in sepsis, the investigators used data from brain autopsies of 170 patients who had died in their hospital during a 4-year period and had given permission for the use of their autopsy material in research at some time prior to death. All individuals who had material for further testing, and did not have evidence of confounding diseases such as CNS disease or some dementias, were selected as potential cases or controls. There were 36 individuals in this pool. Cases were those who were determined to have sepsis, based on clinical and laboratory hospital records and post-mortem cultures of spleen, kidney, or lung, providing a total of 13 cases.

26.1.3 Identifying Controls

Controls may be identified from any of the sources noted above. In many ways the identification of controls is more difficult than the identification of cases. Ideally, the controls should represent the same population as the cases and satisfy the same inclusion and exclusion criteria as the cases, with the exception of the outcome. Although there may be exceptions in special circumstances, in general you would want as potential controls only people who would be identified as potential cases if they had the disease.

In practice, when cases are identified through a health care provider, there are advantages to identifying controls from the same population – that is, people who are being seen at the same facility for a health condition at the same level of seriousness. This will generally make other participant characteristics more comparable.

Example 26D: Example 7C described a study to determine if lack of exercise is associated with the onset of Type II diabetes in adults younger than 40 years. Cases were identified and recruited from the diabetes clinic in a public hospital. Controls would be matched (Chapter 27) to the cases on sex and age within 5 years. Since the investigators wanted the controls to be identifiable as cases if they had the disease, they wanted to select as controls individuals who used the hospital for their own medical care as well. One possible control group was patients in other clinics in the hospital. Because they were using the hospital for one condition, it is likely that they would use it for other conditions as well. Thus, they would have been identified as cases if they were detected with diabetes. Such individuals would likely be similar to the cases in terms of income, education, access to care, and so forth. However, they all have some other condition, and these other conditions might be associated with exercise or lack of exercise as well. Another possible control group is parents of children being treated in the hospital clinics. Such individuals are likely to use the hospital for their own care, and would likely be similar in overall demographic factors, access to care, general knowledge, and health behaviors as patients in hospital clinics, so that they would have been identified as cases if they had diabetes.

However, using controls from a facility or practice is not always appropriate.

Example 26A (continued): As cases were recruited through community resources and advertisements in newspapers in different languages, this would be the appropriate method for identifying controls as well. For this study, which was investigating food groups, a major potential confounding factor would be ethnic group. Thus, the controls would need to be recruited with an ethnic distribution similar to that of the cases.

Controls need to represent participants who have the same chance to be included in the study as the cases do.

Example 26D (continued): Several commonly used control groups would be inappropriate for this diabetes study. Sometimes investigators use individuals who are employed at the hospital and are free of diabetes or related diseases as controls, as such controls are usually easy to obtain. However, there were many potential confounders between the cases and this potential control group. The potential control group had a higher income, were better educated, and had access to better medical care, as well as potentially a healthier diet and more awareness of the importance of exercise. Another possible control group would be individuals recruited from the general population of the catchment area for their hospital. However, such a control group might differ in terms of income, education, and access to medical care from the cases who actually use the hospital. Thus, neither of these groups would be appropriate controls for this study, since neither group was likely to have the same chance of being identified as a case if they had diabetes.

In addition, the availability and reliability of records for the controls should be equivalent to that of the cases. If these conditions can be met, then cases and controls need not come from the same source. You may, for example, identify cases from a registry but recruit controls from the general population from which the registry is drawn.

Example 26B (continued): In this study, cases were identified from public records that were created to cover the area defined by the rapid case ascertainment system. Thus, controls had to be recruited from the general population of the same area. A technique called random digit dialing was used to do this (Section 13.3). The controls were frequency-matched to the cases, which means that overall the distribution of some prespecified characteristics (such as age, sex, and race) is similar for cases and controls (Section 27.5).

When controls also have medical problems, you have to ensure that they still meet the specified inclusion and exclusion criteria for controls. In particular, you must be confident that the controls do not have the condition of interest.

Example 26C (continued): There were 23 potential controls who had autopsy results, no CNS or dementia, and did not have evidence of sepsis from clinical, laboratory, and autopsy results. This is the perfect control pool since they all would have been included as cases if they had had evidence of sepsis. To ensure complete separation of the controls from the cases, however, an additional six potential controls who had some suggestion of sepsis were excluded, ensuring that sepsis at time of death was very unlikely in any of the controls. Thus, there were 17 individuals left in the control group.

Example 26D (continued): Because of the frequency of undiagnosed diabetes in the general population, once controls were identified, they were given a standard diabetes screening test to ensure that they did not have diabetes.

26.2 Inclusion and Exclusion Criteria for Controls

For concurrent controls, control participants are selected and evaluated at the same time and, like the cases, according to documented inclusion and exclusion criteria. Selection of controls must be done without knowledge of the specific exposure(s). As discussed earlier, control participants may be recruited from the general population or may be selected from an existing patient population, such as hospital records. However, there are two sets of criteria: one for the cases and one for the controls. In general, these two sets would be the same except that they would be opposite in the criterion that define having the outcome of interest. But just this difference may not be sufficient to have a good control group. There may be other conditions that the controls might have that would confound the comparison.

Example 26D (continued): Controls were also excluded if they had impaired glucose tolerance, a precursor to diabetes, detected during the screening test.

There is a tendency to think that since you have defined the conditions for cases very clearly, you can skimp on the definitions for the controls, perhaps defining them as not having the outcome of interest. Often inclusion criteria include the very generic phrase "normal, healthy controls." As discussed in Section 12.2 this sounds pretty clear, but what is "normal"? Or "healthy"? How "normal" or how "healthy"? Many people would say that anyone who volunteers for a clinical study is unusual. Others might say no one is normal. These terms should be thought of not as absolutes, but rather in terms of your investigation. Sometimes healthy refers not only to current status but also to prior personal and family history.

Example 26E: In a study of depression the investigators wanted to test whether participants with depression have a higher rate of a specific polymorphism than do participants who are not depressed. A participant with a family history of depression might not be suitable for this study as a control, even if the participant has never had any mental illness. But this same family history would not necessarily affect this participant's suitability for a study where the outcome was pulmonary disease.

How will you measure "normal" or "healthy"? Will you do a physical examination? If so, what will be included? If your screening includes laboratory measurements, what tests will you use, and what range of results is acceptable? Will it be an absolute range or the normal limits for the laboratory doing the tests? Even if you only measure height and weight, what are the limits on normal? A normal body mass index might be defined as 18–25, as 18–27 (which would include overweight people, at least by some criterion), or even as 18–30. Is 18 too low? It might be if you are trying to recruit controls for a study of patients with anorexia. Are there diet restrictions or requirements? Is someone who exercises several hours a day, as serious athletes do, normal? Are you planning to ask about medications and over-the-counter drugs? What about participants taking vitamins? Are all vitamins acceptable, or do you want to exclude participants taking megavitamins? Does medication free mean no aspirin? No oral contraceptives? What about herbal remedies?

Another commonly used term is "standard." But what are your standards? This is a particularly important point when diet is a factor. What is a "standard diet"? What is the fat content of a "high-fat" diet? How will this be measured? Similarly, what is a "normal" amount of exercise? At what level does alcohol intake become enough to exclude an individual from the study?

In some studies the use of a "normal, healthy" control group may introduce biases and is therefore inappropriate. In studies that depend on the participant's recall of events or behavior prior to the outcome becoming apparent, a control group may consist of participants with an unrelated but similarly serious outcome, on the theory that they would be more like the cases in the effort they put in to recall information which should reduce recall bias (Section 17.1.4).

Example 26F: Example 17J discusses a case-control study assessing various prenatal exposures in infants born with a specific serious birth defect. The use of "normal, healthy infants" as controls is likely to overestimate the association, since the parents of such infants are unlikely to put the same effort into recalling prenatal events as cases would. A more appropriate control group would involve infants with other serious birth defects, as their parents would be more likely to make the same effort to recall prenatal exposures as the parents of cases. One concern, however, is that these control birth defects might also be associated with some prenatal exposures. If several different types of birth defects are included as controls, this concern would be reduced, as it would be unlikely that all the birth defects would be associated with the same prenatal exposure.

In studies of genetic causes of disease, a control group could consist of participants who are similar to the cases in lifestyle factors, such as diet, exercise (or lack thereof), and smoking, even when these are considered "bad" behavior. Some studies require the participation of individuals who are currently abusing alcohol or using illegal street drugs. These studies raise extensive ethical issues and must be undertaken with extreme caution to protect the rights and safety of the participants.

26.3 Special Situations

26.3.1 Multiple Control Groups

In some situations it is useful to have multiple control groups, on the theory that each of the different control populations might have biases compared to the cases, but these biases would likely be different so that if consistency of results is found, this would strengthen the evidence for the association being real.

Example 26G: In a case-control study of a rare serious childhood illness, multiple control groups were used to avoid potential confounders. One control group was composed of children seen at the same emergency room as the cases, as this would control to some extent for local access to medical care. A second control group was composed of children being treated in the same hospital as the case, as cases were routinely moved to tertiary care institutions because of the severity of the disease. This group was included to attempt to control for severity of illness and potential recall bias. A third group was composed of children from the same classroom as the child, to attempt to minimize any socioeconomic and ethnic differences between cases and the control group. Finally, a fourth control group was obtained from the community using random digit dialing, to control for potential community factors. All four control groups led to similar results, so there was strong and consistent evidence for the exposure-outcome relationship.

26.3.2 Case-Control Studies within Cohort Studies

In large cohort studies, case and control groups may be selected as subgroups of the full cohort of participants. Often a case-control study is a substudy of a cohort study; this is called a "nested case-control study."

Example 26H: The National Collaborative Perinatal Project was a large cohort study of more than 58,000 pregnancies and their outcome in 12 centers in the years between 1959 and 1974. Children were given extensive neonatal examinations and follow-up examinations at regular intervals up to 8 years of age. In addition to examining association between prenatal events and outcome within the total group, subgroups of the total population were used for specific substudies. For example, to examine the risk factors for cerebral palsy (CP), a case-control study included all the infants with CP and a control group of up to three matched infants for each affected child.

As all the prenatal exposure information was collected concurrently during the pregnancies, the use of normal infants in the control group is appropriate as there would be no concern about recall bias.

26.3.3 Historical Controls

Occasionally it is not possible to recruit concurrent controls for a study, and you must use information from individuals that were evaluated in the past, referred to as historical controls. In the best circumstances these controls are an actual group of participants that were evaluated at some time in the past and for whom you can retrieve the individual data – such as participants who were systematically studied in your center for an earlier study following a defined protocol. Sometimes only summary statistics are available in the literature, so that you have an implied control group.

There are many problems with historical controls that can lead to false conclusions and biased studies. It is difficult, sometimes impossible, to determine if the controls and the study participants were similar on factors that could confound the analysis. You as the investigator have no control over the methods that were used to collect data for the control group. Since the groups were selected at different times and possibly in different geographical areas, differences between the groups may be due to factors such as improved disease surveillance techniques, life style changes, changes in definition of disease, changes in the population demographics due to immigration, and so forth.

Example 26I: Assume you wanted to determine if a public health information campaign had a beneficial effect on some parameters of public health in a community by comparing current statistics to statistics from five years ago. However, during that period, there was significant economic improvement in that area that led to greater employment, and the number of uninsured individuals dropped dramatically because of legal changes. Thus, even if you see an improvement, you cannot determine if the education program had an effect on general health.

Results in observational studies are often compared to published norms. These are another type of historical control group, and the same problems apply. It is important to know exactly what population was used to generate the norms, since they may not be applicable to participants in your study. Often data generated in academic centers on "normal healthy controls" are based largely on the student population, who are younger, healthier, and more active than a typical patient cohort.

26.4 Should the Sizes of the Groups Be the Same?

In Appendix B we discuss the importance of sample size (total number of participants in the study) and how an appropriate sample size is required to give you adequate power – that is, a good chance of showing that the differences between the groups or the associations that you propose are statistically significant. If the cases are sparse or difficult to find, then increasing the size of the control group will increase the power, as was done in Example 26H. The increase in power plateaus after 3–4 controls per case. For a fixed total sample size, a study in which the groups are of approximately equal size will give higher power than one in which groups are very unequal. Therefore, it is often the best use of resources to have equal numbers of cases and controls if possible. If the number of cases is limited but controls are readily available and it is relatively easy to retrieve the data required for controls, increasing the control group size may not be much of a problem. In the rare situation when it is substantially easier to obtain cases than controls, a larger number of cases may be appropriate.

26.5 Ethical Issues

In studies involving control groups, the selection of controls is key to the scientific validity of the study. This is most critical in a case-control study, since the investigator is specifically picking both cases and controls for comparison. As we have noted before, if a study lacks scientific validity, it is not ethical, since you are wasting the time and effort of participants to acquire potentially faulty information. Bias in selecting controls will compromise the validity of the study. You must take particular care that it is not introduced inadvertently. You must ensure that the participants in a case-control study, both the cases and the controls, are selected without knowledge of their exposure and do not differ in ways that might confound the major comparisons.

It is not ethical to study individuals who are practicing self-destructive behavior, such as alcohol abuse, and not in some way act to encourage the individuals to modify their behavior during or after the study. This latter is, of course, true no matter what the individual's role in the study is.

KEY POINTS

- All participants in case-control studies must be selected without knowledge of their exposures.
- Control participants are necessary to support the assumption of a link between an exposure and an outcome in a case-control study.
- In a case-control study the controls are selected to meet specific criteria. These should be the same criteria as that used for cases, except that they do not have the outcome of interest.

- Terms such as "normal," "healthy," and "standard" must be specifically defined for each particular study.
- Every effort must be made to avoid systematic differences between cases and controls that would bias the outcome of the comparison.
- Equal group sizes are the most efficient use of resources, but unequal size may be necessary when there are only a limited number of either cases or controls available.
- If there is no alternative, historical controls and published norms may be used in place of a concurrent control group, but they have many problems and may lead to invalid results.

27

Matching in Observational Studies

In Sections 25.4 and 26.3.1 we described the use of multiple cohorts and multiple control groups, respectively. For cohort studies, cohort characteristics, except for the factor of interest, should be as similar as possible. For case-control studies, the cases and control groups should be as similar as possible, with the exception of the outcome. Even if the inclusion and exclusion criteria (Section 26.2) are the same except for specific items relating to the group being recruited, the groups may not be comparable on key prognostic variables and thus the comparisons may be biased. In this chapter, we describe how to make the groups more similar using matching. Matching means that participants in one or more groups are selected at least partially on their similarity on certain characteristics to participants in another group. Matching may be done either by matching individuals or by matching the distribution of the characteristics in the groups, called "frequency matching." We focus our discussion on case-control studies, as matching is most commonly used in them and the selection of the control group is a critical decision for the validity of the study. Matching may also be appropriate in a comparative cohort study.

27.1 Why Match?

In interventional studies the investigators rely on randomization to make the study groups equivalent on prognostic factors, eliminating prognostic bias (Section 17.1.1). If the factors are very important, then stratified randomization can be used (Section 21.3.1). In observational studies, when groups are being compared, it is also important to ensure that the groups do not differ on important prognostic factors. Sometimes the investigators can rely on homogeneity within the populations or a very large sample size that should allow the prognostic factors to be distributed equally across all groups so that their effect can be assessed and incorporated in the analysis. However, if the groups studied differ on critical factors in addition to the characteristic used to identify the group (exposure in comparative cohort studies; outcome in case-control studies), then the exposure-outcome relationship may be affected by these other factors. This problem is called confounding (Section 16.2). Matching in an observational study is a way to reduce confounding.

Example 27A: You plan to do a case-control study in elderly individuals with a condition that becomes more common and tends to worsen as people get older. Cases would be recruited from a clinic, but controls would be recruited from the general population. Controls would tend to be younger then the cases, no matter what age range is used as the inclusion criterion, because older people are more likely to have medical and mobility issues, decreasing the chance of them volunteering as controls. Reducing the upper age limit on the cases would reduce the generalizability of the study, but the potential distribution of ages could still be different between the two groups and could still confound differences in the exposure(s) of interest between the two groups. Using matching to have a similar age distribution of cases and controls would reduce this concern.

27.2 Who Are You Matching?

Matching requires one group be identified as the index group and the other group(s) matched to this index group. In a case-control study the index group is the cases, while in the comparative cohort study the index group is the cohort which has the exposure of interest. In both designs, we use the terms "index case" for individuals in the index group and call the groups matched to the index group the "controls." For simplicity, we assume there is only one control group. In practice there may be multiple control groups, especially in a case-control study, with each control group matched independently to the index group for different characteristics. Within each control group, there may be multiple participants matched to a single index case.

Example 27B: In a case-control study of vaccine side effects the investigators have a large database of members from an HMO. Given the large number of potential controls and small number of cases (individuals with side effects), the investigators designed the study to have up to five individually matched controls for each case. Potential cases and controls were then contacted and invited to participate in the study.

Using multiple controls is a way to gain statistical power (Section B.7) if the number of participants in the index group is relatively small. Usually the number of controls per index case is five or fewer, but larger numbers have been used. It is not necessary for each index case to have the same number of controls, since there are statistical methods to analyze data even with varying numbers of controls.

27.3 When Is Matching Done?

The basic definition of matching assumes that the process occurs during the recruitment phase of the study. The variables used for matching and the matching criteria are defined before the study begins. Participants are recruited into the index group as they become available, but participants in the control groups must match the index group to be included in the study. Frequently both the index group and the controls are recruited from a larger pool of available individuals in a cohort study, rather than specifically for the study.

Example 27C: In a case-control study of a particular birth defect, cases were infants born with this defect in a group of regional hospitals. The controls were infants born in the same hospitals during the same period. The mothers were matched on age, parity, and ethnicity. In addition, the infants had to match on sex and gestational age.

Example 27D: An investigator proposed to do a record review of variables associated with the occurrence of nosocomial infections in the surgical unit of a large hospital. Records of all surgeries are available from the hospital database. All patients who had evidence of post-surgical nosocomial infections will be selected. Once they are identified, up to 5 controls, matched on sex and surgery type, and similar in age and date of surgery will be selected from the remaining individuals in the file.

In some studies matched subgroups are created in the analysis phase of a study, after information on all the participants is available and the database is complete. This method is frequently referred to as post hoc matching. This is frequently done with data from a large cohort study which has information on the matching variables for all the participants. This should be part of the study design and the specific details of the matching procedure defined in the protocol.

Example 27E: The Framingham Heart Study, initiated in 1948, was designed as a longitudinal investigation of constitutional and environmental factors influencing the development of cardiovascular disease in men and women free of these conditions at the outset. The original study enrolled more than 5,000 participants for the first examination and at this writing is enrolling and testing a third generation of participants. In addition to the primary analyses, participants and data from this study were used for case-control, case-cohort, and matched cohort studies of other outcomes. For example, to study the causes of cognitive decline after stroke, investigators identified a group of 74 cases from the study cohort who had suffered a stroke during a 13-year period as cases and a control group of 74 participants, matched on age and sex, who had not had any cardiovascular events. The groups were compared on several variables thought to be associated with cognitive function, including pre-stroke measures.

If post hoc matching is not part of the basic design, it may introduce problems of credibility, since it may seem that the choice of variables and participants included in the control group was driven by the data rather than scientific theory.

Example 27F: Investigators completed a cohort study in children of the effects of an exposure on a specific outcome after 5 years. The results of the study were neither statistically significant nor clinically important. The investigators examined the data further and noticed that if they selected a subgroup that had the outcome and matched its members to specific controls, they would have a statistically significant difference. They were advised that if they published this analysis, it could be greeted with skepticism, since it was data driven. It could be followed up in a subsequent study designed to investigate the hypothesis, however.

27.4 Individual Matching

Individual matching is the most common method used in case-control studies and in comparative cohort studies when the cohorts are drawn from a larger population. The matching process must be the same for all index cases, and all controls must be matched and all index cases must have a match to be included in the analysis. You cannot mix matched and unmatched individuals in either group. If you believe that individual matching will be too difficult with the available population, then you might consider frequency matching (Section 27.5). If you begin a study planning on using individual matching, then determine that it is too difficult to find controls and would like to switch to a frequency matched design, then you should work with a statistician or other knowledgeable person to determine whether switching to frequency matching is a good choice in terms of practicality and validity.

27.4.1 Defining Matching Criteria

To do individual matching, you must first identify the variables on which to match and define the standards for matching on each variable that you have selected. The criteria for each variable can specify an exact match or an interval for the match, such as age plus or minus 5 years (this is sometimes referred to as "list matching"). Usually the width of the matching interval depends on the potential effect of the variable in the population to be studied, so you might allow a wider discrepancy in age when you are studying middle-aged adults than you would if you were studying young children or very old individuals. Sometimes you must specify standards for how values for the variable are defined, much as you did when defining inclusion and exclusion criteria for the study pool. Thus, if you wish to match on ethnicity, you must define your ethnic groups and specify how you will determine if a participant is a member of one of them.

Example 27D (continued): Patients will be matched on sex, age, date of surgery, and surgery type. Matching on sex is clear. The age criterion specifies a difference of 5 years or less in either direction, while the date of surgery was matched to within 30 days. The "surgery type" must be more specific. The investigator could specify a very close match, such as location, procedure, and extent of invasiveness (severity, spelled out in the protocol), which might make it very hard to match all the cases. Alternatively, a general match only on severity might be done to make matching easy, or a combination of general location of surgery and severity used.

Sometimes the matching criteria are combined into a score based on the variables of interest. It may be determined by a computer model or by your or others' best estimates of the importance of certain factors. The score will be computed for all participants, including the index cases, and the control's score must be within some range of the index case's score to be considered a match for the index case. Alternatively, the score may be a difference score, based on the differences between the index case and the control on each variable.

Example 27G: Researchers have developed scores that quantify a woman's risk of breast cancer based on many factors, including age, family history, reproductive history, and life style factors. In a case-control study of the role of an industrial exposure as a possible cause of breast cancer, this risk score could be used to match participants who could then be compared on the exposure.

A mathematical model called the propensity score is used in many studies to try to balance groups on variables that might be confounded with the outcome of interest. It combines several variables to predict the probability that participants belong to a specific group. The process of developing the model can be complex and requires a fairly large number of participants, so that it is not suitable for small studies. It also requires that data on the matching variables be available for participants and potential controls before the specific controls are selected, so it is not usually appropriate for prospective studies.

Example 27H: In a matched-cohort study performed by a health insurance group to investigate the effects of a heart failure care support program, a cohort of 277 patients who had had heart failure and participated in the program was compared to a matched cohort of patients who also had had claims for heart failure but lived in a different state that did not have the program. A propensity score was used for matching. The variables in the formula included demographic characteristics as well as medical service utilization, prescription drug use, and procedures performed during the year prior to enrollment. This propensity score was used to try to eliminate the possible confounding effects of factors, such as an individual's tendency to use medical services, when estimating the effect of the heart failure care support program.

27.4.2 Choosing between Eligible Controls

Additional methods for selecting controls must be specified when controls are selected from a pool of eligible participants and matched to index cases. If you are selecting from a list of participants that match on distinct characteristics, as opposed to a score, then the simplest method is to identify a subgroup of all controls that meet the matching criteria for an index case and then randomly select the required number of controls from this subgroup. If the matching criterion is a score, then you may select all participants who meet the specified limits on the score and proceed to randomly select the required number from this subgroup. Alternatively, you could select the "best" controls for each index case, where best would be defined as a score closest to the index case's score or smallest difference score. Again, if there are more potential controls with the same score than needed for the study, then you should select randomly from this group.

When you are matching from a pool, it often turns out that one control participant will match more than one index case. This is a common problem in matched designs. Sometimes this can be resolved using the closest match if the matching is based on a score. Another method is to randomly assign the control to one index case. But this may result in an imbalance in the number of controls per index case. Suppose the design calls for three controls per index case. Index case A has six potential controls and index case B has three potential controls, of which two are also in A's subgroup. If those two controls are randomly assigned to either A or B, then B could wind up with only one control. Ideally you would just assign both of the shared controls to B, but what if there was also an index case C who needed them, and so forth. Algorithms to optimally assign controls can get very complex, and often require multiple iterations of the matching process.

Example 27I: In a multi-center cohort study of births over a 10-year period, an index group of children born with cerebral palsy was identified. Then up to three matched controls were selected for each case, using the following criteria: same sex, date of birth within six months, estimated gestational age within one week, birth weight within 250 grams, same site of birth, mother's age within 3 years, and same parity (defined as 1, 2–3 or > 3). The initial algorithm resulted in a large number of overlapping matches for each case, so the criteria were modified to use a modified distance score. For each criterion, equality was scored as 0 and differences were scored from 1 to 3 depending on the scale. Then cases were rematched based on minimum scores, which reduced the overlap. A file was created, consisting of cases and controls where there were three controls per case and no overlap problems. Then the remaining potential controls in the database were reassigned to try to get three controls per remaining case. At the end, some cases were manually reviewed by someone not connected with study and with no knowledge of any of the variables other than those in the matching criteria, to form additional matched sets.

You can also get control participants who are good matches to more than one index case when you are matching during the recruitment phase, but this is usually easier to resolve. You would need to specify in the study design how the new control would be assigned. Usually, the control would be matched to the first suitable unmatched index case in the study.

27.5 Frequency Matching

Frequency matching, often referred to as "matching on distribution," is simpler than individual matching. Frequency matching means that the summary statistics for the variable you are matching on will be similar in all groups. Thus, if sex is an important confounding variable, then matching on distribution means that each group would have the same percentage of females. If age were important, at a minimum the groups should have a similar mean age and standard deviation, or median and range. On variables like age, the groups are often matched more closely by defining classes (e.g., age in 5 year bands). This does not require that all classes have the same number of individuals, only that the distribution in each group is the same. The frequencies to be attained are based on the index group available. This means that the investigator must examine the recruitment statistics periodically to assure that the balance is maintained, and if necessary, focus on recruiting controls with specific characteristics. It is also useful to plan to recruit at least some of your controls after all the cases are enrolled.

Example 27J: In a case-control study, the acceptable age range is 25 to 70. The design specifies 100 cases and 200 controls to be recruited over 2 years. At the end of one year, the sample of affected cases is 75% female and, for each sex, 60% of the cases are 55–70 years old and only 10% are 25–40 years old. However, the controls are 50% female and have only 40% in the older group and 25% in the younger group. The investigators can assume that the age and sex distribution in the affected group will not change. Therefore, they need to modify the recruitment strategy to try to recruit more female controls and more controls of both sexes in the older group and fewer in the younger group.

Frequency matching does not reduce the between-group variability as much as individual matching, but it is often easier to achieve, particularly when there is more than one control group. Moreover, it usually does not require special methods for analyzing the results.

27.6 Practical Issues

27.6.1 Overmatching

Overmatching is used to describe a study where too much matching has been used. One type of overmatching occurs when the matching criteria are related to the exposure to be tested, so that the effect of the exposure is eliminated, or heavily diluted, by the matching.

Example 27K: Investigators were studying the effect of air quality on the development of childhood asthma. The cases were children who developed asthma in the first 10 years of life. The controls were children free of asthma or other respiratory problems, who were matched for age (within 2 years), sex, and socioeconomic status. In the city where the investigators were recruiting their population, poorer individuals were more likely to live in more polluted areas. Therefore matching on socio-economic status is overmatching and would make the cases and controls more similar in exposure than they should be.

27.6.2 Excessive Matching Criteria

Another potential problem occurs when you include matching criteria that have no effect on the variables you are studying. In the example of surgical infections (Example 27D), there is no information that infections are associated with ethnicity, therefore matching on ethnicity would only make it more difficult to find participants without improving the study. Similarly, adding criteria that are strongly associated with existing matching criteria will also increase the difficulty of finding participants without making the study better. Examples of this type of excessive matching include matching on both body weight and body mass index or on both age and Tanner stage in children.

27.6.3 Special Problems

There are several problems that occur when matching is a part of a study. The most common problem is that recruitment becomes more difficult and may lead to some available index cases being excluded from the study. If the individuals are being selected from a large database, then this may not be a problem.

Example 27L: This study compared the growth and medical history of low birth weight children to normal birth weight children. The controls were matched to the cases on sex, ethnicity, and date of birth within three months. All the participants were drawn from a clinic in a major medical center and all the information was drawn from existing medical records. Parents were asked for permission to use their child's data in the study. Although the final database might not include some cases or controls who could not be matched, all parents were asked to participate, because the assessments were from records and could be done when enrollment was complete and did not require any extra effort from the parents of the children. At the end of the study, cases and controls were matched using the techniques described in Section 27.4.2, and those cases that could not be matched were not used.

However, if you are recruiting participants specifically for the study, then you may have to reject what might otherwise be very good control participants for the study if they do not match any index cases, or may have to reject index cases if you cannot find a match for them.

Example 27M: In a case-control study to determine if individuals who developed depression after age 55 had lesions in a specific area of the brain, the cases were patients at the investigators' clinic. The controls were recruited from the general population and were to be matched to the cases on age, sex, marital status, and socioeconomic status. Control selection began after half of the cases had been recruited and evaluated. The controls had been asked to allow access to their medical history and to complete a questionnaire on marital status and socioeconomic status which was needed for matching. Potential controls who did not match any of the current cases were asked if they could be contacted at a later date when someone with their characteristics was needed. The investigators found that some individuals were agreeable to this but others were insulted at being rejected and refused, feeling that the effort they had put into the study had been wasted.

Finally, there can be very real problems finding appropriate controls, and you may need to reassess what control population to use if you use matching.

Example 27N: A case-control study assessed the physical fitness 5 years after surgery of children who had had heart valve replacement in the first 10 years of life. The investigators' original plan was to use siblings of the child who were close in age as controls. However, they realized that this would mean that many of the cases could not be used because they did not have such siblings. Therefore, to use the maximum number of cases possible, the investigators decided to switch to using controls from the general population who were not related to the cases.

27.6.4 Data Analysis

Although data analysis is not part of this text, you should be aware that procedures for comparing individually matched groups are different from those comparing unmatched groups. There are well-known basic procedures if one control is matched to one index case. However, if multiple controls are used for a single index case, then more complex analysis procedures are required, particularly if the number of controls varies between index cases. We strongly recommend that if you are thinking about doing a matched study, that you discuss the analysis with a statistician before starting the study. This is less of a problem if the groups are matched on frequency, but the input of a statistician will greatly enhance your study, no matter what the design.

27.7 Ethical Issues

It is very easy to give the impression of bias in a matched study. The criteria for selection of controls must be defined before the study has begun and be strictly followed, so that a potential control meeting the matching criteria is automatically included in the study. The rules for resolving multiple possible pairings must be objective and clear. Post hoc matching is open to the accusation of being data-driven – that is, that the control group is selected to enhance differences between the groups. To counter this possibility, control participants could be selected through an automated system, with random selection from available controls.

Many studies include clinical interviews, self-report instruments, and other testing not required for usual treatment. These assessments involve both cost to the study and inconvenience for the participants. These resources are wasted if an index case cannot be matched, or a control not used at the end of the study. Depending on the effort required by the participant and the risks of the study procedures, it might even be potentially unethical to attempt to recruit individuals (especially controls) that are unlikely to be included in the analysis.

KEY POINTS

- Matching is used to enhance the comparability of different groups in non-randomized studies.
- Matching implies that there is an index group (cases in a case-control study; exposed in a comparative cohort study), and participants in other groups are matched to the index group.
- Matching may occur during recruitment or after all the participants are recruited.
- Matching may be to specific individuals or groups may be frequency matched.
- For individual matching, a matching criteria specifies which variables are used for matching and how they are combined to determine how close a match is.
- There must be decision rules for assigning controls to an index case when more than one pairing is possible.
- Frequency matching matches the groups on the distribution of key characteristics.
- The investigator should avoid matching on factors that may obscure the effect of the exposures of interest.
- The investigator should avoid having such stringent matching criteria that recruiting for the study is very difficult.

28

Blinding in Observational Studies

Although blinding is typically thought of as something done in interventional studies, it can and should be used in observational studies as well. This reduces the chance of biasing the results, since judgment is needed when extracting or collecting data to be used in observational studies. There are multiple ways that investigators may be blinded to aspects of the participant's history to reduce bias. We describe these first for written records, then situations in which participant contact is necessary, and finally for the situation where only a single investigator is involved in a study, which is typical in a record review.

28.1 What Can Be Blinded?

The standard for interventional studies is the double-blind study, in which neither the participant nor those involved in assessing the outcome know which intervention the participant is receiving. This is not possible in an observational study, since the participant knows at least the exposure or the outcome, and often both. Thus, the focus of blinding in an observational study is on blinding those involved in the assessment of the participants. In an ideal world of scientific research, all exposures and outcomes would be measured by precise and reproducible criteria and would not require subjective judgment. Unfortunately, we do not live in such an ideal world, and so the protocol needs to specify how, precisely, blinding is to be done to minimize the potential for bias in the results. There are three basic features of a study that could be blinded to those involved in the data abstraction and collection: the exposure information, the outcome information, and the actual hypothesis underlying the study that links the exposure and outcome information.

28.2 Blinding of Written Records

When only written records will be used, different assessors can be used to review the exposure information and the outcome information. In the simplest situation, one set of records would contain the exposure information and another set of records would contain the outcome information.

Example 28A: This is a cohort study of individuals who worked in a chemical plant during 1970–1990. The objective was to determine if workers who had "high" exposure to a specific chemical had a reduced respiratory function at age 60 compared to workers in the same factory who were either not exposed to this chemical or had only short-term or minor exposures. The raters reviewed the work records of each individual and classified them as high, moderate, or low exposure based on their job description, work areas, and time in these jobs. Different raters reviewed the participants' medical records for signs of deterioration in respiratory function. The raters reviewing the work records were blinded to the participants' outcomes; the raters reviewing the medical records were blinded to the participants' exposure.

Often, however, there is not a clean separation of the exposure and the outcome information. In that case the documents must be copied and the information must be redacted, either by blacking out the information with a heavy pen or cutting away that part of the document. Two sets of documents are needed: one with the exposure information redacted and one with the outcome information redacted. There should be a designated person involved in doing this task, and this person should not be involved in the subsequent data abstraction of either the exposure or the outcome information for any of the records they reviewed in full. Like in Example 28A, there should then be different assessors for the redacted exposure information and the redacted outcome information, to minimize the possibility of assessor bias when abstracting the data.

28.3 Blinding When Assessors Have Contact with Participants

If the assessors will have contact with the participants as well as doing record extractions, then any participant identification should also be removed and a different study identification number used for the written records and the information directly obtained from the participants.

Example 28B: In this cohort study, exposure information can be obtained from work records, as in Example 28A, but participants must be contacted to obtain current medical information. In such a case, the work records should be given one set of study IDs, while a second set of study IDs would be used for the personal interviews so that the interviewers would not be aware of their exposure information. An investigator not involved in abstracting either the exposure information or interviewing participants (usually the study statistician) would generate both sets of numbers and then maintain the linkage between the two so that the exposure and outcome data could be combined after all the data were collected.

If the information will come from a personal interview, then the rater would be asked not to discuss the topics that are the objects of the blind. One good way to do this is to develop a script for the interview and instruct the rater not to digress from it. The rater should be instructed on ways to keep the interview on track without alienating the participant. These methods may be used to blind the participant's status from the rater. However, this is not always possible in an interview; it may be obvious from the physical appearance or setting of the interview what the status is, particularly in a case-control study. Sometimes an interview can be done by telephone, which may help blind the rater to the participant's status.

In some studies, to enhance objectivity in the interview, the interviewer may be blinded to the hypotheses of the study, or may be blinded as to what the important exposures or outcomes are.

Example 28C: In a study of the relationship between environmental exposures and lung cancer, the investigators had the interviewers inquire about multiple environmental exposures as well as a residential history. They also measured basement radon levels and outside air particulate matter. Although the primary hypothesis for the study was that radon levels would be associated with increased rates of lung cancer, the interviewers were told only that the study was about the relationship of environmental factors and disease, and the consent information was similarly vague for the participants in the study.

28.4 What to Do When Blinding Is Not Possible

Sometimes, when a record review is being done by a single investigator, blinding is not possible without additional help. A colleague might copy records for you and systematically black out the outcome information in one set of records, and the exposure information in the other set of records, but finding someone to help you with this might be difficult. In this case, we would first recommend that you do the blinding of the records, and enlist two colleagues, one to abstract the outcome data, and the other to abstract the exposure information. Even this, however, might not be possible for you to arrange.

You are then faced with a quandary: either do not do the study, or do the study without blinding. If you proceed to do the study, then you must make sure that you are abstracting the exposure and outcome information as objectively and rigorously as possible. There are several ways to improve the reliability of your doing this, although none can completely eliminate the possibility of subconscious bias.

Although online medical records might have the information you need already coded for certain common exposures (e.g., smoking and alcohol consumption), often records need to be reviewed manually. You should first review a fraction of the records to determine the various ways in which the exposure information and the outcome are recorded. You then should prepare a detailed set of rules that document how information may be reported and how it is interpreted and coded for the study. Then, you must apply the rules rigorously. You must document each specific case in which a decision that is not fully supported by these rules has been made and why the specific decision was made. Often, a pattern of exceptions occurs, which would cause you to revise your formal coding rules. These formal coding rules provide details of how decisions are made for the majority of records and form the basis for part of the methods section of the manuscript. The complete rules might be included as supplementary material in the final publication. Equally important, the list of exceptions allows you to go back after all the coding is done to review all the special cases at one time to ensure that they are being coded consistently.

Example 28D: An investigator has to work alone on a record review. The study is to determine whether specific aspects of a particular procedure (the location of a stent) are related to subsequent adverse outcomes. Although the online medical record allows participants to be identified by the procedure of interest, it does not contain information either about the potential risk factors for the adverse events or the precise placement of the stent, which must be obtained from the medical record for each patient. The investigator systematically reviews the medical history information for all visits prior to the procedure and prepares details of how different risk factors are identified in the record. Only after coding all the potential risk factors that may confound the results as well as the location of the stent, does the investigator then retrieve information about the specific adverse outcomes for the patient, which can be obtained based on procedure codes from the online medical record. This is a reasonable approach to obtain the exposure information separate from the outcome data, minimizing potential bias in abstracting the data.

28.5 Ethical Issues

A biased study has little or no value, no credibility, and wastes time and resources for everyone involved. Deliberately biasing results is unethical and may be illegal. But the more worrisome problem to us is subconscious bias. If an investigator is aware of some information, such as exposures, this may color the assessment of other information, such as outcomes. In our experience, investigators tend to bend over backwards not to let the knowledge affect their judgment about the outcome, but this is still a bias. The investigator subconsciously uses a bit more stringent criterion to ensure that an adverse outcome is present before coding it as present. Blinding raters to whatever values are not required for them to make their assessments is the best way to reduce bias. Blinding enhances the credibility of the study, so the study can potentially have a larger impact – which makes the extra effort involved worthwhile.

KEY POINTS

- Blinding should be used in observational studies whenever possible.
- The preferred technique is to separate the data abstraction or collection of exposure information from the data abstraction or collection of outcome data.
- There should be formal procedures for data abstraction and scripts prepared if participants are interviewed.
- Efforts should be made to blind the data abstractors and interviewers as much as possible to the hypothesis underlying the study.
- If blinding is truly impossible (not just difficult), rigorous written rules are essential and must be followed to minimize bias in data abstraction. All exceptions to these rules need to be noted when they occur and then reviewed after all data abstraction is completed to minimize potential biases and ensure consistency of data abstraction.

Part VI

PRACTICAL ISSUES

29

Acquiring High Quality Data

The validity of a study depends on many things, from hypotheses that are based on sound science, to a study design that will test these hypotheses without bias, to appropriate, well-defined methods for measuring the study variables. It also depends on the quality of the data that are collected and analyzed. The results of a study are only as good as the information that goes into it, and even the most advanced technology and statistical methods will not make up for poor quality data. During the implementation phase of the study, data quality must be maintained by use of appropriate methods to collect and record the study data so that it is accurate and complete. These procedures should be developed when designing the study. Resources for data collection must be included in the study budget and time must be allowed in the study schedule to ensure that the data being collected are of high quality.

29.1 Creating a Study ID

Even before you collect any data, you need to develop a method of assigning a Study ID to the participant. The Study ID is a unique number to identify the specific participant in the study. A Study ID is meaningless except as a link to the person's identify for this specific study. To preserve the participant's confidentiality, this should be a unique number that is not related to any number associated with the participant, such as age, date of birth, or social security number. This number would not be used in other contexts (such as in the health care medical record number, encounter number, etc.) to identify the participant.

The Study ID should be used for all data collection, even when the information is collected as part of the screening process and the individual may never become part of the study. If some of the measurements are to be done by raters outside the study group, such as blood tests and interpreting MRI scans, the participant should be identified only by the Study ID. Sometimes you may be using information from a written report that was generated outside your group, not as part of your protocol. In this case someone would have to add the Study ID to the record and remove or black out the participant's name and any other personal identifiers.

The link between Study ID and the person's identity should be kept in an encrypted computer file or a locked cabinet or drawer with limited access, following standards required for protecting confidential personal identifiers at your institution. The same procedures should be used for recording and keeping other identifying information, such as social security number or address. Computer records of personal information should be created by a single person and be encrypted and password protected and follow whatever procedures are required at your facility. Any subsequent information, should it be paper copy or a computer file, should exclude all personal information and use only the Study ID to identify the participant. If you need to keep a source document with the participant's name, such as a consent form, then it too must be kept in a locked cabinet following the procedures specified at your institution.

29.2 Methods for Data Collection

Sometimes the data you need already exists and will be accessible either in written format, as in a chart, or on a computer file. It is important to ensure that you will have access to these data and what the terms of this access are when you write the protocol. One requirement will almost always be to ensure that you will protect the confidentiality of the participant. This is already discussed in detail in Section 29.1. If the data already exist, the major issues involve data abstraction (if from paper records) and record verification, which are issues we focus on in Chapter 30. Here we focus on the collection of primary data.

29.2.1 Questionnaires

The general term "instrument" for data collection includes both actual questionnaires, computer input by the participant, and structured interviews by an interviewer. Instruments collect data in a structured manner, usually with precoded response options for most questions. When a participant directly enters data into a computer, the data entry format will still be based on a paper form, even if data are never collected on paper.

Information collected via questionnaires may be completed by the study participant or by a study team member interacting with the participant. When a team member is involved, we refer to that person as an "interviewer." Historically, the questionnaire was a paper form completed in pencil and then entered into the computer or a typed record. In many studies, paper forms are still used. Forms may also be completed on a touch screen or another electronic device including a smartphone. Using electronic devices requires additional resources for the devices themselves (especially if provided to the participant) and software to collect the information. There already exists some public domain software for this for different computer platforms, and we expect that this will become even more widely used on tablets and smartphones. For some participants, computer interaction is a bonus because they like or are intrigued by computers, but some people are intimidated by them and may require guidance and some instruction or training. The advantage of such direct entry is that the data entered by the participant requires no data transcription into a computer file. The disadvantage of this approach is that there is no possibility of correcting or validating the data later, so that inconsistencies cannot be resolved. For this reason, the software used should check the data while it is being entered to ensure that the data are valid and, as far as possible, consistent across the different questions being collected during the visit. If possible, this data validation would include consistency with other responses from the participant over time. Data checking is discussed in Section 30.5.

Example 29A: When a new patient shows up at a medical office, he is generally asked to complete a questionnaire with his demographic data and some medical history including current medications. Often other questionnaires about symptoms and problems are collected at the same time.

The information collected in Example 29A is mainly objective or measurable and limited to the questions on the form, although there may be multiple responses to single questions, such as current medications. You may use an instrument like this to collect basic information when you are evaluating a potential participant for inclusion in the study. Very often, you can use the entry form in your institution and just add the extra information you need for this first step. This has the advantage of saving time. With an instrument that has been in use for a long time, inconsistencies should have been corrected, except for your additions.

Other instruments may collect objective or subjective responses, or both. For subjective data, additional precautions are needed to ensure that the interviewer collects as unbiased data as possible, which is discussed extensively in Section 29.2.2. The study may, and almost always should, use data collection methods (questionnaires, structured clinical evaluations) that have been developed and validated by others if such data collection instruments exist. For example, the Hamilton scale for depression, the Beck Depression Inventory, or the Center for Epidemiological Studies Depression Scale may be used to measure the extent of depression and related symptoms. There are a large number of existing validated scales to measure many psychological states or traits. We recommend that you use a published and generally accepted scale for measuring subjective information.

If a question has several choices but only one can be selected, this must be clearly and prominently stated. For paper forms, we believe it is better to ask the participant to circle a choice than to write the number in a box next to the question. We have found that even when asked to enter the number of the choice, participants will often circle it anyway and not always enter it; moreover the handwritten entered number can be hard to read, and potentially the circled answer and the number entered may be different. When this happens, and if there is no way to determine which response is correct, this item must be considered missing data. This problem should not occur when direct data collection using a computer is done, as usually the option would be selected from a drop-down list.

In designing a questionnaire you must remember that it is intended both to pose questions and record responses, and to be used as input to a database. Therefore, it must be designed with both in mind: easy for respondents to understand and complete, and structured for ease of data entry, especially when entered directly by the participant, or by scanning a paper document.

The characteristics of the study participants should be considered. If the questionnaire is too long for the participants, they may simply not complete it or answer without thinking. Although there is no right answer for how many questions is too many, our basic rule of thumb is "when in doubt, throw it out." A question should be included only if you are sure that you need it. It is better to be missing an interesting secondary variable then to be missing the most important data for the study. Participants may also be reluctant to come for follow-up visits if repeating the question-naire is part of the protocol, and losing participants completely is even worse than missing some potentially interesting information.

The level of the language in the questionnaire should be geared to the participants. If the study participants will be drawn from a popula-tion with a low education level, then the wording of questions should be geared to that level. Sometimes a pictorial scale, in which the participant just marks where she feels she is on a line from none to a maximum, may be easier for the participant. For small children and possibly some adults, a more elaborate pictorial scale may be used.

Example 29B: The Wong-Baker Faces Scale for assessing pain in chil-dren consists of a series of six cartoon faces with expressions ranging from a happy face (no hurt) to a crying, frowning face (hurts worst). Children can pick which face most clearly reflects how they feel. A numeric scale from 0 to 10 by twos is used to code the child's response. For adults, typi-cally either a 10-point scale or a 10-cm line, called a visual analog scale, is used as one measure of pain.

In an interview, a member of the study staff obtains the information by talking with the participant. Sometimes the interview is based on a questionnaire and the interviewer reads the questions and asks the participant to select from the responses. This is usually done instead of providing the participant with a written form when the investigators feel that the individual may have some problem completing a written form, and is common in settings where literacy is low (such as some international studies). Even though the actual questions and allowable responses are fixed, the attitude of the interviewer and the way the question is asked can affect the answer, so very often interviewers are asked to work from a script and undergo training to ensure consistency.

Example 29B (continued): Even though the Wong-Baker Faces scale is pictorial, for very young children an interviewer is needed to complete the form. The children are unable to read the questions and instructions for the use of the form, but they are able to point to the picture about how they feel when an interviewer asks them.

Participants should always be told that they can skip a question if they do not want to answer it. Some questions may be offensive to certain people, and they will just not answer them. This may lead the participant to abandon the questionnaire or even abandon the study. If this is a possibility, then this should be discussed before giving the questionnaire to the participant, both to try to convince the participant of the importance of answering the question truthfully and to reinforce that the participant can skip the question if they wish and continue answering the other questions.

If the study population includes many participants who do not speak English as a first language, then the questionnaire must be translated into the most common other languages for use by those participants. This is usually verified by asking someone who is not familiar with the instrument to translate it back into English, and then comparing the initial and back-translated version. There are Spanish-language versions of many instruments in use today, as well as versions in other languages, and we expect more will become available.

29.2.2 Open-Ended Data Collection by an Interviewer

Although interviewers may be used to complete standardized questionnaires, data collection by an interviewer often is free-form – that is, open questions and open answers that are coded after the interview. Such an interview should still be structured – that is, covering specific topics and questions of interest – but should not direct the responses. In a free-form interview, or a free-form question, the interviewer asks general questions and participants respond with the information in their own words. In either case the interviewer may expand upon the question or the participant's answer to help clarify the participant's responses. The additional information or prompts provided by the interviewer need to be specified to minimize the potential for the interviewer to bias the responses of the participant.

For some structured interviews, once the interview is completed, the results can be summarized using a scoring or rating manual. This requires training the raters in how to complete the score sheet. If multiple raters are involved, then tests for consistency between raters must be run and, if discrepancies are found, additional rater training is required.

Example 29C: In a study of mental illness the research assistants were asked to conduct a structured interview and use the results of this to complete a standard form assessing depressive symptoms. When the study began, the first dozen interviews were videotaped, and then all the research assistants were asked to view the videos and complete the form for each participant. The results were then compared and, if there were discrepancies, further training was initiated.

Sometimes, however, the investigator is using the interview to develop an understanding of a problem. In this case, even if a previously used questionnaire is being used in the study, the focus is on identifying the themes in the participants' responses. When there are open-ended answers, the interview should be recorded and then transcribed. The first few transcripts then are reviewed and an initial set of concepts for the responses prepared. This should be done both by the investigator and either another investigator or the most senior of the research staff, and the concepts compared and discrepant results for each interview resolved. Then an initial coding of the responses is developed, which may need to be revised after further interviews find that some respondents' answers do not fit into the codes already identified. There is software available to help with coding of qualitative interviews.

Example 29D: An investigator intends to develop interventions to help improve linkage to HIV care in a specific immigrant population, and then test their effectiveness. The first step in this project was to interview participants (in their native language, by bilingual interviewers) to understand the issues that the participants saw affecting their ability to link to HIV care. After an interview was completed it was transcribed, and the investigator and interviewer separately identified themes within the interview. Additional participants were interviewed until no new themes were being identified in the interviews. At that point all the interviews were coded to identify the themes that each participant had mentioned and the results summarized over all participants to identify the most frequently mentioned problems and potential solutions identified by the participants for these problems.

Collecting information by an interviewer has the advantage that the interviewer can encourage and help the participant provide the information. An interviewer can explain the meaning of questions, can give additional information if necessary, and, in some cases, ask questions to help the participant remember some things, such as events in his or his family's health history. But this advantage can also create problems. If there are differences in the ability of different interviewers to obtain information, then the validity of your data may be compromised. This problem can be minimized by cross-training of the interviewers. The interviewers must also be trained to maintain a balance between helping the participant remember and prodding until the participant comes up with a false memory.

Example 29E: In a structured interview, the interviewer is trying to determine if there is any history of Type II diabetes in the participant's family. A participant is a little vague about some family members, but remembers one uncle who "took pills" and complained a lot about a low-sugar diet. After prompting by the interviewer using prompts pre-specified in the interviewer manual, the participant thinks he remembers the word "diabetes" being mentioned. The interviewer has to decide if this is definite enough to be considered an indication that the uncle had diabetes. The interviewer may ask the participant more questions, but must be careful not to steer the participant to a preferred response.

Ideally, the interviewer manual would provide detailed guidance on how to judge whether this is an indication that the relative had diabetes.

The interviewer must also be trained to avoid being judgmental.

Example 29F: Food intake questionnaires use different methods to define portion sizes. Simple weights or measurements are usually not sufficient, since most people do not weigh or measure their food, and guesses are usually very inaccurate. Some questionnaires use pictures of portions for reference, such as a small, medium, and large serving of pasta. The interviewer may help but not direct the individual to pick the best description. The interviewer should avoid comments both about the person's weight and the size of the portions selected. In addition, many people lie about this information: heavy people often select smaller portions than they really eat. Even if the interviewer doubts that the person actually eats the size selected, the interviewer cannot question the response. Sometimes, after the interview is completed and the participant has left, the interviewer completes an assessment about the reliability and validity of the responses.

If the participant does not speak English, then the interviewer should be bilingual in English and in the language of the participant. If that is not possible, then a trained translator might be used, but this poses potential problems as there may be nuances in the intended questions that may not be conveyed in the translation. Sometimes an individual will offer to bring a friend or relative to translate. We strongly recommend against this. Frequently the friend or relative may not strictly translate what is asked or what is said but instead may simplify a question, or try to guess what the interviewer would like for an answer or what the participant really means, rather than what the participant actually says. Sometimes you have to reject participants who are otherwise good candidates for a study because you cannot communicate with them accurately.

29.2.3 Other Types of Procedures Done by Study Staff

In addition to questionnaires and interviews, study staff may do other assessments or run specialized laboratory assays available only for a research project. These may include specific tests of muscle function, strength assessment, and tests of endurance, as well as specialized assays. For these tests, the protocol should have sufficient detail to ensure that the tests are applied consistently throughout the study. For a laboratory test, these may include the manufacturer, name and stock number of reagents to be used, tubes used for interim storage, dilution, time in solutions, centrifuge speed and time, time to cure, and temperature at all times in the processing and during storage.

Even commonly used procedures, such as measuring height and weight, should be spelled out in the protocol. What method is used to measure length in a baby? When during the day is weight measured? What instrument, often identified by name and model, is used for weight measurements? Is the participant fasting? How much and what type of clothing is a person weighed in, normal indoor clothing or a hospital gown? If normal indoor clothing, are sweaters and jackets to be removed?

The study staff may need to be trained in the particular methods for the assessment, and time should be allowed for practice sessions before the study begins. The assessor must be able to communicate easily with the participant. If more than one assessor is involved, then there must be cross-training to ensure that assessments are consistent. Some tests come with a complete manual on how to perform the test, often including a video example.

Example 29G: A study in elderly individuals used a five- item test to assess mobility. The first three items measure the ability to stand (from hardest to easiest test). The participant and the assessor decide which of these three tests to use, and only that test is tried. The entire assessment, including the last two items, takes less than 5 minutes. The manual of procedures included two pages of instructions for the study staff to perform these assessments correctly. This included details such as when to say "stop" during some of the tests, where the assessor is supposed to stand while doing the assessment, and so forth, as well as coding instructions for participant refusal or the assessor deciding that performing a specific assessment was not appropriate for a particular participant. Despite this level of detail, Example 18I illustrates how different study coordinators interpreted these instructions differently.

Sometimes, even with the most rigorous training, there still could be a very subjective aspect to an assessor's judgement about a test. In that case, ideally a single assessor would be used for the study. If that is not possible then a single assessor should be used for all of a participant's visits, to minimize assessor variability over time. In either case, it would be essential that the assessor be appropriately blinded, either to the participant's treatment group in an interventional study or to the participant's exposure or outcome as appropriate in an observational study.

29.2.4 Tests Done by Non-Study Staff

This section refers to various tests which are available for all patients at your institution and are used for your participants during a study. One example would be a standard chemistry panel drawn to ensure safety during a study testing a new medication. Other examples include tests such as imaging studies, a standard electrocardiogram, or a cardiovascular stress test.

The role of the test in the study determines how detailed the test description has to be in the Manual of Procedures (MOP; Section 29.3). If the data is a primary or secondary outcome of the study, there should be enough detail provided so that the precise test can be replicated over time at each site. For example, an MRI study would include all the details of how the specific MRI tests are performed and analyzed so that an imager would be doing the test exactly the same way on every occasion for every participant. This would include details of the specific device which would be used for testing. In contrast, if specimens have to be shipped to a specific laboratory for a specialized assay, there would be little if any detail about how the test is performed at the specialized laboratory. The study protocol would include very detailed instructions for how the specimens are collected, stored, shipped, and tracked, however. For some outcomes such as safety measurements, a simple statement that the analysis is done at an approved laboratory or specific commercial laboratory would be adequate.

Even if a test is done precisely, however, there are often subtleties in the interpretation of the results which is why often only a single individual or group might be reading all the images for a study or interpreting all the electrocardiograms.

29.3 The Manual of Procedures (MOP)

We have mentioned in multiple places in this chapter that procedures need to be spelled out in detail. As mentioned in Example 29G, a form collecting at most five pieces of information had two pages of instructions on how to administer the test. This is not at all atypical. The methods section of a grant application describes in very broad terms what will be done and how it will be done, but in our experience such material is never sufficiently detailed for study staff to actually perform a study.

Detailed specifications of all the procedures in the study should be collected in a document. We prefer calling this the "Manual of Procedures" (MOP), although other terms, such as "Manual of Operations," "Study Manual," and "Study Implementation Guide," are also used. No matter what it is called, the MOP will specify all the data sources, data collection instruments, instructions for administering the instruments, and instructions and scripts for interviews. The MOP is usually maintained as a loose-leaf notebook that is provided to each member of the study team. There are often changes to procedures as the study is implemented so a loose-leaf binder allows for easy page replacement. We strongly recommend that every page contain a version number and date, as often only a page or two will be changed at a time. All changes need to be implemented by all members of the study team to ensure that they are collecting data consistently so that the results will be valid at the end of the study.

29.4 Ensuring Validity in a Multi-Site Study

If the data is measured at different sites, then methods to ensure data consistency across sites should be specified in the MOP and procedures implemented to ensure consistency across sites. All the concerns when there is more than one rater or interviewer in a study are multiplied when the study involves multiple sites.

Example 29H: In a multi-site study in the United States, one of the lab values was bilirubin, but the specific procedures for obtaining bilirubin were not specified in sufficient detail in the MOP. Some sites reported total bilirubin, others reported direct and calculated indirect bilirubin (which together add to total bilirubin), and other sites reported conjugated and unconjugated bilirubin using methods such that the total was not equivalent to the total bilirubin.

The problem in Example 29H would not have happened if the MOP had been more specific on the methods for measuring bilirubin. Similarly, if the study had been done at only a single site, even if the MOP was not specific, this would not have been a problem unless the laboratory had changed testing and reporting methods during the course of the study.

We recommend that there be at least one meeting or Web seminar for multi-site studies involving all the principal investigators and their senior research assistants or study coordinators to review the protocol and the procedures involved. If questionnaires are involved, the interviewer manual needs to include especially detailed instructions. We recommend that the research staff watch videotaped interviews and then practice with research staff from other sites to ensure that the interviews are being administered consistently. We cannot overemphasize the level of detail required in a multi-site MOP.

Example 29I: In a multinational study, one of the questions was participant age. After all the data was collected, it was observed that the age at the study site in one country was slightly higher than the other sites. After discussion, it was discovered that in that country, age at birth is 1, which eliminated much of the discrepancy.

This problem can also arise when a study involves immigrants from different countries.

29.5 Ethical Issues

If the integrity of the study data is not assured, then the results of the study may be questionable and the validity of the study may be compromised. Therefore, you need to plan how data will be collected before the study starts. This includes planning who will collect the data, how it will be collected, and how much time it will take to collect the data, both for an individual participant and for the staff involved. The burden on the participant is a major concern when collecting data, and every effort should be made to collect only the minimum data necessary. Adding "just one more questionnaire" which might provide interesting and potentially useful information sounds reasonable – until you think about the total time it will take the participant to complete all the questionnaires. You need to consider whether it is feasible for the study staff to manage and coordinate the data collection. If it takes 75 minutes for a staff member to do all the activities required for a visit, and participants are scheduled every 90 minutes, there is a great deal of pressure to stay on schedule, rather than to spend time interacting with the participant as a person. As discussed in Section 24.3, we believe that these interactions are key to adherence and retention of participants in a study. When planning the study, resources, both human and financial, need to be considered to ensure that data can be collected reliably. If this is not done, then the time and effort of all individuals associated with the study, especially the participants, is wasted, which raises ethical concerns.

The privacy of the participants must be protected by restricting access to identifiable data whenever it is collected. This includes personal information from individuals when they are being screened for inclusion in the study, and eventual exclusion from the study does not eliminate this responsibility. A Study ID, described in Section 29.1, should be used for all data collection, even when the information is collected as part of the screening process and the individual may never become part of the study.

KEY POINTS

- Maintenance of data quality is essential for a valid study.
- Maintaining participant confidentiality is critical, even if they are not enrolled in the study.

- A Study ID should be used to link all personal information with other information, even screening data.
- Data quality depends on carefully and completely described measurement procedures. These should be collected in a Manual of Procedures (MOP) that will be available to all study personnel.
- The burden of data collection on participants should be minimized.
- Questionnaires must be designed to promote accurate responses.
- Some information may come from structured interviews. To assure consistency of results, interviewers should work from a script.
- For qualitative interviews, where the questions and answers are both open-ended, interviews need to be recorded and consistent rules developed for coding responses.
- Procedures for questionnaires or interviews must include methods to use with non-English speakers if they are eligible for the study.
- If multiple raters will be used, there should be cross-training and testing done to ensure consistent evaluations for all participants.
- The techniques and equipment for all procedures must be described in sufficient detail that they can be replicated over time.
- Adequate resources (both financial and human) are needed to maintain data quality.

30

Data Management

The results of a study are only as good as the information that goes into it, and even the most advanced technology and statistical methods will not make up for poor quality data. In the previous chapter we discussed ways to obtain quality information from varied sources. In this chapter we assume that the information will be stored on a computer file to be organized, displayed, and analyzed. There is a substantial possibility of introducing errors during this process, so that methods for reducing the error rate and verifying that the data are correct are critical.

30.1 Basic Approaches to Data Storage

We begin by defining the terms that will be used in this chapter. A "database" is a collection of information stored on computer media, organized in such a way that a computer program can quickly select desired pieces of data. Software is the computer code that controls everything that the computer does. The terms "program" and "software" are used interchangeably. The process of creating a database from varied data collection instruments and organizing and maintaining it is known generally as "data management." This may include creating new variables from the input data, such as computing BMI from height and weight. A single piece of information in a database is referred to as a "field;" a "record" is a defined set of fields, and a "file" is a collection of specific records. A field is often called a "variable" as it contains the value of a specific variable that was collected during the study. The database may consist of a single file or a series of files that can be linked with software. We will not discuss database design, since this requires special expertise, as does the analysis of the data.

There are two basic approaches to storing data in a database. A single file of records with the same fields is easily created using a spreadsheet (such as Microsoft Excel®). Alternatively, a series of different but linked files can be stored in a relational database (such as Microsoft Access®) in which the linking is denoted by a particular variable (such as the Study ID; Section 29.1) which is present in each record in each file. In our experience, most investigators who are working on their own seem to prefer spreadsheets because they can begin entering data immediately, the organization is straightforward, and the software is relatively easy to use. Relational databases are more complicated to design and use. They generally require that the user learn about the software and develop a plan to organize the data before beginning data entry. This generally requires that either the user has previous training with the database program or that he get the support of a computer specialist. However, just as you should never jump in and collect data from participants without carefully thinking through the data needed and the data collection process, you also have to think about how to organize and store your data. In our experience, this is one of the major weaknesses with investigators using spreadsheets: they just jump in and enter data, rather than first thinking about data organization.

Example 30A: An investigator has imaging results for 12 variables at each of 24 sites in the body in each of 18 patients. This is a total of 288 (12 variables per site x 24 sites) variables, plus 8 variables for the Study ID and some demographic characteristics, for a total of 296 variables. The investigator enters the data and proudly presents the statistician with a spreadsheet with columns A through KJ entered, for each of the 18 patients in the study. Since the investigator actually wanted each of the variables summarized and related to the others within the site, separately for each site, all analyses were site specific. The statistician points out that the investigator should have created two spreadsheets: one with the Study ID and demographic variables with 18 records (one for each patient), and a second spreadsheet with the 12 variables for a site, plus the Study ID and a site identifier (total 14 variables), with 432 records (18 participants x 24 sites), which would make the data processing, analysis, and preparation of tables much less time-consuming, and thus much less expensive for the investigator. Here we are using two spreadsheets instead of a more complex relational database structure, but reaping the same benefits of the more complex structure.

Sometimes it is sensible in terms of data entry and validation to use multiple spreadsheets, as in Example 30A, but at some point the investigator may want to present results using data from both spreadsheets. Combining data from different spreadsheets can sometimes be done by manipulating spreadsheets within the spreadsheet program, but if the spreadsheets can be imported into an analysis program, then that program should have the ability to combine information from multiple spreadsheets based on key fields such as the Study ID.

If the investigator is using software to collect data directly from participants, then this software may impact the approach to data storage. Most such software provides output in a format that is compatible with a spreadsheet, but such formats can generally be read into a database program as well.

Spreadsheets and relational databases are appropriate for different types of data. A spreadsheet is most appropriate when there will be a single record for each person. The record will consist of a number of individual fields (variables or data items) storing the information about the participant.

Example 30B: An investigator wants to do an outcome study of patients who received a specific treatment in the hospital clinic in the past year. Unfortunately, the hospital does not have a record system that can provide the data to the investigator directly, so the investigator uses the hospital records to locate the patients, extracts demographic data from the intake record, and then finds outcome measures at the end of the year. He enters the data in a spreadsheet and uses the spreadsheet functions to determine basic statistics, such as sex distribution, age, and serum markers, and to plot the serum markers against age. The data is verified manually for accurate data recording (see Section 30.5), and basic statistics, such as ranges, are used to help identify potential errors, such as outliers, which are values outside the expected range.

In contrast to the relatively simple organization of data in a spreadsheet, a relational database allows for different types of information to be stored in different files, linked together using what is called a "key" variable (the Study ID, and often additional variables) to link the different tables together. This organization allows for much more complex data storage than in a spreadsheet. As Example 30A showed, however, sometimes several spreadsheets can be used to mimic this basic structure. Setting up a relational database may require a substantial amount of learning time and possibly the assistance of a data management professional.

Example 30C: This is a study of the long-term effectiveness of an educational program for participants with Type II diabetes. The participants attend a series of lectures on nutrition, proper use of medications, monitoring glucose, and dealing with unforeseen events. The participants have a complete physical and are tested on their knowledge at intake and at the end of the program. During the course of the study all medical events and drugs are recorded. Both diabetes-related events and events that might not be related are recorded. The number of events is not fixed and will vary considerably between participants. The investigators had funding to pay a database specialist, who set up a relational database that allowed for multiple events per participant.

As illustrated in Example 30A, however, it would also be possible to set this up using spreadsheets with some thought and attention.

Example 30C (continued): The spreadsheet approach would require that there be separate sheets for (1) participant demographics, (2) knowledge at intake and end of the program (with an additional variable to show the time of the event), (3) results of the physical examination, (4) medical treatments (with additional identifiers for the start and stop of the medications, and (5) each event (with an additional identifier for the date and number of the event).

A relational database program may be used to store a simple database with a single file if there is a compelling reason to use it. This might arise if extensive data checking has to be done at the time of data entry, which is extremely difficult to implement in a spreadsheet program.

Data analysis programs, such as SAS® and Stata®, also will have some data management capabilities, depending on the program. However, these programs often require a significant learning time and assistance from a knowledgeable user and are not recommended for simple data storage. Many of these programs have added a menu-driven option, which is intended to make them easier to use.

30.2 Documenting the Data

30.2.1 Data Organization and Coding

One problem with using a spreadsheet is that it is easy to begin to enter data, without planning how the data will be analyzed, which affects how it should be stored, as illustrated in Example 30A. In our experience, this is a common mistake that invariably causes much of the data entry to be done again (and again, and again).

It is much better to think ahead about how the data is to be organized, what the valid values are, and how missing data will be treated. This would include not just the values on the questionnaire or ranges of values in biological tests but also any recodes that were added by the database program, such as missing value codes. The acceptable values or range of values for the input variables should be documented and available to the database staff and the users of the database. These would include not just the values on the questionnaire or ranges of values in biological tests but also any special codes that were added. The most common special code is 9 or several 9's that are used to signify missing data. Sometimes these are written down by the study staff before the data is submitted for data entry; other times the data entry staff is instructed to put them in. All special codes must be documented so that future users of the data will understand them and most importantly account for them properly in the analysis. Even if you are the only person doing the data entry and planning to do your own data analysis, you should prepare appropriate documentation, since you can forget these details.

Example 30D: Data analysts were working with a file about newborn conditions. It had been created by a team in a different section of the institution. They were told 99 was the code for the missing data. They began by producing summary statistics for each variable, excluding the 99's. They found that they had a surprisingly high average age for fathers. When they looked at the data, they found there were a large number of fathers who were 88 years old. They contacted the study team who informed them that they had used 88 for missing data when the parent refused to give an age.

30.2.2 The Code Book

The detailed information about the data is often collected in a code book. The typical code book will consist of a series of tables, one for each type of record. Usually it will contain, at a minimum:

- the variable name as it is in the computer (which would be the column heading in a spreadsheet, or the name in the relational database);
- the variable definition, which may just be the name of the field from the data collection instrument;
- the size of the field (number of characters) if in a relational database;
- the source of the variable on the data collection instrument or, if the field is a recode, the sources and, sometimes, the algorithm for recoding;
- the allowable values, which may be a range of values or a list of codes with the meaning for each code; the missing value code(s), and, if more than one missing value code is used, the meaning of the different missing value codes.

The code book may also contain notes on the data, if appropriate, usually separate from the table.

Example 30E: A table from a code book might look like this.

Field Name	Source	Field Size	Values	Missing Datacode
Study ID		4	Numeric	None allowed
Sex	Document	1	1: Female	9
			2: Male	
Age	Document	2	18–65	99
Age Group	Recode of Age	1	1: 18–35	9
			2: 36–50	
			3: 51–65	
FBS	Fasting Blood Glucose	3	Number 50–450	999

Note that we have used 9, 99, and 999 as missing value codes. Such codes are common, but it is essential when the data is analyzed that they be explicitly excluded from any summary statistics.

30.3 Selecting a Data Storage Program

Although specific programs are likely to become ever more complex, and eventually simpler programs will become available, the basic options (a spreadsheet, a relational database, and a data analysis program) are likely to endure. Here are some suggestions on how to choose an appropriate program.

- First of all, find out what software and support is available to you from your institution. Software can be expensive, but many institutions have IT groups that provide software at low or no costs. Some grants will support software purchases.
- Select the least complicated type of software that will serve your purpose. It may be appealing to use a highly thought of package, such as SAS®, but that may have two disadvantages. First, there may be a steep learning curve that will take up time you should be spending on other aspects of the study. Second, the more complicated the program, the more likely it will require some programming to run, and the more complicated the program, the more rules you must obey and the more frustrating it can be when things do not work.
- Unless you know the program very well, make sure there is someone who can help you in case you have a problem. This could be another member of your research group, a helpful colleague, or, if you are lucky, an IT group at your institution. Such groups may provide free or low-cost services, or may be run on a full cost-recovery basis, making them similar to other consulting resources.

Example 30F: SAS®, the Statistical Analysis System, is a very well-known and widely used system for data analysis. It has many features, including data management features, a structured query language, and up-to-date statistical methods. It is expensive, but some institutions have a site license making it available to researchers at a very nominal annual cost. However, it takes substantial time to learn and become proficient in its use. Moreover, the latest statistical procedures may be far more than you need for your study, and are likely to require a great deal of specialist knowledge to use appropriately. R (www.r-project.org) is a free statistical package used by many statisticians engaged in statistical research, but it also requires a substantial time commitment to become proficient with it. However, there are many publications on how to use both these programs for basic data analysis, which may be all you need.

Remember that most data analysis programs will compute whatever statistics you ask for, but that does not mean that those are the right statistics to describe your data or test your hypotheses.

Example 30G: A 4-point rating scale is used to assess severity of disease, with 0 meaning no disease, 1 used for slight disease, 2 for moderate disease, and 3 meaning severe disease. Any software program will happily calculate a mean severity of the numeric values. There are multiple possible distributions that would give any particular mean score. If the mean score was 1.500 it could be that 50% of the group have mild disease (coded as 1) and 50% have moderate disease (coded as 2). Another possibility is that 75% of the group have mild disease (coded as 1) and 25% have severe disease (coded as 3). In the most extreme case, 50% of the group have a score of zero (no disease) and 50% have a score of 3 (severe disease), the mean would still be 1.500. Calculating the frequency of the codes is far more meaningful. In the last case, the distribution shows that half the population actually do not have the disease at all.

30.4 Methods of Data Capture

If the data is in written format, you need to have it entered into the computer, which, if there is a lot of data, may require the help of data entry staff. If the data is structured, as in an intake form with clearly marked fields, you can enter data directly from the form. Often, when existing documents are being used rather than special forms for a study, you do not want to convert all of the data on a document to a computer file. You can either mark up the document showing the fields you want to keep or, if that would be unacceptably messy or hard to follow, manually transfer the data you need to a new form with a clear format. This will reduce errors in entering the data into a computer but may introduce errors in copying.

Data entry may be by key entry, scanned documents, direct transfer from measuring equipment to a data file, or by direct entry from the participant or interviewer. Key entry is the most susceptible to error. Scanning equipment has become more accurate over time but is still susceptible to error, particularly if some responses are handwritten. Often software must be adapted for an application and this must be validated before being put into use, usually by applying it to a small test data set designed to have some tricky problems. Direct transfer of a data file is usually error free technically, but often the data still must be reviewed for content errors, such as assay errors. There may also be transmission errors, although technical procedures can be used that would identify when this occurs.

Since the advent of portable computers and tablets, data collected with questionnaires or interviews can be directly entered into a computer file. Some studies also collect data on smartphone apps, and we expect that this will become more common in the future. It is essential to have the software verify that the data values are acceptable – such as within a given range of numbers – as it is entered and notify the person entering the information if there is an error. It is obviously an advantage for accuracy to have any errors or inconsistencies identified immediately so that it can be corrected on the spot. This is particularly important if the data is being directly entered by a participant, as there will be no source document that can be used if there are inconsistencies in the data entered. There may be a disadvantage, however, if the flow of the interview would be interrupted by error messages or if it reminds the individual being interviewed that his answers are being collected. If the data entry process is sufficiently awkward or time-consuming, the participant may drop out of the study – the last thing you want.

Example 30H. In a cross-sectional study of sexual behaviors in men who have sex with men, a smartphone app was used to collect data anonymously. Most of the data were simple yes or no questions, but there were questions about number of partners and frequency of activity. If a person reported no partners in the previous week, the questions about the activities in the previous week were skipped. If a person reported partners, but answered 0 to frequency of each specific activity, then the option "other activities" appeared which was a fill-in to try to obtain some information. Individuals entering a number of partners, but reporting no activities at all were queried, after the initial data was saved, pointing out that the data was not consistent, and asking if they wished to revise any of their answers.

The approach to data collection needs to be determined before data is collected, as changes during the course of the study may affect data quality and reliability. For this reason we recommend that there always be a small pilot phase in any study to test all the procedures before data collection of participants begins.

30.5 Verifying Data

No matter what method is used to get the data into a computer file, you must verify that the data in the data file are correct – that is, that it accurately represents the collected data. If source documents exist, there are several different types of verification that need to be done. The first level involves checking source documents before they are submitted for conversion to a database, while the second level involves comparison of the data in the database to the source documents. This step is important even if the data entry software also checks the data, because an error that leaves the value within the valid range will not be detected by the software. For example, in Example 30E both a correct age of 45 and a data entry of 54 are valid values. For directly entered data, once the procedures to capture data have been tested and validated, you are assured that the data in the data file accurately represents the data entered, so these two steps can be skipped. Similarly, these steps may be omitted if the source of the data and the methods of data capture are very reliable, such as transfers between computers.

The third level is an examination of the contents of the database itself to identify any implausible values that are not due to errors in the coding or in the transfer to the database. This step is needed no matter what the source of the data or how it is captured into the database.

The first level of verification, if needed, may consist of a knowledgeable individual reading the source documents to make sure they are complete and only valid codes are entered. If the data entry document has been derived from a source, such as a laboratory report, a more time-consuming comparison of coded sheets to source documents may be required. This would also be needed if the data is abstracted from preexisting documents and entered onto a study-specific form to make data entry easier. In small studies this is often done by the person responsible for the data collection; in larger studies it may be done by another individual, sometimes a senior staff member, but more typically another person involved in the data collection.

Comparison of the data in the database to source documents may be done in several ways. Manual editing is the oldest and most obvious method of verification. It may be done by visual comparison with the source documents. This is the simplest way but also the slowest, the most labor intensive, and the most prone to errors. It may be useful for small files such as Example 30A. Preferably, two people will do this: one will read the data from the computer file while the other compares it to the source documents. Another approach is to have the data reentered by another individual, usually one known for accuracy, into a separate file. Software is available to compare two files, often while the data is being reentered. This is usually quicker than visual comparison but is still time-consuming and is only useful for data that was key entered.

Example 30I: An investigator was doing a record review of patients who presented at the emergency room with possible appendicitis, to determine what factors influenced the decision to perform surgery. The investigator abstracted information from hospital charts for one year, and then asked a colleague to verify his data extraction (first-level verification). A research assistant entered the data into a single computer file and the investigator verified this by comparing the data to his original records (second-level verification).

Computer programs can be used to validate data for consistency no matter what the source was. These may detect errors in the data transfer and also may detect errors in the source. During the data capture phase, simple field edits may check for valid codes and valid ranges (called "range checks") and comparability between fields. For example, participants may be asked to skip some questions on a form if the answer to a certain question is No. These instructions are known as "skip patterns."

Example 30J: A general medical history form that was given to all potential participants in a study included several skip patterns. Section 1 of the form collected for demographic information, such as sex. Section 2 of the form collected history of pregnancy and childbirth. Men were instructed to skip this section. The first question of Section 2 asked how many pregnancies the person had, and, if the answer was 0 the person was told to go on to Section 3. Otherwise, details of each pregnancy were collected. Editing software can be programmed to validate that no one who was identified as Male in Section 1 filled out any part of Section 2, that a woman who said she had 0 pregnancies skipped the rest of Section 2, and that a woman who said she had at least one pregnancy completed basic information in Section 2 for exactly the number of pregnancies reported.

We recommend that all fields be given numeric codes if possible. Using letters may cause multiple problems, such as the frequent confusion of uppercase and lowercase letters. It is not uncommon to find four genders in a file: M, F, m, and f. This is also true for other alphabetic information: Aspirin and Apsirin are not the same to a computer.

Once the data is in the database, summary statistics such as means, extreme values, frequencies and cross-tabulations can be used to detect discrepancies in the data that might not be detected by range checks for the third level of validation. Not only single values but also calculated values such as age or BMI may be used to detect inconsistencies between variables. Unlikely age values indicate a potential error in either the date of birth or the date of measurement, but may be real. A very large or very small BMI can be due to an error in weight or height, but is sometimes real. When the summary statistics show questionable results, the records that have the unlikely values need to be identified and then the source documents examined to determine whether the errors are in the data transfer (which can easily be fixed) or in the original source data.

Example 30K: In a study of testosterone replacement therapy, participants underwent strength testing at baseline and after 6 months of treatment. The test included the maximum amount of weight that a participant could lift one time (1RM). When the data was examined, the 1RM distribution for both baseline and 6 months were within the range of values specified for the study, but when the percent change at 6 months was examined, there was one very extreme value, about 600% improvement, while the next biggest increase was only about 100%. When the original record was examined, it showed that the recorded value for the participant at baseline was at the low end of the range whereas the recorded value at six months was at the high end. After checking the man's height and weight at baseline, the investigators decided that the baseline value was most likely correct. Since there was no other data suggesting that the 6-month value was reasonable (such as a note that the participant had started a serious exercise program), the investigators concluded that the 6-month value and thus the change measure calculated from it were incorrect and need to be treated as missing values.

If errors are found, they should be corrected if possible. If the error is a data entry error, then it may be corrected from the source document. If the data comes from the source document, then sometimes it can be corrected by going back to other records or to the participant and sometimes by common sense. In Example 30J the error might be incorrect sex or an incorrect number of pregnancies, and sometimes could be corrected; for example, study staff would usually know the participant's sex.

Example 30L: If a participant's age, computed from date of birth and visit date, is unrealistically low or high, you can usually tell from the dates which is likely to be the incorrect one. If the error is due to an invalid date of birth, which was recorded in the study records, you may still be able to get the correct date of birth from other records or by asking the participant. If there is an invalid visit date, you may be able to get the correct visit date from other study records, such as the date of laboratory tests.

If a variable cannot be corrected, then it must be considered missing data. In Example 30K, examination of the participant's other physical characteristics suggested that the baseline value was correct, but review of the other data at 6 months suggested that value was an error. It was not possible to retest the participant because neither the baseline nor the 6-month conditions could be duplicated. Unfortunately, the error was on the source document so there was no way to determine the correct value.

Data verification should be done without knowledge of the participant's role in the study, as otherwise such knowledge might bias the reviewer when it is necessary to decide whether a value is acceptable. In an interventional study, the reviewer should not know the treatment group for participants while the data is being validated. In a case-control study, the reviewer should not know whether the participant is a case or a control, and in a cohort study, the reviewer should not know any of the outcome variables when validating the exposure data. Ideally, the reviewer would not know the value of any other variables except those necessary to determine if the value is truly an error or just an outlier.

Example 30K (continued): The reviewer has to know the before and after 1RM values and the physical measurements for the participant to determine whether the percent change is an error, and possibly identify which of the before or after variables is an error. Information indicating the participant's treatment, including side effects, is not needed for this and should not be known to the reviewer.

Even the best staff member will make errors in coding or entering data, and errors in mechanical data capture can occur. But if verification shows an unacceptably high error rate, then steps to correct this should be initiated. These may include further training of the staff, modification of the data collection instruments, or upgrading of scanning equipment or programs.

30.6 Preserving Confidentiality

In Chapter 29 we discussed the importance of preserving the individual's confidentiality. The first step is to assign them a Study ID number (Section 29.1), which is meaningless except as a link to the personal information. All the documents that are used to create a data file should be identified by the Study ID number only. The link between Study ID and the person's identifying information should be kept in a secure computer file separate from the other data, or a locked cabinet or drawer with limited access. Needless to say, you must continue this security when creating the database. All documents will be identified by the Study ID number only, particularly if they will be sent to other groups to be processed. Records on the data file should not contain any identifying information. We recommend that computer records of personal information be maintained in a separate file created by a single person, password protected, and stored on encrypted hardware using methods approved at your institution, separately from all other data. If images are involved in the study, then it is essential that any stored images have patient identifiers removed before storage, or that they be stored with the other personal information and not as part of the general data file.

After a study is completed, there is often a requirement to archive the data to assure that questions about the data can be investigated even after the results are published. The archiving requirements are sometimes specified by sponsors or by legal requirements. Whenever the data is archived, participant confidentiality must always be preserved.

Participants also have the right to withdraw consent at any time. When this occurs, the participant may have the right to withdraw permission for the use of any data collected during the study if this right has been specified in the consent form. Given that multiple backups of the data should have been made to ensure that data is never lost, it will be impossible to physically delete the participants' data from backup data sets. The data, however, would have to be removed from the primary data set and should not be used in any analysis of the study.

There is also an increasing movement for data sharing. This has been required for all large studies sponsored by the U.S. National Institutes of Health since 2003. Journals are beginning to impose requirements on availability of data as well, and may insist that the data be available as a condition of publication. When such requirements are imposed, the investigator must remove an extensive list of potential personal identifiers, specified in the Privacy Rule (Section 2.1.2). Additional information may also have to be withheld depending on the specifics of the study if it could potentially be used to identify an individual. This process produces a de-identified data set intended to protect participant confidentiality.

Finally, there is also the problem of hackers breaking into business or institutional files. It is important that the database be protected from unauthorized entry. In addition to password protection, your institution should have procedures to protect and backup the files in their system. You want to ensure that these procedures are applied to your files automatically.

30.7 A Note on Programs

Although the previous sections mention specific programs as examples for different types of data storage programs, we remind you that between the time this is written and the time you read it, new programs may be available for your use. The basic concepts, however, should still hold.

30.8 Ethical Issues

In this chapter we are concerned with maintaining the quality of the data as it is transferred to a computer for analysis. This activity can present several opportunities for errors, and methods for validating the data must be used. If the integrity of the study data is not assured, the results of the study may become questionable and the validity of the study may be compromised. Therefore, it is necessary to decide how these activities will be done when planning the study and assure that there are adequate resources (financial and technical staff) so that these activities can be carried out correctly.

You must continue to protect the confidentiality of the participants through this step, and make sure that even if material is transferred between functional groups, such as investigator and data entry staff, or images to a central reader, that participant privacy is protected. Participant privacy must be protected even after the study is completed. If data needs to be shared, then resources and technical support to create de-identified data sets must be considered when planning the study.

KEY POINTS

- Maintenance of data quality is essential for a valid study.
- Data quality depends on carefully and completely described measurement procedures when the data is collected.
- The study data used for analysis must be verified.
- Data may be verified in several ways:
  - review of the data entry documents before data entry;
  - verifying that the data on the database is the same as the data in the source documents; and
  - verifying that the data in the database is consistent and plausible.
- Data should be corrected if possible, but uncorrectable data must be treated as missing data.
- Steps to protect participant confidentiality should be included in the data management plan.
- Maintaining data quality through data processing and analysis requires resources that must be included in the protocol budget.

STATISTICAL CONCEPTS

Hypothesis Testing

This book is about designing compelling clinical research. This involves a rigorously defined hypothesis to be addressed using an appropriate study design with appropriate measurement techniques and observation times so that at the end of the study you will be able to draw compelling conclusions. These conclusions require that the hypothesis be tested using appropriate statistical methods for the study design adopted and the measurements made. We introduce the basic concepts of hypothesis testing in this appendix.

A.1 The Criminal Trial as an Analogy for Hypothesis Testing

A common analogy to hypothesis tests is a criminal trial. Table A.1 presents the results of a jury trial to make the analogy clearer. In Table A.1, the columns are the truth, known only to the defendant: innocent or guilty. The rows are the verdict: not guilty or guilty. The cells of this 2x2 table are whether the jury's decision was correct or incorrect. We call an incorrect verdict an "error" in the table to strengthen the analogy.

There is a truth (either the defendant is innocent or guilty), but only the defendant actually knows this. There is also a verdict (either not

Table A.1. Verdicts versus Trial

	Truth	
Verdict	Innocent	Guilty
Not guilty	Correct	Error
Guilty	Error	Correct

guilty or guilty), which is the decision the jury makes without knowing the truth. No matter which verdict the jury returns, it may be correct or incorrect. Thus the jury may decide the defendant is guilty even though the defendant is actually not guilty, or the jury may return a verdict of not guilty even though the defendant is guilty. A trial occurs because the prosecutor hopes to prove the defendant guilty. The jury is supposed to assume the defendant is not guilty until proven otherwise.

For the jury, there is no way to know whether the verdict (decision) is correct or incorrect except in exceptional circumstances. Conceivably, a guilty defendant might admit it after the jury returns a verdict.

Example A1: A jury returns a verdict of not guilty. Since under U.S. law a defendant cannot be tried twice for the same crime, the incredulous defendant, whose story during the trial was that it was all a mistake, shouts out, "Thank you, you fools! I got away with it."

Example A2: A jury returns a verdict of guilty. The defendant spends multiple years in jail, until another person, close to dying, confesses to the crime to clear his conscience.

Unfortunately, Example A2 is much more likely to be how legal errors are discovered.

A.2 Hypothesis Testing

Hypothesis testing is similar to a trial. We have two hypotheses, either of which could be true:

- the null hypothesis (a straw man, which you hope to disprove)
- the alternative hypothesis (which is what you hope to prove)

which is similar to a trial of whether the defendant is not guilty or guilty. There are also two decisions that we can make using statistical testing:

- fail to reject the null hypothesis
- reject the null hypothesis

which is similar to the jury deciding on not guilty (or, in certain systems not proven) and guilty.

Table A.2 Decisions versus Truth

	Truth	
Decision	Null Hypothesis	Alternative Hypothesis
Fail to reject null hypothesis	Correct	Error
Reject null hypothesis	Error	Correct

The hypothesis testing situation is shown in Table A.2. Like Table A.1, the columns are the truth, the rows are the decisions, and the cell entries are the accuracy of the decision.

A study occurs because the investigator hopes to show that the alternative hypothesis is true. Like a jury, the investigator starts with the presumption that the null hypothesis is true. The investigator makes the decision based on the results of a statistical test.

Here the defendant on trial is the null hypothesis, while the verdict is the decision made from statistical testing. Just as a trial occurs not to prove that someone is innocent but to try to prove that the person is guilty, you do an experiment in the hopes of rejecting the null hypothesis. Usually the null hypothesis is that there are no differences between two or more groups, between a group and a hypothesized value, or that there is no association between an exposure and an outcome. The alternative hypothesis is what you hope the data will show – for example, that there is a difference between the two groups. Usually the alternative hypothesis is the opposite of the null hypothesis.

The alternative hypothesis can be either two-sided or one-sided, depending on whether you are interested in any difference or only a difference in a specific direction – such as only being interested if the result in one group is larger than in the other. Even though you are thinking of a one-sided alternative most of the time, this may cause you to miss an important unexpected (and sometimes unwelcome) finding, so a two-sided alternative is recommended for almost all studies.

Example A3: In the study in Example 22A, two oral treatments are compared for the treatment of Type II diabetes. The sponsor of the trial (who makes the new treatment) hopes that the new treatment is superior to the current treatment in controlling HbA1c. Therefore, this is a superiority trial, and the null hypothesis is that there is no difference between the two treatments, while the alternative hypothesis is that there is a difference, which is a two-sided approach. Although the sponsor is interested only in showing that their new treatment is better, if it turns out that the new treatment is worse, the company should not miss that information.

Example A4: In an early study of a new exercise program for building strength in elderly individuals, the investigator is only interested if the new intervention is more effective than the standard exercise program. If the new program is not better, the investigator will try to develop an alternative program. Here the investigator decides to use a one-sided significance test and is willing to miss evidence that the program is actually worse than the standard exercise program being offered.

The analogy between a trial and an experiment is not perfect, however. In a trial, usually there are at least two advocates: one trying to convince the jury that the defendant is guilty and one trying to convince the jury that the defendant is not guilty. In an experiment, you have a single investigator who is trying to find the truth even though hoping for a certain outcome.

In a randomized interventional study, the null hypothesis is usually that two quantities (such as the mean blood pressure or the mean time to recovery) are the same in the two groups. In practice, the null hypothesis is interpreted to mean that there is no clinically important difference between the two groups. If measurements are sufficiently precise or enough observations are made, a difference (however trivial) can always be found.

Hypothesis testing has an advantage over a criminal trial in that it is possible to specify the probability of the errors mathematically. The significance level, usually denoted α, is called the "Type I error." It is the probability that you reject the null hypothesis based on your experiment if the null hypothesis is actually true. This is equivalent to finding an innocent person guilty. Probabilities vary from 0 (impossible) to 1 (certain). Traditionally, the significance level is 0.05 for a two-sided significance test. This implies that one time in 20 you will reject the null hypothesis even though it is true. The actual test statistic is calculated after the study is completed. It is based on the study design and the statistical test used for the analysis. This is chosen by the investigator and should be specified before the experiment starts.

The other type of error, failing to reject the null hypothesis when the alternative hypothesis is true, is called a "Type II error." The probability of this error is denoted by β. Unlike the Type I error, which is specified by the significance level, the probability of a Type II error depends on a specific value of the expected effect if the alternative hypothesis is true. The value $1 - \beta$ is called the "power" of the study. It is the probability that you will detect a statistically significant effect for this specific value of the alternative hypothesis, which itself is an important part of the design of the study.

Calculating power is more difficult than simply specifying a significance level, as power is calculated for a specified expected difference or effect size, the expected variation in the data, and a specific sample size. The power changes if any of these factors change. Power increases if the effect size is bigger, if the variation in the data is smaller, or if the sample size is bigger.

It is sometimes helpful to use the analogy of power as the chance of detecting a signal in a noisy message. The ability to detect a signal increases as the signal gets stronger or the noise in the message gets smaller. The effect size is the signal you want to detect, which is why power increases as the effect size gets bigger. The noise in the signal is proportional to the variability but decreases as the sample size in the study increases. Power increases as the noise gets smaller: the variation in the data gets smaller, or the sample size gets bigger.

Traditionally when designing a study, one is expected to have 80% power or higher, and the sample size needed to give you the desired power is calculated based on the specific values used for the alternative hypothesis. This is discussed in more detail in Appendix B.

Hypothesis testing is done after the experiment is completed to determine whether the results are statistically significant. The formal hypothesis testing framework is shown in Table A.3. Again, the columns are

Table A.3. The Formal Hypothesis Testing Framework

	Truth	
Decision	Null Hypothesis	Alternative Hypothesis
Fail to Reject Null Hypothesis ("Not statistically significant")	Correct 1-α	Type II Error β
Reject Null Hypothesis ("Statistically significant")	Type I Error α	Correct (Power) 1-β

truth, the rows are decisions, but now the cells include both whether the decision is correct and formal names and notation for the errors.

In designing an experiment, you specify both the Type I error, α (usually 0.05, two-sided), and the desired power (1-β) for a specific effect.

Example A3 (continued): To design a study the sponsor needs to make assumptions about what the effect size will be and what the variability in the measurement would be. If the sponsor chooses a large effect size (such as a 1.0% reduction in HbA1c compared to standard treatment [10.9 mmol/mol in IFCC units]), then the study would be smaller than if the sponsor chooses a small effect size (such as a 0.4%, 4.4 mmol/mol) for the same power and estimated variability in the measurements.

The third major element in hypothesis testing is the P-value. Sometimes the P-value is confused with the significance level (α), but they are not the same thing. The P-value is calculated from the data after the study is completed and then compared to the significance level (α), which was specified when the study was designed. The P-value is the probability that the results of the statistical test or something more extreme would have been observed if the null hypothesis is true and the other assumptions of the statistical test are correct. As the P-value is a probability, it ranges from 0.0 (impossible) to 1.0 (certain). There are many assumptions involved in statistical tests and one of the most important is that there are no systematic biases in the data. The P-value calculated will not be valid if there is bias in the study.

A.3 Determining Statistical Significance

Hypothesis testing is a formal method of determining statistical significance. After collecting the data, you determine statistical significance using a simple process:

- First, you apply a statistical test to the observed data to calculate what is called the "test statistic." The statistical test is determined by the study design and the nature of the data, as different statistical tests are used for different types of outcomes (such as discrete variables, continuous variables, and time-to-event variables).
- Second, you determine the P-value by comparing the test statistic calculated from your data to the distribution for the test statistic assuming that the null hypothesis and other assumptions are true. The P-value calculation depends on whether your alternative hypothesis is one-sided or two-sided, but not on the specific value of the alternative hypothesis you selected. If you are doing a one-sided test, then only differences in the correct direction can give a small P-value. For the conventional two-sided test, the direction of the difference does not matter.
- Third, you compare the P-value calculated from the data after the study ends to the significance level, α, specified before the study started. If the P-value is smaller than the significance level, the results are called "statistically significant." If the P-value is not smaller than the significance level, then the results are considered "not statistically significant."

If the P-value is smaller than the significance level, then you "reject the null hypothesis" and have found a statistically significant difference.

Example A5: In a randomized double-blind parallel group study comparing two different hypnotics for sleep, the sponsor used validated objective procedures to assess sleep duration to ensure accurate measurement of the outcome. The new hypnotic had a longer mean sleep duration than the standard of care and the P-value was smaller than the α=0.05 (two-sided) specified in the protocol. Since the randomized, double-blind design eliminated the most common types of biases, the P-value calculated was likely to be a valid measure of the effect of the intervention. Thus, the sponsor was able to reject the null hypothesis that the mean sleep duration was the same in the two groups.

Example A6: An investigator did a pilot study testing a new treatment to delay progression of chronic renal failure to end stage renal disease, Participants were randomized to standard of care plus the new treatment or standard of care alone. This was an open-label study because the investigator did not have access to placebo medication. The endpoint was estimated glomerular filtration rate (eGFR) obtained from standard laboratory results. The use of an objective endpoint reduces, but does not eliminate, concern that the study was not blinded. The P-value was greater than the traditional $\alpha=0.05$ (two-sided). Therefore the investigator failed to reject the null hypothesis that the change in eGFR was the same in the two groups.

It is important to look at precisely what the results mean. In Example A5 the decision is to reject the null hypothesis. As the new hypnotic had a longer mean sleep duration than the standard of care, the sponsor could conclude that there was a statistically significantly longer mean duration of sleep with the new hypnotic compared to the standard of care.

The interpretation is more complicated in Example A6. The results are not statistically significant, so the decision is formally stated as "Fail to Reject Null Hypothesis." The decision is not called "Accept Null Hypothesis," because that is not the decision. Failing to reject is not the same as accepting. It means that there is not enough evidence in the study to reject the null hypothesis.

If the results of the study are not statistically significant, you need to determine the utility of the study by recalculating the power for the alternative hypothesis specified before the study began using the variability observed in the experiment. If this post hoc power is sufficiently high, then you can conclude that there is good evidence that the difference between the two groups, if any, is not as large as you hypothesized. If the power is not large, however, then it is very difficult to conclude anything. This is shown in Figure A.1.

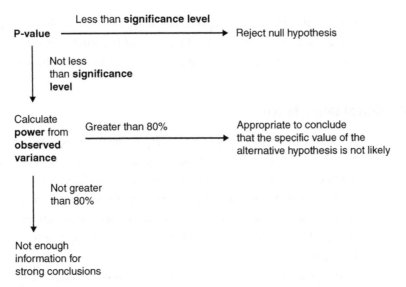

Figure A.1.

Example A3 (continued). The sponsor decided to design the study to have 80% power assuming that the treatment effect would be a 1% difference in HbA1c. At the end of the study, the P-value was greater than the significance level (α) specified before the study began, so the sponsor concluded that the results failed to reject the null hypothesis. The variability was even smaller than the estimate used when planning the study, but the difference found was only 0.4%. As the variability was even smaller than their initial estimate, the study had more than 80% power to detect a 1% difference between the two groups if such a difference existed. The sponsor has to conclude that the difference, if any, is less than the 1% which was assumed when designing the study.

Example A6 (continued). The investigator had not done a formal power calculation for the pilot study, which was approved by the local Institutional Review Board (IRB) without a formal sample size justification. She went to a statistician for assistance to calculate the power for the study. The statistician explained that you calculate post hoc power for the alternative hypothesis specified before the study began. As she did not have a pre-specified alternative hypothesis, they explored the issue further. The statistician learned that other studies with a 20% difference in eGFR had been considered clinically important, so used that value as the alternative hypothesis. Based on the sample size of the study and the observed variability, the power of the study was under 20%. Her study, while interesting, could not make any firm conclusions.

A.4 Clinical Importance

Although this Appendix is called Hypothesis Testing, it is essential to keep in mind why we are testing hypotheses. We are trying to assess whether the effects we find in a study are statistically significant or not. If the effects are statistically significant, then there is reasonable evidence that the results are not due to chance, although this would be expected to be the case for 1 claim out of 20, using the traditional 0.05 Type I error.

The goal of your study is not solely to have a statistically significant effect, however. You are hoping to show an effect that matters, that is important for clinical care. The term "clinical importance" is used to denote this concept. Always remember that statistical significance is not the same as clinical importance. Statistical significance implies that an observation is unlikely to have occurred by chance if the assumptions underlying the analysis are true. A statistically significant result occurs because the effect (signal) is large compared to the noise (little variability in the data or a large sample size). Statistical significance does not imply that the observation matters or is important. Similarly, an observation may be very important clinically but may not be statistically significant. A result is not statistically significant because the effect (signal) is small compared to the noise (more variability in the data or a small sample size.) Statistical significance does not imply clinical importance, and clinical importance does not imply statistical significance.

Example A5 (continued): The new hypnotic was statistically significantly ($P < 0.000001$) better than the standard of care in mean sleep duration, but the difference was only 7 minutes: 8 hours 26 minutes in the standard of care arm versus 8 hours 33 minutes of sleep on average with the new treatment.

Example A6 (continued): The result was not statistically significant ($P=0.18$), but the estimated difference between the two groups was even larger than what would be considered a clinically important effect: no change in eGFR during the course of the study in the experimental group, while eGFR decreased by 25% in the control group, about the amount expected for this population for the length of the study. These results would be clinically quite important if real, since it could delay progression to renal failure. Because this difference, even though clinically important, might be a chance finding, it needs to be confirmed in another – and larger – study.

A.5 Ethical Issues

There are several different ethical issues involved in hypothesis testing, calculating a sample size, and designing a study. Here we will focus on the ethical issues of hypothesis testing, although we must emphasize that using unreasonable assumptions when planning a study raises ethical concerns about doing the study at all, since the study has little chance of achieving its goal. This point is discussed further in Appendix B.

There are two major issues when considering hypothesis testing. First, one always needs to consider the potential for bias in a study as a possible explanation of any significant findings. Failing to do this, in our opinion, is equivalent to accepting a result because you like the way it came out. Investigators always attempt to explain results that they do not like (a negative finding), and this same effort must be made to rule out other explanations of positive findings to maintain scientific integrity.

The second issue is what might be termed "desperately seeking significance." This is a common phenomenon that we have often observed over the years. After the study is over, there is a natural hope to find statistically significant results. Such results make the effort of the study feel more worthwhile and, we admit, make publication of small studies easier. Nonetheless, if the basic results of the study are negative after appropriate analysis, that result needs to be accepted and published. One should not, as some investigators do, attempt to find subgroups that are significantly different so that one can report significant results. For example, we are aware of reports that a treatment works in men 40–44 years old. This is data dredging, equivalent to changing your null hypothesis after looking at the data. If you do tests of 20 different subgroups, each with a Type I error of 5%, then you would expect to reject the null hypothesis one time by chance. If you do 60 independent tests, then you would be expected to have three statistically significant results by chance. Testing until you find something statistically significant, and then reporting it without discussing all the tests that were done, is deliberately misleading at best.

KEY POINTS

- Hypothesis testing is a formal method to determine the statistical significance of the results of a study.
- There are three basic elements in a hypothesis test:
  - a null hypothesis, which is what you hope to disprove: usually that there is no difference between the groups;
  - an alternative hypothesis, which is what you hope to prove. The important aspect for hypothesis testing is whether this is a one-sided or two-sided alternative hypothesis, as this has implications for the P-value calculated from the data; and
  - the Type I error (α) that determines the probability that you will reject the null hypothesis even though it is true. The Type I error is specified before the study is done.
- There are two decisions you can make at the end of hypothesis testing: to fail to reject the null hypothesis, or to reject the null hypothesis.
- The decision is made by comparing the P-value, calculated from the data after the study is completed, to the Type I error (α), specified before the study began.
  - If the P-value is less than α, you reject the null hypothesis.
  - If the P-value is more than α, you fail to reject the null hypothesis. This is not the same as accepting the null hypothesis. No matter which decision you make, you can be correct or you can be wrong.
- When the study is designed, you should define the value of the effect you hope to observe and make sure that your study has a high probability (power) of detecting this effect if it exists.
- Statistical significance is not the same as clinical importance.

- Statistical significance implies that a finding is unlikely to have occurred by chance if the assumptions for the calculations are true. Statistical significance does not imply that the finding matters or is important.
- Clinical importance implies that a finding matters. Clinical importance does not imply that the finding is real, however, as it could be nothing more than a chance result.
- Statistical significance does not imply clinical importance, and clinical importance does not imply statistical significance.

Appendix B

Determining the Sample Size for a Study

In Appendix A we introduced the basic framework for hypothesis testing. Here we discuss sample size, which is a critical aspect of study design. We have placed this as the last material in the book because sample size should be considered only after you have worked on the basic design of your study and thought about the key features including who you would hope to study, what measurements you hope to collect, and how you will minimize the potential for bias in your study. Most importantly, you have to ensure that the study, once completed, will give meaningful results, whether they are what you hoped for or not.

B.1 Why Sample Size Matters

In Appendix A we discussed how to interpret the results of a study in terms of whether the results are statistically significant, and, if not, whether the study had reasonable power to detect the predefined difference. Both the significance level and the planned power for the study are specified when designing the study.

A major factor affecting the power of the study is the number of participants in the study, that is, the sample size. If the study is too small, there will not be enough information for strong conclusions and the work involved in the study will be wasted.

Example B1: In Example A6, an investigator found what could be a clinically important effect in slowing the progression of eGFR decline in patients with chronic renal failure, but the results were not statistically significant (P= 0.18), so the investigator could not rule out that this difference might have been a chance finding. The investigator, in discussion with the statistician, decided that a 20% difference in eGFR was a reasonable alternative hypothesis for a clinically important effect. If the investigator wanted to design a study to detect a difference of 20% in eGFR assuming the standard deviation observed in her study, then the study would need to be about seven times as large to have had adequate power (80%) for this alternative hypothesis,

Equally, however, if a study is far bigger than it needs to be to make compelling conclusions, then too many participants have been exposed to the risks of the study, no matter how minimal, which is again unethical. Moreover, a very large sample size may lead to an effect being statistically significant even when it is clinically unimportant, which may exaggerate the usefulness of a new treatment.

Example B2: In Example A5, a manufacturer of a new sleeping treatment did a very large study, with 10,000 participants per group, to show that their new medication is more effective than an existing medication, and succeeded in showing a statistically significant difference (P< 0.000001) for a very small effect (7 minutes average sleep time). It is possible that the company designed the study for a very small effect size, or a much more variable endpoint, but it is also possible that the study was much larger than it needed to be so that the small effect could be claimed as statistically significant with an exceedingly small P-value.

So the goal of determining the sample size is to find the "just right number," not too small and not too big, to have a reasonable chance to detect the effect of interest as statistically significant, but not to recruit far more participants than needed.

B.2 Calculating a "Just Right Number"

In theory, there is one, and only one, "just right number" of participants. The basic elements of the calculation are the following:

- the type of endpoint (continuous, binary, ordered categorical, unordered categorical), which dictates the statistical test you will need to use;

- the magnitude of the difference that matters (the alternative hypothesis);
- the noise in the endpoint (the standard deviation);
- the statistical characteristics of the study
  - what is considered statistically significant (the Type I error or α; conventionally, this is 0.05, two-sided);
  - how confident you want to be that, if the difference and the variability are what you specified, you will detect the difference as statistically significant (the power of the study). Traditionally power should be at least 80% and often 90% is desired.

Power is equal to $1-$Type II error, where the Type II error is the probability that the alternative hypothesis is true but the statistical test fails to reject the null hypothesis. The calculations also involve the study design and assumptions about how many additional participants are needed so that at the end of the study you have the number you need after some participants drop out.

Example B3. An investigator determines that a study requires 100 participants to complete the study, and expects that as many as 20% of the participants might drop out. The investigator needs to recruit 125 participants, so that after allowing for 20% of the 125 participants dropping out, there will be about 100 participants completing the study.

In this chapter we assume the most common study type: a parallel group interventional study, trying to show that one intervention is different from (superior to) the other, so that the null hypothesis is that the two interventions are the same. There are other goals for some studies: showing that two interventions are similar (called an "equivalence study"), or showing that one is not too much worse than another (called a "non-inferiority study"), but both are beyond the scope of this material. Once all these decisions have been made, you or the statistician who is working with you can put them into a computer program that calculates power and sample size, and there you have it: the unique "just right number" given your assumptions.

B.3 The Problem with the "Just Right Number"

The two big assumptions involved in calculating this "just right number" are the magnitude of difference that matters and the variability of the endpoint. In theory, the magnitude of difference that matters is the smallest difference that would be clinically important; a smaller difference would not matter clinically. Unfortunately, such a difference cannot be rigorously defined and differs for different investigators.

Example B4: An investigator wants to study whether a treatment improves survival in extremely premature infants (born before 32 weeks). The investigator feels that if this improves survival by 1%, it will be a clinically important difference given what is known about the side effects and complications of the therapy. This means that for this investigator a potential benefit from therapy of 1% improvement in survival would be sufficient to outweigh what is known about the risks (the side effects of the treatment; the complication of administering the treatment to premature infants), and that if that benefit is found, the therapy should be used. Other neonatologists, however, might weigh the benefits and risks differently. A neonatologist who considers the risks as unimportant compared to an increase in survival might well consider a smaller improvement in survival, perhaps even 0.1%, as clinically important. In contrast, a neonatologist who considered the risks particularly worrisome might feel that a much larger improvement in survival, such as 5%, would be necessary for the treatment to be clinically worthwhile. Thus the clinically important difference might be 1%, 0.1%, or 5% depending on an individual's views about the importance of the side effects and complications compared to an improvement in survival.

Despite the problem with determining such a difference, it is essential to specify one when planning a study to calculate the "just right number."

Example B4 (continued): After much discussion with colleagues, the investigator decides that the potential risks of substantial long-term morbidity mean that a larger improvement in survival is necessary for the treatment to be useful. Thus, the investigator decides that the clinically meaningful difference should be a 5% difference and consults a statistician to review the design and for an appropriate sample size. After reviewing the design proposed (a parallel group randomized double-blind interventional study), the statistician asks what the survival rate currently is, which the investigator estimates from his experience as 70–80%. The statistician suggests that the investigator review the clinic records to get a better estimate for the patients likely to be included in the study, but calculates the sample size for this range to give the investigator a rough idea of the needed sample size. Since the difference is relatively small, the sample sizes are large: 2,582 total for 70% versus 75% and 1,890 total for 80% versus 85%, for 80% power and an alpha level of 0.05 (two-sided). The investigator is rather shocked by this and blurts out that he was thinking of a study of 100 or 200 infants total, since even 200 infants would require two or three years for him to recruit.

Here we see the nub of the real sample size problem: we can calculate the "just right number" under a set of assumptions, but that may not be at all feasible for a study.

B.4 Legitimate Ways to Reduce the "Just Right Number"

There are many legitimate ways to decrease the "just right number." Perhaps the easiest thing to consider is altering the endpoint to make it more sensitive. Instead of a yes or no variable, one can use a more sensitive measure.

Example B5: In a study to see whether a new agent increased platelet count, the investigators originally proposed a double-blind randomized placebo controlled study to see whether a drug raised platelet count above a prespecified criterion (a yes-no variable) compared to no treatment. Given the expected effect of the drug (50% above this criterion in the treated group versus 30% in the control group population), the sample size needed was 103 per group for 80% power and alpha=0.05, two-sided. If the endpoint were changed to the increase in the actual change in platelet level, which was expected to be 50,000 in the experimental group compared to 30,000 in the control group, with a standard deviation of 40,000, then the sample size would be reduced to 64 per group for the same Type I and II errors. Although this reduces the sample size, it is important to note that this also changes the question being answered. In the first case the question is whether there was a difference in the proportion of participants achieving a specific level, while in the second the question is whether there is a difference in the change in the number of platelets.

Another way to decrease the sample size is to reduce the variability of the measurements. There are two components to the variability: variability between individuals and variability in the measurement itself. It is usually simpler to reduce measurement variability than variability between individuals.

The most important way to reduce variability in measurements is to ensure that all assessors are following the same procedures and making measurements the same way. In Section 29.3, we talked about the importance of the Manual of Procedures (MOP) and of specifying standardized procedures for data collection. However, even with the most completely described procedures, there may still be variability between the assessors.

Variability between investigators in multi-center studies may be due to differences between institutions. Another source may be when there is considerable variability in making the measurement. Even automated procedures to measure diastolic blood pressure have considerable variability when measuring the same person several times, reflecting the variability of blood pressure in an individual. One way to reduce the variability in the measurement is to increase the number of times you make a measurement, and use the average value, since mathematically this should have a smaller error around the true value.

Example B6: Because of variability in blood pressure readings, when assessing changes in blood pressure over time, it is conventional to measure blood pressure several times during the course of each visit when it is a major outcome in a research study. The average of several blood pressure measurement during a single visit will usually be a more precise measure than a single blood pressure reading of an individual's blood pressure. An even more precise measurement, using a Holter monitor, can be used to obtain an average blood pressure over 24 hours. This, however, has a substantial cost and is very inconvenient for participants.

However, even the most systematic process will not eliminate the inherent variability between different individuals. For this, it is necessary to try to make the population more homogeneous.

Example B7: Intra-ocular pressure is variable in an individual around their true average pressure over time. Sometimes the measured value will be higher than the true underlying value and sometimes lower, even if the measured value is the average of several measurements. Averaging will reduce the variability around the true value at the time of measurement but will not reduce the day-to-day variability in pressure within a person. Thus, when recruiting glaucoma patients for a study, it is common to require two measurements of intra-ocular pressure on different days, both of which show that the potential participant has glaucoma, before considering that the inclusion criterion is met. If intra-ocular pressure was assessed only on one day, there would be a chance that the participant met the criterion only because that measurement happened to be a high value around their true value, but that they did not have glaucoma. When measured on different days, the chance that the patient is erroneously considered to have glaucoma is substantially reduced, making the participant population more homogeneous.

Another way to reduce the variability in the outcome measurement(s) is to reduce the variability between participants by narrowing the inclusion criteria, for example by restricting the age range or limiting enrollment to patients with a particular stage of the disease, to create a more homogeneous population in the study. Although factors such as these are often limited for good reasons, a narrowly defined study population can limit the generalizability of your results to the population of interest. This is discussed in detail in Chapter 11.

Finally, the statistical characteristics can sometimes be modified to reduce the required sample size. Sometimes it is legitimate to use a one-sided test of statistical significance, as illustrated in Example A4, where the investigator would redesign the exercise program if it did not show a benefit. The investigator would not be able to show that the new exercise program actually produced worse results using a one-sided significance test, but was not concerned about this. This might be a risk you are prepared to accept, but is it scientifically defensible? Importantly, using one-sided significance tests often raises problems when you go to publish your results if they are positive.

You could also use lower power when designing the study. This increases the chance that even if your assumptions are correct, you might fail to show the observed difference as statistically significant. This risk might be acceptable when you are going from what is considered high power (90% or more) to something still considered acceptable (80% or more), but if you decrease power below 80%, you really run the risk of not being able to conclude anything.

B.5 The Magical Thinking Way to Reduce the "Just Right Number"

All the procedures in Section B.4 require additional work to reduce the sample size. Some investigators, however, approach the problem not from what number they need, but from what number they want.

Example B4 (continued): The statistician provided sample sizes for the range of survival that the investigator felt was appropriate, but suggested that the investigator review the clinic records to get an accurate estimate of survival without the treatment. The investigator does so and reports that survival is 78% in the population he is interested in studying. The statistician does a quick calculation and obtains a total sample size of 2,050 individuals for the study for an estimated difference of 5% (80% power, alpha=0.05, two-sided). The investigator asks what the sample size would be if the difference is 10%, and the statistician calculates a total sample size of 480. The investigator then says, "OK, what about a 15% improvement?" for which the statistician calculates a total sample size of 188. The investigator is now happy! He has a justification for the size of study he wanted to do: the 100 to 200 infant study he was looking for. If he assumes that he has a breakthrough and will increase survival by 15%, he can now justify the number! The statistician points out that the investigator was initially hoping for a 5% survival, and that just changing a number to get the sample size the investigator wanted does not make it likely to happen, but to no avail. The investigator has what he wanted: a mathematically justified sample size, even though the assumptions are extremely implausible.

Our experience is that investigators usually report as their initial expected difference the amount that they hope the intervention could accomplish, and that the changes described in Example B4 may be made to justify a feasible sample size, even if there is no hope that the difference could be close to this big. Doing a study when it has virtually no chance of being successful is unethical.

B.6 An Alternative Way of Thinking about Sample Size

Instead of manipulating the assumptions until you are able to justify the sample size you want to use and pretending that these are the values that you think you can achieve, think about what information a specific sample size would be able to give you at the end of the study. This means that given the sample size and realistic assumptions about the variability of the measurement, you can calculate what difference you can reasonably expect to detect, and what power you have for the difference you believe really exists.

Example B4 (continued): At this point, fortunately, the investigator decided to step back and think about the project further. Was this difference in survival plausible for the intervention he was testing? He had originally been thinking that a 1% difference would be good enough, and then been persuaded that a 5% difference would be necessary to have convincing results of the benefit of therapy. Now the investigator is saying that the study is looking for a 15% difference in survival, far beyond what he had hoped for when he started out thinking about the study. The investigator admits to himself that he does not believe that his new intervention has any chance of achieving such a dramatic improvement. Rather than give up completely, however, the investigator decides to focus on different endpoints, such as the duration of time on mechanical ventilation and the total duration of hospitalization rather than the binary endpoint of survival.

Here, the investigator is doing precisely what we would recommend. Clearly, survival is too ambitious an endpoint, but you can focus on a more immediate (and easier to influence) short-term endpoint. Ideally, you should develop an experiment that might be able to get a hint of whether the intervention is beneficial on another endpoint, one that might be predictive of survival.

Sometimes, however, despite a tiny sample size, a study can be worthwhile.

Example B8: An investigator specializing in a very rare disease had a total of 12 patients with the syndrome, which he estimated was approximately half the total cases in the United States. He was interested in testing a relatively simple intervention to see whether this improved things for these patients, and estimated that either 7 or 8 of his patients would agree to participate. Despite the fact that the study would only be able to detect a very large difference as statistically significant, he decided to proceed with the study using a crossover design, so that at the end of the study he would be able to recommend the treatment to those participants who benefited from it. If the study had an overall significant effect, he would then recommend it to his patients who had not participated in the study.

B.7 Ratio of Sample Sizes between Different Groups

Most interventional studies use equal sized groups, as this gives the highest power for the total sample size studied. Occasionally, unequal randomization (often 2 in the experimental arm to 1 in the control arm) is used to make an interventional study more appealing to potential participants, as they have a higher chance of being assigned to the experimental group (which they assume will be better, although the purpose of the study is to see it this is true).

In case-control studies, however, it is often the situation that cases are difficult to find and recruit while controls are plentiful. In this situation, increasing the size of the control group will increase the power, although the increased power will be less than if the study consisted of equal-sized groups with the same total number of participants. The increase in power plateaus after 3–4 controls per case. If it is relatively easy to retrieve the data required, such as when the data is in a computer database, increasing the sample size may not be much of a problem. If a study requires a significant personnel effort or cost for each case or control participant, however, then an effort should be made to keep the groups as close together in size as possible to get the maximum power for the effort.

B.8 Calculating the "Just Right Number"

Despite all the caveats about the "just right number" we have given, you do need to specify a sample size when planning the study. At www.cambridge.org/9780521840637, there is further information about the underlying calculation of the sample size and links to obtain software for sample size calculation and websites with sample size calculators.

B.9 Ethical Issues

Almost any sample size can be rigorously justified if one makes assumptions such that the mathematics gives the answer desired. The mathematics will be correct, and under the assumptions you put in, you will have a "just right number." However, if the assumptions are unrealistic then the effort in making the sample size calculation is wasted and the "just right number" calculated is useless. Yes, the new experimental therapy in Example B4 might show an improvement in survival from 78% to 93%. But is this plausible? If it is not, then you have little chance of making any definite conclusions and have done something that, at the very least, is intellectually dishonest.

Unless there is a reasonable chance that a study will have a conclusion, the ethics of the study are at best questionable. A study that does not have a reasonable chance of answering the questions being asked is a waste of everyone's time and energy. Participants are being exposed to a risk, no matter how small, in any study. Unless there is a reasonable chance that their time, energy, effort, and sacrifice will lead to credible conclusions for the study, the study is unethical.

KEY POINTS

- Sample size is an important issue when planning a study.
- There is a tendency to focus on justifying a feasible number of partici-pants, and make assumptions so that this number comes out of the sample size formula as the "just right number."
- The mathematics leading to this "just right number" will be correct, but if the assumptions are implausible, or frankly nothing more than manipulation to justify a feasible number, then the study has little chance of being useful.
- A better approach when there are feasibility issues is to focus on what information the study can provide, and whether this information makes the study worth doing.

Index

Note to index: An *f* following a page number designates a figure; a *t* following a page number indicates a table.